T0228936

Sleep Issues in Women's Health

Editors

KATHRYN ALDRICH LEE
FIONA C. BAKER

SLEEP MEDICINE CLINICS

www.sleep.theclinics.com

Consulting Editor
TEOFILO LEE-CHIONG Jr

September 2018 • Volume 13 • Number 3

ELSEVIER

1600 John F. Kennedy Boulevard • Suite 1800 • Philadelphia, Pennsylvania, 19103-2899

http://www.theclinics.com

SLEEP MEDICINE CLINICS Volume 13, Number 3
September 2018, ISSN 1556-407X, ISBN-13: 978-0-323-61412-2

Editor: Colleen Dietzler
Developmental Editor: Donald Mumford

Sleep Medicine Clinics (ISSN 1556-407X) is published quarterly by Elsevier Inc., 360 Park Avenue South, New York, NY 10010-1710. Months of issue are March, June, September and December. Business and Editorial Offices: 1600 John F. Kennedy Blvd., Ste. 1800, Philadelphia, PA 19103-2899. Customer Service Office: 3251 Riverport Lane, Maryland Heights, MO 63043. Periodicals postage paid at New York, NY and additional mailing offices. Subscription prices are $203.00 per year (US individuals), $100.00 (US students), $486.00 (US institutions), $245.00 (Canadian and international individuals), $135.00 (Canadian and international students), $540.00 (Canadian institutions) and $540.00 (International institutions). Foreign air speed delivery is included in all *Clinics* subscription prices. All prices are subject to change without notice. **POSTMASTER:** Send change of address to *Sleep Medicine Clinics*, Elsevier Health Sciences Division, Subscription Customer Service, 3251 Riverport Lane, Maryland Heights, MO 63043. Customer Service: **Tel: 1-800-654-2452 (U.S. and Canada); 314-447-8871 (outside U.S. and Canada). Fax: 314-447-8029. E-mail: journalscustomerservice-usa@elsevier.com (for print support); journalsonline support-usa@elsevier.com (for online support).**

Reprints. For copies of 100 or more of articles in this publication, please contact the Commercial Reprints Department, Elsevier Inc., 360 Park Avenue South, New York, NY 10010-1710. Tel.: 212-633-3874; Fax: 212-633-3820; E-mail: reprints@elsevier.com.

Sleep Medicine Clinics is covered in *MEDLINE/PubMed (Index Medicus).*

Printed in the United States of America.

PROGRAM OBJECTIVE

The goal of *Sleep Clinics of North America* is to keep practicing physicians up to date with current clinical practice by providing timely articles reviewing the state of the art in patient care.

TARGET AUDIENCE

All practicing physicians and other healthcare professionals.

LEARNING OBJECTIVES

Upon completion of this activity, participants will be able to:

1. Review sleep disordered breathing in pregnancy and the role of circadian rhythms in postpartum sleep and mood
2. Discuss sleep and sleep disorders in the menopausal transition and impact of poor sleep on physical and mental health in older women.
3. Recognize management strategies for restless legs syndrome/Willis-Ekbom disease during pregnancy.

ACCREDITATION

The Elsevier Office of Continuing Medical Education (EOCME) is accredited by the Accreditation Council for Continuing Medical Education (ACCME) to provide continuing medical education for physicians.

The EOCME designates this enduring material for a maximum of 15 *AMA PRA Category 1 Credit*(s)™. Physicians should claim only the credit commensurate with the extent of their participation in the activity.

All other healthcare professionals requesting continuing education credit for this enduring material will be issued a certificate of participation.

DISCLOSURE OF CONFLICTS OF INTEREST

The EOCME assesses conflict of interest with its instructors, faculty, planners, and other individuals who are in a position to control the content of CME activities. All relevant conflicts of interest that are identified are thoroughly vetted by EOCME for fair balance, scientific objectivity, and patient care recommendations. EOCME is committed to providing its learners with CME activities that promote improvements or quality in healthcare and not a specific proprietary business or a commercial interest.

The planning committee, staff, authors and editors listed below have identified no financial relationships or relationships to products or devices they or their spouse/life partner have with commercial interest related to the content of this CME activity:

Lakshmy Ayyar, MD; M. Safwan Badr, MD, MBA; Fiona C. Baker, PhD; Ann M. Berger, PhD, APRN, AOCNS, FAAN; Diane B. Boivin, MD, PhD; Joseph Daniel; Dilorom M. Djalilova, BA, BSN, RN; Signe K. Dørheim, MD, PhD; Benicio N. Frey, MD, MSc, PhD; Kari Grethe Hjorthaug Gallaher, MD; Corrado Garbazza, MD; Kalpalatha Guntupalli, MD; Mary Katherine Howell, MS; Stella Iacovides, PhD; Dalton W. Janssen, BSN, RN; Alison Kemp; Laura Kervezee, PhD; Clare Ladyman, BSc, PGDip; Laura Lampio, MD, PhD; Kathryn Aldrich Lee, RN, CBSM, PhD; Teofilo Lee- Chiong Jr, MD; Mauro Manconi, MD, PhD; Jennifer L. Martin, PhD; Ellyn E. Matthews, PhD, RN, AOCNS, CBSM, FAAN; Päivi Polo-Kantola, MD, PhD; Tarja Saaresranta, MD, PhD; Fidaa Shaib, MD; Joan L. Shaver, PhD, RN, FAAN; Ari Shechter, PhD; T. Leigh Signal, PhD; Anastasiya Slyepchenko, HBSC; Katie L. Stone, PhD; Kristin Urstad, PhD; Qian Xiao, PhD; Salam Zeineddine, MD.

The planning committee, staff, authors and editors listed below have identified financial relationships or relationships to products or devices they or their spouse/life partner have with commercial interest related to the content of this CME activity:

Ihori Kobayashi, PhD: receives research support from Merck & Co, Inc.

UNAPPROVED/OFF-LABEL USE DISCLOSURE

The EOCME requires CME faculty to disclose to the participants:

1. When products or procedures being discussed are off-label, unlabelled, experimental, and/or investigational (not US Food and Drug Administration [FDA] approved); and
2. Any limitations on the information presented, such as data that are preliminary or that represent ongoing research, interim analyses, and/or unsupported opinions. Faculty may discuss information about pharmaceutical agents that is outside of FDA-approved labelling. This information is intended solely for CME and is not intended to promote off-label use of these medications. If you have any questions, contact the medical affairs department of the manufacturer for the most recent prescribing information.

TO ENROLL

To enroll in the Sleep Medicines Clinic Continuing Medical Education program, call customer service at 1-800-654-2452 or sign up online at http://www.theclinics.com/home/cme. The CME program is available to subscribers for an additional annual fee of USD $140.

METHOD OF PARTICIPATION

In order to claim credit, participants must complete the following:

1. Complete enrolment as indicated above.
2. Read the activity.
3. Complete the CME Test and Evaluation. Participants must achieve a score of 70% on the test. All CME Tests and Evaluations must be completed online.

CME INQUIRIES/SPECIAL NEEDS

For all CME inquiries or special needs, please contact elsevierCME@elsevier.com.

SLEEP MEDICINE CLINICS

THE CLINICS ARE AVAILABLE ONLINE!
Access your subscription at:
www.theclinics.com

Contributors

CONSULTING EDITOR

TEOFILO LEE-CHIONG Jr, MD
Professor of Medicine, National Jewish Health,
University of Colorado Denver, Denver,
Colorado, USA; Chief Medical Liaison, Philips
Respironics, Pennsylvania, USA

EDITORS

KATHRYN ALDRICH LEE, RN, PhD, CBSM
Professor Emerita, Department of Family
Health Care Nursing, UCSF School of Nursing,
University of California, San Francisco,
San Francisco, California, USA

FIONA C. BAKER, PhD
Senior Program Director, Human
Sleep Research Program, Center for
Health Sciences, SRI International,
Menlo Park, California, USA; Honorary
Professorial Research Fellow, Brain Function
Research Group, School of Physiology,
University of the Witwatersrand,
Johannesburg, South Africa

AUTHORS

LAKSHMY AYYAR, MD
Houston Pulmonary, Sleep & Allergy
Associates, Baylor College of Medicine,
Houston, Texas, USA

M. SAFWAN BADR, MD, MBA
Professor of Medicine, Division of Pulmonary
Critical Care and Sleep Medicine, Department
of Internal Medicine, Wayne State University,
University Health Center, Detroit, Michigan,
USA

FIONA C. BAKER, PhD
Senior Program Director, Human Sleep
Research Program, Center for Health
Sciences, SRI International, Menlo Park,
California, USA; Honorary Professorial
Research Fellow, Brain Function Research
Group, School of Physiology, University of the
Witwatersrand, Johannesburg, South Africa

**ANN M. BERGER, PhD, APRN, AOCNS,
FAAN**
College of Nursing, University of Nebraska
Medical Center, Omaha, Nebraska, USA

DIANE B. BOIVIN, MD, PhD
Director, Centre for Study and Treatment of
Circadian Rhythms, Douglas Mental Health
University Institute, Professor, Department of
Psychiatry, McGill University, Montreal,
Quebec, Canada

DILOROM M. DJALILOVA, BA, BSN, RN
PhD Student, College of Nursing, University of
Nebraska Medical Center, Omaha, Nebraska,
USA

SIGNE K. DØRHEIM, MD, PhD
Department of Psychiatry, Stavanger
University Hospital, Stavanger, Norway

BENICIO N. FREY, MD, MSc, PhD
Women's Health Concerns Clinic, St Joseph's
Healthcare Hamilton, Associate Professor,
Department of Psychiatry and Behavioural
Neurosciences, McMaster University,
Hamilton, Canada

KARI GRETHE HJORTHAUG GALLAHER, MD
Department of Psychiatry, Stavanger University Hospital, Stavanger, Norway

CORRADO GARBAZZA, MD
Doctor, Clinical Research Physician, Sleep and Epilepsy Center, Neurocenter of Southern Switzerland, Civic Hospital, Lugano, Switzerland

KALPALATHA GUNTUPALLI, MD
Professor, Baylor College of Medicine, Houston, Texas, USA

MARY KATHERINE HOWELL, MS
Doctoral Student, Department of Psychology, Howard University, Washington, DC, USA

STELLA IACOVIDES, PhD
Lecturer, Faculty of Health Sciences, Brain Function Research Group, School of Physiology, University of the Witwatersrand, Johannesburg, South Africa

DALTON W. JANSSEN, BSN, RN
PhD Student, College of Nursing, University of Arkansas for Medical Sciences, Little Rock, Arkansas, USA

LAURA KERVEZEE, PhD
Department of Psychiatry, Centre for Study and Treatment of Circadian Rhythms, Douglas Mental Health University Institute, McGill University, Montreal, Quebec, Canada

IHORI KOBAYASHI, PhD
Research Assistant Professor, Department of Psychiatry and Behavioral Sciences, Howard University, Washington, DC, USA

CLARE LADYMAN, BSc, PGDip
Doctoral Candidate, Sleep/Wake Research Centre, College of Health, Massey University, Wellington, New Zealand

LAURA LAMPIO, MD, PhD
Senior Research Fellow, Department of Pulmonary Diseases and Clinical Allergology, Sleep Research Centre, University of Turku, Turku, Finland; Trainee, Department of Obstetrics and Gynecology, Helsinki University Hospital, Helsinki, Finland

KATHRYN ALDRICH LEE, RN, PhD, CBSM
Professor Emerita, Department of Family Health Care Nursing, UCSF School of Nursing, University of California, San Francisco, San Francisco, California, USA

MAURO MANCONI, MD, PhD
Professor, Head, Sleep and Epilepsy Center, Neurocenter of Southern Switzerland, Civic Hospital, Lugano, Switzerland

JENNIFER L. MARTIN, PhD
Associate Professor, Department of Medicine, David Geffen School of Medicine, University of California, Los Angeles, Los Angeles, California, USA; Associate Director for Clinical and Health Services Research, Geriatric Research, Education and Clinical Center, VA Greater Los Angeles Healthcare System, VA Sepulveda Ambulatory Care Center, North Hills, California, USA

ELLYN E. MATTHEWS, PhD, RN, AOCNS, CBSM, FAAN
Department of Science, College of Nursing, University of Arkansas for Medical Sciences, Little Rock, Arkansas, USA

PÄIVI POLO-KANTOLA, MD, PhD
Professor, Department of Obstetrics and Gynecology, Turku University Hospital, University of Turku, Senior Research Fellow, Department of Pulmonary Diseases and Clinical Allergology, Sleep Research Centre, Turku, Finland

TARJA SAARESRANTA, MD, PhD
Acting Professor, Department of Pulmonary Diseases and Clinical Allergology, Sleep Research Centre, University of Turku, Chief Specialist in Pulmonary Diseases, Division of Medicine, Department of Pulmonary Diseases, Turku University Hospital, Turku, Finland

FIDAA SHAIB, MD
Associate Professor, Baylor College of Medicine, Houston, Texas, USA

JOAN L. SHAVER, PhD, RN, FAAN
Professor, Biobehavioral Health Science Division, University of Arizona College of Nursing, Tucson, Arizona, USA

ARI SHECHTER, PhD
Department of Medicine, Center for Behavioral Cardiovascular Health, Columbia University, New York, New York, USA

T. LEIGH SIGNAL, PhD
Associate Professor and Associate Director, Sleep/Wake Research Centre, College of Health, Massey University, Wellington, New Zealand

ANASTASIYA SLYEPCHENKO, HBSc
Women's Health Concerns Clinic, St Joseph's Healthcare Hamilton, Neuroscience Graduate Program, McMaster University, Hamilton, Canada

KATIE L. STONE, PhD
California Pacific Medical Center Research Institute, San Francisco, California, USA; Department of Health and Human Physiology, Department of Epidemiology, University of Iowa, Iowa City, Iowa, USA

KRISTIN URSTAD, PhD
Associate Professor, Faculty of Health Sciences, University of Stavanger, Stavanger, Norway

QIAN XIAO, PhD
California Pacific Medical Center Research Institute, San Francisco, California, USA; Department of Health and Human Physiology, Department of Epidemiology, University of Iowa, Iowa City, Iowa, USA

SALAM ZEINEDDINE, MD
Sleep Medicine Fellow, Division of Pulmonary Critical Care and Sleep Medicine, Department of Internal Medicine, Wayne State University, Harper University Hospital, Detroit, Michigan, USA

Contents

Menstrual Cycle Effects on Sleep 283

Fiona C. Baker and Kathryn Aldrich Lee

Subjective and objective sleep changes occur during the menstrual cycle. Poorer sleep quality in the premenstrual phase and menstruation is common in women with premenstrual symptoms or painful menstrual cramps. There is increased sleep spindle activity from follicular to luteal phase, potentially progesterone related. Luteal phase changes also include blunted temperature rhythm amplitude and reduced rapid eye movement sleep. Women with polycystic ovary syndrome should be screened for sleep-disordered breathing. Short sleep duration is associated with irregular menstrual cycles, which may affect reproductive health. Menstrual cycle phase and menstrual-related disorders should be considered when assessing women's sleep complaints.

Impact of Shift Work on the Circadian Timing System and Health in Women 295

Laura Kervezee, Ari Shechter, and Diane B. Boivin

Women who do shift work are a sizable part of the workforce. Shift workers experience circadian misalignment due to shifted sleep periods, with potentially far-reaching health consequences, including elevated risk of sleep disturbances, metabolic disorders, and cancer. This article provides an overview of the circadian timing system and presents the sex differences that can be observed in the functioning of this system, which may account for the lower tolerance to shift work for women compared with men. Recent epidemiologic findings on female-specific health consequences of shift work are discussed.

Sleep Health in Pregnancy: A Scoping Review 307

Clare Ladyman and T. Leigh Signal

Using scoping review methodology, this article investigates the literature on sleep duration, continuity/efficiency, timing, daytime sleepiness/alertness, and perceived sleep quality in each trimester of a healthy pregnancy. Data suggest significant variability in sleep between women, with less evidence to support major changes in sleep health across trimesters. There is a need for further research on this topic to better inform women and their health providers.

Management Strategies for Restless Legs Syndrome/Willis-Ekbom Disease During Pregnancy 335

Corrado Garbazza and Mauro Manconi

Restless legs syndrome/Willis-Ekbom disease is a common disorder during pregnancy that may have a significant impact on the health of affected women, leading to negative consequences in the short and long term. An accurate diagnosis helps to recognize the syndrome and choose the optimal therapeutic strategy, based on the characteristics and needs of the patient. This article summarizes the main treatment options recommended by the consensus clinical guidelines of the International Restless Legs Syndrome Study Group and provides a short guide to the management of restless leg syndrome during pregnancy in clinical practice.

> Sleep-disordered breathing (SDB) in pregnancy can present as snoring and/or obstructive sleep apnea (OSA), and the prevalence is increasing owing to the increase in maternal obesity. Pregnant women often present with fatigue and daytime sleepiness rather than the classic symptoms. Habitual snoring, older age, chronic hypertension, and high prepregnancy body mass index are reliable indicators of an increased risk for SDB and should trigger further testing. The gold standard for diagnosis of OSA is an overnight laboratory polysomnography. Although there are no studies linking SDB to poor fetal outcomes, fetal well-being remains paramount throughout the course of pregnancy.

> Women often experience sleep disturbances and worsening sleep quality throughout pregnancy and postpartum. Circadian rhythms are closely linked to sleep problems and mood disorders. This systematic review provides a summary of studies of circadian rhythms and associated sleep problems and maternal distress, among postpartum women. Articles were identified through a systematic literature search. Circadian rhythm disturbances were strongly correlated with depression, social factors, and mothers' exposure to light postpartum. Future research should include larger, prospective studies as well as randomized controlled trials for measuring the effect of circadian rhythm interventions on postpartum mental health outcomes.

> Chronic pain and sleep disturbances are intricately intertwined. This narrative review provides comments on observations related to pain, stress immunity, and sleep. Sleep evidence is reviewed from studies of select conditions involving pain (ie, functional somatic syndromes and autoimmune) that are predominant in women. Chronic pain and poor sleep encompass persistent stress-immune activation with systemic inflammation, cellular oxidative stress, and sick behavior indicators that increase morbidity and threaten quality of life. In painful conditions, sleep impairments are nearly ubiquitous, and exaggerated combined effects should not be underestimated or ignored, nor should crucial implications for clinical practice and research.

> Sleep deficiency is common and distressing for women with breast cancer throughout the care continuum. This article describes the scope and quality of evidence related to exercise interventions to improve sleep in women with breast cancer. Fifteen studies met the criteria, and 12 were judged to be of excellent quality. The most frequent intervention was walking, primarily during the time of chemotherapy. Eleven studies reported postintervention improvement in sleep deficiency. Most yoga, qigong, and dance intervention studies reported no differences between groups. Emerging evidence exists for the effectiveness of aerobic exercise to improve various sleep outcomes in women with breast cancer.

> After exposure to traumatic stress, women are at greater risk than men for developing symptoms of some psychiatric disorders, including insomnia and nightmares. Sleep disturbance is one of the most refractory symptoms of posttraumatic stress disorder. Women were included in a few studies that examined the efficacy of psychological or pharmacologic interventions for trauma-related sleep disturbances. Studies demonstrated preliminary evidence for efficacy of cognitive behavioral therapy for insomnia, imagery rehearsal therapy, and combinations of these techniques in treating insomnia and nightmares in trauma-exposed women. Prazosin as an adjunct to ongoing treatment is a potentially efficacious strategy for treating trauma-related nightmares in women.

> Sleep disorders are common among women veterans and contribute to poor functioning and quality of life. Studies show that women veterans are particularly prone to insomnia, sleep-disordered breathing, and insufficient sleep. Standard cognitive behavioral therapy for insomnia should be viewed as first-line therapy for insomnia disorder, and women veterans should be screened and treated for sleep-disordered breathing. Behavioral and lifestyle factors contributing to insufficient sleep should also be addressed. Challenges exist in diagnosing and treating sleep disorders in women veterans, in part because of high rates of psychiatric comorbidities, such as posttraumatic stress disorder and depression.

> The menopausal transition is associated with an increase in insomnia symptoms, especially difficulty staying asleep, which negatively affects quality of life. Vasomotor symptoms are a key component of sleep disruption. Findings from polysomnographic studies are less consistent in showing disrupted sleep in menopausal transition independent of aging; further prospective studies are needed. Hormone therapy alleviates subjective sleep disturbances, particularly if vasomotor symptoms are present. However, because of contraindications, other options should be considered. Further work is needed to develop preventive and treatment strategies for alleviating sleep disturbances to ensure better health, quality of life, and productivity in midlife women.

> Many aspects of sleep and circadian rhythms change as people age. Older adults usually experience a decrease in sleep duration and efficiency, an increase in sleep latency and fragmentation, a high prevalence of sleep disorders, and weakened rest-activity rhythms. Research evidence suggests that women are more likely to report aging-related sleep problems. This article presents epidemiologic and clinical evidence on the relationships between sleep deficiency and physical and mental outcomes in older women, explores potential mechanisms underlying such relationships, points out gaps in the literature that warrant future investigations, and considers implications in clinical and public health settings.

Preface
Sleep and Women's Health Across the Lifespan

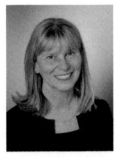 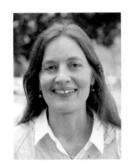

Kathryn Aldrich Lee, RN, PhD, CBSM   Fiona C. Baker, PhD

Editors

In women, sleep interacts with reproductive health, and sleep disorders can emerge within the context of reproductive stages. Substantial research has occurred since the last *Sleep Medicine Clinics* issue about sleep in women, guest edited by Dr Helen Driver in 2008.[1] However, evident from the reviews in this current issue, the field of sleep and women's health remains an active and complex area with many unanswered questions. We are pleased to offer this broad series of reviews, showing fundamental relationships between sleep and reproductive stages, as well as emerging knowledge about women's sleep in special populations (military) and in the context of traumatic stress exposure. These selected authors used their research and clinically focused expertise to identify knowledge gaps for future research and provide clinicians with a solid understanding of current issues surrounding sleep and women's health.

In addition to reviewing knowledge about sleep in the context of reproductive stages (menstrual cycle, pregnancy, menopause), this special issue includes reviews of research on circadian rhythms and shift work. The article by Kervezee and colleagues addresses sleep problems for women in the workforce, particularly related to shift work. As you read their review, we invite you to think about how similar shift work sleep issues may be for new mothers during postpartum adjustment to parenthood.

While pregnancy and postpartum are relatively brief periods in a woman's lifespan, these reproductive phases represent monumental physical and psychological changes with implications for health and potential for sleep disturbances that may be temporary or permanent if nothing is done to intervene. During child-bearing and child-rearing years, women's sleep is often sacrificed for other priorities, including parenting responsibilities and working outside the home. It was striking to us that so little is known about how bedtimes change during postpartum, which can effectively result in mothers being cast in the role of shift worker, but with no days off from parenting.

It is often during child-rearing years that chronic health conditions emerge. If sleep has been relatively good during reproductive age, a chronic illness can quickly change sleep or further compound a preexisting sleep problem. The role that stress and inflammation plays in sleep disorders is reviewed by Shaver and Iacovides, setting the stage for health issues that arise when women experience trauma, particularly women military Veterans at risk of posttraumatic stress disorder. These review articles highlight the need for research on sleep in civilian and military populations of women who experience trauma, whether it be domestic violence or trauma in the workplace.[2,3]

Even without a traumatic event or onset of a chronic illness, normative menopausal transition often brings fluctuations in sleep patterns without much guidance about expectations for onset, intensity, resolution of symptoms, or coping mechanisms. Insomnia is prevalent in the context of menopause, often linked to

Sleep Med Clin 13 (2018) xv–xvi
https://doi.org/10.1016/j.jsmc.2018.06.001
1556-407X/18/© 2018 Published by Elsevier Inc.

disruptive hot flashes that require consideration when treating sleep disturbances in this population. As discussed in the final article, sleep is a critical component of healthy aging, and emerging research on aging women links sleep disruption with memory-related disorders as well as poor health.

In closing, we would like to thank our expert contributors to this special issue. They covered the topics in great depth and clearly addressed the issues from clinical perspectives that are important in health care. We also thank the many others who conduct research on women's sleep issues, and encourage initiatives like the Society for Women's Health Research Interdisciplinary Network on Sleep.[4] While we say "many others," there are still so few, and we warmly welcome the next generation of researchers and clinicians interested in this topic to join forces to move the science forward.

Kathryn Aldrich Lee, RN, PhD, CBSM
Department of Family Health Care Nursing
UCSF School of Nursing
University of California, San Francisco
Box 0606, Room N411Y 2 Koret Way
San Francisco, CA 94143-0606, USA

Fiona C. Baker, PhD
Human Sleep Research Program
Center for Health Sciences
SRI International
333 Ravenswood Avenue
Menlo Park, CA 94025, USA

E-mail addresses:
Kathryn.Lee@ucsf.edu (K.A. Lee)
Fiona.baker@sri.com (F.C. Baker)

REFERENCES

1. Driver H. Sleep and disorders of sleep in women. Sleep Med Clin 2008;3(1):xiii-iv.
2. U.S. Department of Veteran Affairs. Women Veterans Health Care. Available at: www.womenshealth@va.gov. Accessed April 17, 2018.
3. Yablonsky AM, Martin RC, Highfill-McRoy RM, et al. Military women's health: a scoping review and gap analysis, 2000-2015. Report No. N15-015. Silver Spring (MD): Naval Medical Research Center. Defense Technical Information Center. Final report 2017. Available at: www.DTIC.mil. Accessed April 17, 2018.
4. Society for Women's Health Research. Available at: www.swhr.org. Accessed April 17, 2018.

Menstrual Cycle Effects on Sleep

Fiona C. Baker, PhD[a,b,*], Kathryn Aldrich Lee, RN, PhD, CBSM[c]

KEYWORDS

- Menstrual cycle • Follicular • Luteal • Estrogen • Premenstrual syndrome • Dysmenorrhea
- Polycystic ovary syndrome • Sleep spindles

KEY POINTS

- Self-reported sleep disturbance increases during premenstrual and menstruation phases of the menstrual cycle, particularly in women with premenstrual symptoms or painful menstrual cramps (dysmenorrhea).
- Sleep spindles increase in the luteal phase relative to the follicular phase, possibly due to an effect of progesterone and/or its metabolites.
- Women with polycystic ovary syndrome, particularly if obese, are at risk of sleep disordered breathing, partly due to hyperandrogenism that characterizes this syndrome.
- Poorer sleep quality is apparent in the premenstrual phase in women with severe premenstrual syndrome, yet polysomnographic measures show more traitlike sleep alterations that may be related to altered melatonin rhythms. Light therapy shows efficacy in improving mood symptoms.
- Sleep and reproductive function have a bidirectional relationship such that disrupted sleep is associated with altered menstrual cycles, which could impact reproductive function.

INTRODUCTION

From menarche, or first menstrual period, to menopause that signals the end of reproduction, women experience monthly variations in hormones that regulate reproduction. These hormones have widespread effects outside their direct reproductive functions, including influences on regulating mood, body temperature, respiration, autonomic nervous system, and sleep. This review highlights the effects of the menstrual cycle on sleep, considering both physiologic changes in homeostatic and circadian sleep regulation as well as perceived changes in sleep quality. The authors discuss sleep disturbances in the context of young women and menstrual-associated disorders, including polycystic ovary syndrome, dysmenorrhea, and premenstrual dysphoric disorder. They also consider reverse relationships: how sleep and circadian disturbances impact women's reproductive physiology.

DEFINITIONS AND MENSTRUAL CYCLE PHYSIOLOGY

Most women have menstrual cycle lengths between 21 and 30 days, with menses lasting less than 7 days.[1] The menstrual cycle is divided into a preovulatory follicular phase and postovulatory luteal phase, with the onset of menstrual flow marking the beginning of a new cycle (day 1) (**Fig. 1**).

During the follicular phase, follicle-stimulating hormone and luteinizing hormone (LH) are released

Disclosure statement: F.C. Baker has received funding unrelated to this work from Ebb Therapeutics Inc, Fitbit Inc, and International Flavors & Fragrances Inc. K.A. Lee has nothing to disclose.
[a] Human Sleep Research Program, SRI International, 333 Ravenswood Avenue, Menlo Park, CA 94025, USA;
[b] Brain Function Research Group, School of Physiology, University of the Witwatersrand, 7 York Road, Parktown, Johannesburg 2193, South Africa; [c] Department of Family Health Care Nursing, UCSF School of Nursing, University of California, San Francisco, Box 0606, San Francisco, CA 94143, USA
* Corresponding author. SRI International, 333 Ravenswood Avenue, Menlo Park, CA 94025.
E-mail address: Fiona.baker@sri.com

sleep.theclinics.com

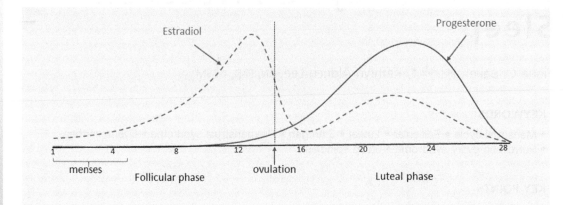

Fig. 1. Changes in estradiol and progesterone across a typical 28-day ovulatory menstrual cycle, where day 1 represents the first day of bleeding.

from the anterior pituitary and act on the ovaries to initiate development of several primary follicles, which produce estrogens, principally estradiol. At the end of the follicular phase, estrogen levels increase, triggering a peak in LH. Ovulation occurs 12 to 16 hours later, around day 14. Following ovulation, the corpus luteum develops, producing progesterone and estrogen, which peak 5 to 7 days after ovulation before declining (in the absence of implantation), resulting in endometrial breakdown and menstruation.

Estrogen and progesterone receptors are widely distributed throughout the central nervous system (CNS), including the basal forebrain, hypothalamus, dorsal raphe nucleus, and locus coeruleus.[2,3] These areas are also involved in sleep regulation, and fluctuations in ovarian steroids across the menstrual cycle can modulate sleep. Indeed, work in rodents shows that sleep patterns fluctuate in concert with natural fluctuations of ovarian steroids; ovariectomy eliminates these fluctuations in sleep, with effects depending on the time of day.[4,5] Although ovarian steroids' mechanisms of action on sleep regulation are not completely clear, both sleep- and wake-promoting areas of the CNS are sensitive to the effects of estrogen. Ovarian steroids could also influence circadian rhythms, including sleep-wake activity, through direct or indirect effects on the master pacemaker: the suprachiasmatic nucleus. The mechanistic framework is, therefore, in place for menstrual cycle–related changes in reproductive hormones to influence sleep and circadian rhythms.

SLEEP AND CIRCADIAN RHYTHMS ACROSS THE MENSTRUAL CYCLE
Self-Reported Sleep Quality

Collectively, studies show that sleep disturbances are more commonly reported by women around the time of menstruation, encompassing the last few premenstrual days (late luteal phase) and the first few days of menstrual bleeding (early follicular phase).[6–9] However, not all studies find a menstrual cycle effect on sleep quality[10] or find only small effects,[11] possibly reflecting between-individual variability in the relationship between sleep and menstrual cycle phase. Van Reen and Kiesner[12] identified 3 patterns: some women show no relationship, others show a midcycle increase in difficulty sleeping, and others show a premenstrual increase in difficulty sleeping. The extent that ovarian hormones directly contribute to perceived sleep disturbance, versus other factors that vary with the menstrual cycle, remains unclear. Changes in progesterone and estrogen, rather than absolute levels, in the late-luteal phase may be a critical factor for sleep quality. Further, symptoms that vary across the menstrual cycle in some women, such as anxiety, depression, headaches, cramps, and breast tenderness, are also associated with difficulty sleeping.[12] Menstrual cycle characteristics are also relevant: women with irregular cycles report more sleep difficulties than women with regular cycles, even when controlling for age, body mass index (BMI), dysmenorrhea, and premenstrual complaints.[13]

Objectively Measured Sleep Quality

Sleep across the menstrual cycle has been studied objectively with actigraphy and polysomnography (PSG). Actigraphy can be easily used to track changes in daily sleep-wake activity in many participants; however, few studies have investigated menstrual cycle–related patterns in sleep. In a actigraphy study of 163 late-reproductive-aged women, there was a significant decline in sleep efficiency (SE) and total sleep time (TST) in the premenstrual week relative to the prior week, with greater effects associated with obesity, financial strain, smoking, and greater apnea hypopnea index,[14] corresponding with studies showing poorer self-reported sleep quality in the premenstrual phase. In a smaller study of 19 women (18–43 years of age), actigraphy SE was positively associated with 1-day lagged estrogen metabolites and negatively with 1-day lagged progesterone metabolites, although effects were weak and self-reported sleep was unassociated with hormone metabolites.[10]

PSG has been used in small numbers of women to compare sleep between discrete menstrual cycle phases, such as midfollicular versus midluteal phase. An exception is the seminal study by Driver and colleagues.[15] Although the sample size was small, sleep was recorded with PSG every second night across an entire menstrual cycle in 9 young women, with phases carefully characterized. They found stable sleep-onset latency (SOL), wakefulness after sleep onset (WASO), and SE across the menstrual cycle.[16] N2 sleep was increased and REM sleep tended to decline in the absence of any change in amount of slow wave sleep (SWS) or slow wave activity (SWA) averaged for the whole night in the luteal phase relative to follicular phase,[15] indicating no change in this marker of sleep homeostasis across the menstrual cycle. Analysis of SWA by sleep cycle, did reveal subtle changes however: higher activity in the first non-REM (NREM) sleep episode and lower activity in the second NREM episode in the midluteal phase compared with the midfollicular phase.[16]

Other studies have mostly confirmed no difference in SWS or SWA between the follicular and luteal phases in young women, although inconsistencies remain (see reviews[16,17]). Others have also found variability in REM sleep with the menstrual cycle phase: REM sleep had an earlier onset[18] and REM sleep episodes were shorter,[16,19] with the amount of REM sleep negatively correlating with progesterone and estradiol levels in the luteal phase.[19] Using a careful ultrarapid sleep-wake cycle procedure, Shechter and Boivin[17] also found that REM sleep was decreased (at circadian phase 0° and 30°) in the luteal phase compared with the follicular phase. This reduction in REM sleep may relate to raised body temperature in the luteal phase.

Finally, most studies support Driver and colleagues'[15] findings of no menstrual cycle variability in sleep continuity PSG measures in young women, although 2 studies found more wakefulness/awakenings in the late luteal phase[20,21] and one study found a steeper increase in progesterone from the follicular to the early to midluteal

phase associated with WASO in the luteal phase.[22] Inconsistencies between studies reflect methodologic challenges, such as small sample sizes, variable cycle length, differences in sampling times across the menstrual cycle, and age-related variability.[16] For example, one study found that women seemed to be more vulnerable to physiologic changes associated with the luteal phase in midlife.[23]

The most dramatic menstrual cycle change in sleep is in electroencephalogram (EEG) activity in the 14.25 to 15.0 Hz (sigma) band corresponding to the upper frequency range of sleep spindles, which is significantly increased in the luteal compared with the follicular phase[15,19,24,25] associated with increased spindle density and duration.[23] Interestingly, midlife women with insomnia showed a blunted increase in sigma EEG activity in the luteal phase, possibly reflecting a weaker influence of the menstrual cycle on sleep EEG in the presence of insomnia.[23] The mechanism for luteal phase increases in spindle activity is unknown; however, it may involve modulation of γ-aminobutyric acid A receptors by progesterone metabolites.[15] Given the supposed sleep-protective function of spindles,[26] increased spindles may function to maintain sleep quality in the presence of luteal phase hormonal changes.[17] Work has begun to explore implications for menstrual cycle variation in sleep spindles, with findings suggesting that spindles could mediate menstrual cycle changes in sleep-dependent memory consolidation.[27,28]

Major findings for PSG measures are summarized in **Table 1**. Upper airway resistance also varies across the menstrual cycle, being lower in the luteal phase in healthy women.[29] The severity of sleep disordered breathing (SDB) may also vary by menstrual phase, which could impact a sleep apnea diagnosis in women. Surprisingly, however, women evaluated for sleep apnea in their self-reported follicular phase had a lower apnea hypopnea index than women evaluated in their self-reported luteal phase.[30] Further studies using a within-subject design are needed.

Circadian Rhythms

Hormonal variations across the menstrual cycle are also associated with changes in circadian rhythms. Body temperature is increased by about 0.4°C[31] due to the thermogenic action of progesterone and has a smaller amplitude due to a blunted nocturnal decline, in the luteal phase compared with the follicular phase.[20] Using an ultrashort sleep-wake cycle procedure to control for light, posture, and food intake, Shechter and colleagues[32] confirmed a reduced amplitude and

Table 1
Summary of evidence comparing objective sleep and related measures during the luteal phase relative to the follicular phase of the menstrual cycle

Variable	Luteal Phase (Relative to Follicular Phase)
SOL	No change
SE	No change
WASO	Most studies in young women show no change Midlife women have more awakenings[a]
SWS and slow wave EEG activity	No change in all-night measures in young women Decreased in midlife women[a]
REM sleep	Decrease in duration of REM sleep episodes
Sigma EEG activity (spindle frequency range)	Increased activity, associated with increased spindle density and duration
Stage 2 sleep	Studies find either increased or no change
Body temperature	Reduced amplitude due to blunted nocturnal decline; no circadian phase shift
Melatonin	No change in phase; 2 of 3 controlled studies find no change in amplitude
Heart rate	Increased (~4 bpm) during sleep, associated with decreased vagal activity
Upper airway resistance	Lower[b]

[a] Data available from only one study.[23]
[b] Data available from only one study.[29]

found no difference in phase for core temperature rhythm in the luteal phase. Melatonin did not differ in acrophase, onset or offset, similar to previous studies that also used controlled conditions.[33,34] Two of these studies also found no menstrual-cycle differences in the amplitude of the melatonin rhythm.[32,34] In one study with controlled conditions, the amplitude of cortisol and thyroid-stimulating hormone rhythms were blunted in the luteal phase[33]; but this finding remains to be replicated.

There are also reports of a raised heart rate (about 4 beats per minute), particularly at night, in the luteal compared with the follicular phase,[16,35–37] although controlled conditions were not used to investigate the rhythms.

In summary, studies using controlled conditions consistently show blunted amplitude of the body temperature rhythm in the luteal phase compared with the follicular phase. Available evidence suggests that melatonin's rhythm is not influenced by the menstrual cycle phase to the same extent as body temperature; however, this remains to be confirmed with additional controlled studies.

SLEEP AND OVARIAN DYSFUNCTION AND ANDROGEN EXCESS (POLYCYSTIC OVARY SYNDROME)
Prevalence, Cause, and Symptoms

The most common endocrine disorder for reproductive-age women is polycystic ovary syndrome (PCOS). PCOS affects 5% to 20% of women, depending on age, type of epidemiologic survey, and diagnostic criteria. There are likely different phenotypes for this syndrome; because polycystic ovaries may or may not be present, discussion about the misleading label of PCOS is leaning toward 3 types: androgen excess with ovarian dysfunction, androgen excess with polycystic ovary morphology, and ovarian dysfunction with polycystic ovarian morphology. The National Institutes of Health estimate that PCOS affects about 5 million women of reproductive age in the United States.[38] High testosterone levels, clinical signs of hyperandrogenism, and irregular menstrual cycles may occur; polycystic ovaries may or may not be present. It is often first diagnosed when a young woman presents clinically with a chief complaint of infertility and laboratory results indicate high serum testosterone or ultrasound reveals an accumulation of cystic, dysfunctional follicles in the ovary.[39] The National Institutes of Health[38] and the Rotterdam Consensus Panel[40] have similar diagnostic criteria (**Box 1**). Long-term health consequences typically result from obesity-related issues and include hyperlipidemia, type 2 diabetes, SDB, and cardiovascular disease.

Although the exact cause of PCOS remains unknown, the abnormal ovarian morphology seen on ultrasound results in the absence of ovarian sources of estrogen and progesterone and leads to irregular menstrual cycles that are likely anovulatory. Theca cells within the ovary continue to secret androgens; the high, unopposed testosterone level is thought to be responsible for clinical manifestations, including

Box 1
Diagnostic criteria for polycystic ovary syndrome

National Institutes of Health[38] (Both of These Criteria Must Be Present)	Rotterdam[40] (Any 2 of These 3 Criteria Must Be Present)
• Presence of oligomenorrhea (fewer than 6 menstrual cycles per year) • Presence of hyperandrogenism (elevated testosterone >2 standard deviations greater than the mean value for the particular laboratory assay)	• Chronic oligomenorrhea (6 or fewer episodes of spontaneous menses per year) • Evidence of hyperandrogenism (either clinical or biochemical) • Polycystic ovaries on ultrasonography

From National Institutes of Health. Final report: evidence-based methodology workshop on polycystic ovary syndrome. December 3–5, 2012; and Rotterdam ESHRE/ASRM-sponsored PCOS consensus workshop group. Revised 2003 consensus on diagnostic criteria and long-term health risks related to polycystic ovary syndrome (PCOS). Hum Reprod 2004;19(1):41–7; with permission.

acne, hirsutism (excessive hair growth on face and body), and alopecia (thinning scalp hair). Excessive weight gain, insulin resistance, snoring, and SDB are also likely to develop; but the time course for these aspects of the syndrome is unknown. Between 50% and 60% of women with PCOS are obese,[41] but adolescents with PCOS are less likely to have SDB than older women with PCOS.[42,43]

Perceived Sleep Quality

Women diagnosed with PCOS often experience sleep problems. Franik and colleagues[41] used self-report measures to compare insomnia in women with and without PCOS. The 95 women with PCOS were 17 to 43 years old and just more than half (53.6%) were normal weight. The prevalence of insomnia was higher in women with PCOS (12.6% scored >10 on the Athens Insomnia Scale and 10.5% scored >14 on the Insomnia Severity Index) compared with controls (3% and 1%, respectively). Although there was no difference in percentage of women in each group with poor sleep quality on the Pittsburgh Sleep Quality Index (PSQI), 25% of the PCOS group reported sleeping less than 6 hours, whereas all controls slept greater than 6 hours per night. It is thought that sleep complaints in

women with PCOS are associated with obesity; however, it is not clear that BMI was controlled in this analysis.

Daytime Sleepiness

Daytime sleepiness would be an expected outcome of poor sleep, but findings are mixed when women with PCOS are compared with controls. Franik and colleagues[41] found no difference in rate of daytime sleepiness (PCOS 7.4%; controls 6.4%), but the cut point for the Epworth Sleepiness Scale (ESS) was not mentioned. Suri and colleagues[44] reported a significant difference in mean ESS scores between PCOS cases (12.5) and controls who self-reported snoring (9.3). They did not control for BMI or SDB and did not report rates of daytime sleepiness based on ESS cut points. The highest rate for daytime sleepiness was reported by Vgontzas and colleagues[45] who used a 4-point scale (none, mild, moderate, severe) and found a high prevalence of daytime sleepiness in women with PCOS (80.4%) compared to controls (27%).

Objective Polysomnography Sleep Comparisons

Two studies that compared PCOS and healthy women's sleep based on one night of PSG had different results. Suri and colleagues[44] compared 50 women with untreated PCOS to controls all studied on the second or third day of the menstrual cycle. The Berlin Sleep Questionnaire was used to screen for SDB, and 58% of the 50 patients with PCOS reported snoring compared with 16% of 100 controls. Based on PSG, only 4% of the 16 controls had SBD, whereas 78% of the patients with PCOS snored and 66% had SDB. After adjusting for BMI and waist circumference, there was no difference in SDB between the two groups. Without adjusting for BMI or SDB, the two groups differed significantly on WASO; patients averaged 55 minutes, whereas controls averaged 38 minutes. SE was similar for patients (84.6%) and controls (87.8%), and they did not differ on SOL (18–23 minutes). REM sleep approached significance, with 56 minutes for patients and 38 minutes for controls ($P = .063$). In contrast, Vgontzas and colleagues[45] also compared women with PCOS with controls in a one-night PSG study without mention of menstrual cycle phase. The 53 patients with PCOS were 16 to 45 years old, with BMIs ranging from 24 to 67 kg/m^2. After adjusting for BMI, both patients and controls had similar REM (percentage of TST), but the PCOS group had longer SOL (44 minutes) compared with controls (30 minutes; $P<.05$). Both groups had longer SOL and less variance[45] compared with the Suri and colleagues' sample.[44]

Sleep Disordered Breathing

It is likely that excessive weight, specifically central obesity, contributes to a high risk for obstructive sleep apnea (OSA) in women with PCOS. In a study of 44 racially/ethnically diverse women (18–40 years old) with PCOS based on the National Institutes of Health's criteria, Mokhlesi and colleagues[46] divided the group into obese (BMI >30; n = 27) and nonobese (n = 17), compared with 34 controls. PSG was not used, and the risk of OSA was based on the Berlin Questionnaire. BMI was the strongest predictor of risk for OSA based on self-reports, but BMI is also a major risk factor in the Berlin Questionnaire. Age was not a significant predictor; when controlling for BMI, neither testosterone level nor PCOS diagnosis were associated with the risk for OSA.[46]

In a recent report of a longitudinal population study in Taiwan, Lin and colleagues[43] noted a prevalence for PCOS of less than 1% of the population. Over time, this group had a higher incidence of OSA than healthy controls after adjusting for age and comorbidities, such as obesity. As shown elsewhere, once BMI is controlled, however, the rates of snoring and SDB are similar to controls[44]; an elevated testosterone level was associated with SDB regardless of PCOS or control group.[44] In contrast, testosterone was not associated with SDB in the 9 patients of PCOS in the Vgontzas and colleagues study[45] but rather with insulin resistance and BMI; however, the BMI cut point was high (32 kg/m²). Of note with implications for treatment, oral contraceptives were used by only 7% of the patients with PCOS with SDB, compared with 20% of patients with PCOS who did not have SDB.

Summary

Few studies have been done using PSG; when there are objective sleep data, it is typically based on one night of PSG with no control for age or menstrual cycle phase. Most sleep research on women with PCOS is focused on SDB, whereby efforts have been made to determine if there is a direct effect of PCOS on SDB or an indirect effect of excess testosterone on central obesity. Despite their relatively young age, women with ovarian dysfunction, androgen excess, and polycystic ovaries are at higher risk of SDB; this risk continues as they age and as their BMI increases. Treatment includes hormonal efforts to lower testosterone levels, which has some evidence of efficacy.[45] Treatment depends on age and phenotype of the syndrome; but oral contraceptives are effective in managing menstrual cycle irregularity, acne, and hirsutism. Metformin is indicated for weight reduction and insulin resistance as well as hirsutism.[47] If present, OSA would be treated with similar protocols for other adults with OSA.

SLEEP AND PREMENSTRUAL SYNDROME
Prevalence, Cause, and Symptoms

Premenstrual syndrome (PMS) is characterized by emotional, behavioral, and physical symptoms that manifest almost exclusively in the late-luteal (premenstrual) phase, with resolution soon after onset of menses. Although many women experience some symptoms premenstrually, up to 18% have severe symptoms that impact daily function.[48] Premenstrual dysphoric disorder (PMDD) is a severe form of PMS evident in 3% to 8% and classified as a depressive disorder in the American Psychiatric Association's *Diagnostic and Statistical Manual of Mental Disorders*, Fifth Edition (*DSM-5*).[48] A PMDD diagnosis requires the occurrence of 5 specified symptoms, of which at least one must be a mood-related symptom experienced in the late-luteal phase, documented for at least 2 consecutive cycles. One of these symptoms is sleep disturbance (insomnia or hypersomnia). The cause of PMDD remains unclear, although symptoms are effectively managed with selective serotonin reuptake inhibitors, anxiolytics, and ovulation-suppressing agents.[49,50]

Perceived Sleep Quality

Women with severe PMS frequently report late-luteal phase sleep symptoms, including insomnia, disturbing dreams, poor sleep quality, daytime sleepiness, and fatigue.[51,52] A recent study used the PSQI to evaluate sleep quality in the past month, not considering menstrual phase, in a sample of female university students (67 with severe PMS/PMDD symptoms and 195 controls).[53] The PMS/PMDD group was more likely than controls to have PSQI scores greater than 5, reflecting poor sleep quality (80.5% vs 56.4%) and higher PSQI scores overall (8.2 ± 3.4 vs 6.5 ± 3.1).[53] PSQI components of sleep duration, SOL, and SE did not differ between groups; however, sleep disturbance, daytime dysfunction, use of sleep medications, and rating sleep quality as poor or very poor were all more prevalent in the PMS/PMDD group.

There may be both trait (across the menstrual cycle) and state (in conjunction with other symptoms) differences in women with PMS/PMDD compared with controls.[51] Traitlike symptoms may then magnify when an additional stressor (eg, hormonal changes associated with menstruation) is present.

Indeed, in one laboratory-based study, women with PMS/PMDD reported more awakenings and felt less refreshed on awakening compared with controls in both the follicular and late-luteal phases and also reported worse sleep quality in their late-luteal phase relative to their own follicular phase.[19]

Objective Polysomnography Sleep Comparisons

Despite evidence of perceived poor sleep quality in the late-luteal phase in women with PMS/PMDD, laboratory studies show little evidence of disturbed PSG sleep parameters specific to this phase. Most studies show no change in SE, arousals, SOL, or sleep EEG in the late-luteal phase relative to follicular phase.[17,19,51] Perception of poor sleep quality in late-luteal phase may be a component of the symptom profile of PMS in the absence of actual sleep disruption, as sleep quality correlated with anxiety in women with PMS/PMDD in the late-luteal phase.[19]

Some studies found differences in PSG measures at both phases of the menstrual cycle, suggesting trait differences in sleep, although the nature of these differences varies between studies.[17,51] Age may influence the severity of sleep disruption in association with symptoms; findings indicate that women more than 40 years old with PMS report more frequent awakenings than younger women[54]; however, PSG studies have not been powered to investigate age-PMS interactions.

Daytime Sleepiness

A few researchers have investigated the second type of sleep disturbance (hypersomnia) listed in the DSM-5 for diagnosis of PMDD. Mauri[55] found that PMS clinic patients reported greater daytime sleepiness in luteal and menstruation phases than other times of the menstrual cycle. Similarly, women with PMS symptoms were sleepier and less alert in the late-luteal phase than in follicular phase, an effect not found in controls in another study.[56] In a survey of 269 young women, women with PMS were more likely to report daytime sleepiness and fatigue premenstrually than controls.[52] Based on objective measures, women with PMS showed psychomotor slowing, with increased lapses and slower reaction times, corresponding with their perceived greater late-luteal levels of sleepiness and fatigue compared with their follicular phase and compared with controls.[57] However, waking EEG measures of alertness and cognitive processing, as well as SOL on the maintenance of wakefulness task, did not differentiate women with PMS when symptomatic, although there were some trait differences.[57]

Altered Circadian Rhythms

Parry and colleagues[58] have conducted several studies to investigate rhythm disturbances under normal sleep and sleep deprivation conditions in PMDD. Although no differences were evident in temperature rhythm between women with and without PMDD during normal sleep, group differences emerged during partial sleep deprivation in the late-luteal phase. Women with PMDD had higher temperature maxima and mesors (rhythm-adjusted mean) than controls. Also, during early sleep deprivation (only sleep 03:00–07:00) compared with baseline in the late-luteal phase, women with PMDD had a delayed acrophase (later time at which temperature peaked), whereas controls had an advanced acrophase.[58] Parry and colleagues[59] also found disturbances in melatonin rhythms and timing of rhythms for cortisol and thyroid-stimulating hormone, suggesting that circadian regulation disturbances may be a factor in PMDD.

In one pilot study on melatonin rhythms in PMDD, the PMDD group had lower nocturnal melatonin levels under controlled conditions at both menstrual phases compared with controls, suggesting a trait difference.[60] A decreased melatonin amplitude in the symptomatic luteal phase was also evident, suggesting an additional sensitivity to the altered ovarian hormone environment (ie, state difference) in PMDD.[60] Women with PMDD also had increased SWS in both follicular and luteal phases compared with controls (similar to other findings[19]), which the investigators hypothesized to be functionally linked to decreased melatonin secretion.[61]

Parry and colleagues[62] have extended their work to investigate differences in response to light between women with and without PMDD. They found that women with PMDD have a blunted phase-shift response to morning bright light in the luteal phase but not in the follicular phase, suggesting less ability to entrain internal rhythms to the external environment and to synchronize other internal circadian rhythms with each other, possibly contributing to mood disturbances that characterize the luteal phase. Given the disturbed melatonin rhythms seen in PMDD, Parry and colleagues[63] have tested appropriately timed light therapy with positive outcomes for mood, although further trials are needed to confirm these effects in larger samples.[50,64]

Summary

Women with severe PMS/PMDD are likely to report poor sleep quality and daytime sleepiness in association with other symptoms in the late luteal phase. However, PSG sleep disruption specific to the symptomatic late-luteal phase is minimal, suggesting that perceived poor sleep and sleepiness may be associated with non–sleepiness-related factors, such as depressed mood or anxiety. Overall, PSG studies indicate traitlike differences in sleep measures; however, the effects are not consistent across studies. A clear disturbance in the circadian rhythm of melatonin is evident in PMDD, both across the menstrual cycle, and specific to the symptomatic phase, which could contribute to the cause of the disorder, and suggests that nonpharmacologic chronotherapies may be effective, with evidence supporting benefit with light therapy.

SLEEP AND DYSMENORRHEA

Dysmenorrhea, defined as painful menstrual cramps of uterine origin, is either primary (menstrual pain without organic disease that typically emerges in adolescence) or secondary (associated with conditions such as endometriosis and pelvic inflammatory disease). The relationship between primary dysmenorrhea and sleep is detailed elsewhere in this special issue (Joan L. Shaver and Stella Iacovides' article, "Sleep in Women with Chronic Pain and Autoimmune Conditions: A Narrative Review," in this issue, 2018). Briefly, evidence indicates that when severe, dysmenorrhea negatively impacts sleep, daytime function, and mood[65–68]; PSG studies also indicate sleep disturbances (lower SE) in association with painful menses.[69,70] Sleep and pain share a reciprocal relationship.[71] Breaking this pain-sleep cycle could be critical for the long-term health of women with primary dysmenorrhea who show increased pain sensitization.[72] One study showed promising effects of a nonsteroidal antiinflammatory drug that alleviated nocturnal pain and restored sleep quality in women with primary dysmenorrhea.[70]

SLEEP AND HORMONAL CONTRACEPTIVES

Combined oral contraceptives (OCs) contain ethinyl estradiol and a synthetic progestin taken for 21 days and a placebo taken for 7 days. During the 21-day period, hypothalamic pituitary ovarian axis activity is suppressed and endogenous estradiol and progesterone levels are low, similar to levels in the follicular phase for nonusers.[73] Across most of the 7-day placebo period, estrogen levels remain suppressed. New formulations contain the minimum steroid doses necessary to inhibit ovulation.[74] Therefore, levels of estrogen and progestin in today's OCs are lower than in older formulations, which needs to be considered when comparing studies.

The few studies that have examined PSG measures in women taking OCs have not found increased sleep disruption or poorer sleep quality; however, sleep architecture is altered. Women had about 12% more N2 sleep on a night during the 21-day period of active pill compared with a night in the 7-day placebo period.[75] They also have more N2 sleep and less N3 (SWS) than naturally cycling women in the luteal phase[75–77] and possibly a shorter REM onset latency.[77] Hachul and colleagues[13] found that women using OCs experienced less snoring, a lower apnea hypopnea index, shorter latency to REM sleep, and fewer arousals. Finally, the use of a synthetic progestin (medroxyprogesterone) was associated with increased upper spindle frequency activity and greater sleep spindle density in women,[78] similar to natural luteal phase effects.

Women taking OCs have increased 24-hour body temperature profiles, similar to the natural luteal phase, probably due to progestin. This increased temperature profile persists during the 7-day placebo period,[76] which contrasts with the rapid decline in temperature, as progesterone levels decline before menstruation in ovulatory cycles. OCs may also influence the melatonin profile, although findings are inconsistent.[20] In one study using a modified constant routine procedure, melatonin levels did not differ between naturally cycling women and women taking OCs, although there was a trend for increased melatonin in the latter part of the night in the OC group.[34]

In summary, OCs alter aspects of sleep architecture as well as body temperature, although their impact on sleep quality seems to be minimal. Given the lower doses of hormones in current OCs, it would be interesting to investigate whether sleep architecture and body temperature changes are still evident.

IMPACT OF SLEEP ON REPRODUCTIVE FUNCTION

Not only does the reproductive cycle influence sleep but sleep can also influence reproductive function.[79] Sleep duration, timing, and quality can influence the reproductive system, with effects depending on reproductive maturity. During puberty, LH is released in a pulsatile fashion during N3, playing a critical role in reproductive regulation.[80,81] In adulthood, direction of the relationship changes in the early follicular phase, with sleep inhibiting pulsatile LH secretion, thought to be critical for recruitment of ovarian follicles.[82]

There are reports of associations between short sleep duration and altered menstrual cycles in both adolescents and adults. Women reporting less than 6-hour sleep were more likely to report abnormal (short or long) menstrual cycle lengths[83]; in a survey of adolescents, short sleep duration ($\leq$5 hours) was significantly associated with an increased likelihood of menstrual cycle irregularity, even after adjusting for confounding variables.[84] There has been a larger body of work investigating the impact of shiftwork on reproductive function in women, given the typical disrupted sleep and circadian patterns in this group. This work is described in detail elsewhere in this special issue (Kervezee and colleagues' article, "Impact of Shift Work on the Circadian Timing System and Health in Women," in this issue, 2018).

SUMMARY

Sleep and circadian rhythms are altered in association with the hormonal changes of the menstrual cycle and in the presence of menstrual-associated disorders. The magnitude of effect varies, particularly for self-reported sleep quality, which worsens in some, but not all, women when premenstrual symptoms emerge. Importantly, women with PCOS have an increased risk for SDB, which should be treated to mitigate health impacts. Potential menstrual cycle variability in sleep quality as well as upper airway resistance should be considered when evaluating reproductive-age women. For research purposes, the impact of the menstrual cycle phase should be kept in mind when data are collected and, ideally, the phase should be documented. When comparing women with men, women of reproductive age should be studied in the early-mid follicular phase before there is potential influence from ovarian hormones.

REFERENCES

1. Wood C, Larsen L, Williams R. Menstrual characteristics of 2,343 women attending the Shepherd Foundation. Aust N Z J Obstet Gynaecol 1979; 19(2):107–10.
2. Shughrue PJ, Lane MV, Merchenthaler I. Comparative distribution of estrogen receptor-alpha and -beta mRNA in the rat central nervous system. J Comp Neurol 1997;388(4):507–25.
3. Curran-Rauhut MA, Petersen SL. The distribution of progestin receptor mRNA in rat brainstem. Brain Res Gene Expr Patterns 2002;1(3–4):151–7.
4. Mong JA, Baker FC, Mahoney MM, et al. Sleep, rhythms, and the endocrine brain: influence of sex and gonadal hormones. J Neurosci 2011;31(45): 16107–16.
5. Mong JA, Cusmano DM. Sex differences in sleep: impact of biological sex and sex steroids. Philos Trans R Soc Lond B Biol Sci 2016;371(1688): 20150110.
6. Baker FC, Driver HS. Self-reported sleep across the menstrual cycle in young, healthy women. J Psychosom Res 2004;56(2):239–43.
7. Kravitz HM, Janssen I, Santoro N, et al. Relationship of day-to-day reproductive hormone levels to sleep in midlife women. Arch Intern Med 2005;165(20): 2370–6.
8. Manber R, Baker FC, Gress JL. Sex differences in sleep and sleep disorders: a focus on women's sleep. Int J Sleep Disord 2006;1:7–15.
9. National Sleep Foundation NSF. Sleep in America 2008 poll. 2008. Available at: http://www.sleepfoundation.org/atf/cf/%7Bf6bf2668-a1b4-4fe8-8d1a-a5d39340d9cb%7D/2008%20POLL%20SOF.PDF. Accessed August 20, 2008.
10. Li DX, Romans S, De Souza MJ, et al. Actigraphic and self-reported sleep quality in women: associations with ovarian hormones and mood. Sleep Med 2015;16(10):1217–24.
11. Romans SE, Kreindler D, Einstein G, et al. Sleep quality and the menstrual cycle. Sleep Med 2015; 16(4):489–95.
12. Van Reen E, Kiesner J. Individual differences in self-reported difficulty sleeping across the menstrual cycle. Arch Womens Ment Health 2016;19(4):599–608.
13. Hachul H, Andersen ML, Bittencourt LR, et al. Does the reproductive cycle influence sleep patterns in women with sleep complaints? Climacteric 2010; 13(6):594–603.
14. Zheng H, Harlow SD, Kravitz HM, et al. Actigraphy-defined measures of sleep and movement across the menstrual cycle in midlife menstruating women: study of Women's Health Across the Nation Sleep Study. Menopause 2015;22(1):66–74.
15. Driver HS, Dijk DJ, Werth E, et al. Sleep and the sleep electroencephalogram across the menstrual cycle in young healthy women. J Clin Endocrinol Metab 1996;81(2):728–35.
16. Driver HS, Werth E, Dijk D, et al. The menstrual cycle effects on sleep. Sleep Med Clin 2008;3:1–11.
17. Shechter A, Boivin DB. Sleep, hormones, and circadian rhythms throughout the menstrual cycle in healthy women and women with premenstrual dysphoric disorder. Int J Endocrinol 2010;2010: 259345.
18. Lee KA, Shaver JF, Giblin EC, et al. Sleep patterns related to menstrual cycle phase and premenstrual affective symptoms. Sleep 1990;13(5):403–9.
19. Baker FC, Sassoon SA, Kahan T, et al. Perceived poor sleep quality in the absence of polysomnographic sleep disturbance in women with severe premenstrual syndrome. J Sleep Res 2012;21(5): 535–45.

20. Baker FC, Driver HS. Circadian rhythms, sleep, and the menstrual cycle. Sleep Med 2007;8(6): 613–22.

21. Parry BL, Berga SL, Mostofi N, et al. Morning versus evening bright light treatment of late luteal phase dysphoric disorder. Am J Psychiatry 1989;146(9): 1215–7.

22. Sharkey KM, Crawford SL, Kim S, et al. Objective sleep interruption and reproductive hormone dynamics in the menstrual cycle. Sleep Med 2014; 15(6):688–93.

23. de Zambotti M, Willoughby AR, Sassoon SA, et al. Menstrual cycle-related variation in physiological sleep in women in the early menopausal transition. J Clin Endocrinol Metab 2015;100(8):2918–26.

24. Baker FC, Kahan TL, Trinder J, et al. Sleep quality and the sleep electroencephalogram in women with severe premenstrual syndrome. Sleep 2007; 30(10):1283–91.

25. Ishizuka Y, Pollak CP, Shirakawa S, et al. Sleep spindle frequency changes during the menstrual cycle. J Sleep Res 1994;3(1):26–9.

26. Steriade M, McCormick DA, Sejnowski TJ. Thalamocortical oscillations in the sleeping and aroused brain. Science 1993;262(5134):679–85.

27. Genzel L, Kiefer T, Renner L, et al. Sex and modulatory menstrual cycle effects on sleep related memory consolidation. Psychoneuroendocrinology 2012;37(7):987–98.

28. Sattari N, McDevitt EA, Panas D, et al. The effect of sex and menstrual phase on memory formation during a nap. Neurobiol Learn Mem 2017;145:119–28.

29. Driver HS, McLean H, Kumar DV, et al. The influence of the menstrual cycle on upper airway resistance and breathing during sleep. Sleep 2005; 28(4):449–56.

30. Spector AR, Loriaux D, Alexandru D, et al. The influence of the menstrual phases on polysomnography. Cureus 2016;8(11):e871.

31. de Mouzon J, Testart J, Lefevre B, et al. Time relationships between basal body temperature and ovulation or plasma progestins. Fertil Steril 1984; 41(2):254–9.

32. Shechter A, Varin F, Boivin DB. Circadian variation of sleep during the follicular and luteal phases of the menstrual cycle. Sleep 2010;33(5):647–56.

33. Shibui K, Uchiyama M, Okawa M, et al. Diurnal fluctuation of sleep propensity and hormonal secretion across the menstrual cycle. Biol Psychiatry 2000; 48(11):1062–8.

34. Wright KP Jr, Badia P. Effects of menstrual cycle phase and oral contraceptives on alertness, cognitive performance, and circadian rhythms during sleep deprivation. Behav Brain Res 1999;103(2): 185–94.

35. Baker FC, Colrain IM, Trinder J. Reduced parasympathetic activity during sleep in the symptomatic phase of severe premenstrual syndrome. J Psychosom Res 2008;65(1):13–22.

36. de Zambotti M, Nicholas CL, Colrain IM, et al. Autonomic regulation across phases of the menstrual cycle and sleep stages in women with premenstrual syndrome and healthy controls. Psychoneuroendocrinology 2013;38(11):2618–27.

37. de Zambotti M, Trinder J, Colrain IM, et al. Menstrual cycle-related variation in autonomic nervous system functioning in women in the early menopausal transition with and without insomnia disorder. Psychoneuroendocrinology 2017;75:44–51.

38. National Institutes of Health. Final Report: evidence-based methodology workshop on polycystic ovary syndrome. December 3–5, 2012.

39. Legro RS, Arslanian SA, Ehrmann DA, et al. Diagnosis and treatment of polycystic ovary syndrome: an Endocrine Society clinical practice guideline. J Clin Endocrinol Metab 2013;98(12):4565–92.

40. Rotterdam ESHRE/ASRM-Sponsored PCOS Consensus Workshop Group. Revised 2003 consensus on diagnostic criteria and long-term health risks related to polycystic ovary syndrome (PCOS). Hum Reprod 2004;19(1):41–7.

41. Franik G, Krysta K, Madej P, et al. Sleep disturbances in women with polycystic ovary syndrome. Gynecol Endocrinol 2016;32(12):1014–7.

42. Helvaci N, Karabulut E, Demir AU, et al. Polycystic ovary syndrome and the risk of obstructive sleep apnea: a meta-analysis and review of the literature. Endocr Connect 2017;6(7):437–45.

43. Lin TY, Lin PY, Su TP, et al. Risk of developing obstructive sleep apnea among women with polycystic ovarian syndrome: a nationwide longitudinal follow-up study. Sleep Med 2017;36:165–9.

44. Suri J, Suri JC, Chatterjee B, et al. Obesity may be the common pathway for sleep-disordered breathing in women with polycystic ovary syndrome. Sleep Med 2016;24:32–9.

45. Vgontzas AN, Legro RS, Bixler EO, et al. Polycystic ovary syndrome is associated with obstructive sleep apnea and daytime sleepiness: role of insulin resistance. J Clin Endocrinol Metab 2001;86(2):517–20.

46. Mokhlesi B, Scoccia B, Mazzone T, et al. Risk of obstructive sleep apnea in obese and nonobese women with polycystic ovary syndrome and healthy reproductively normal women. Fertil Steril 2012; 97(3):786–91.

47. Kamboj MK, Bonny AE. Polycystic ovary syndrome in adolescence: diagnostic and therapeutic strategies. Transl Pediatr 2017;6(4):248–55.

48. Halbreich U. The etiology, biology, and evolving pathology of premenstrual syndromes. Psychoneuroendocrinology 2003;28(Suppl 3):55–99.

49. Rapkin A. A review of treatment of premenstrual syndrome and premenstrual dysphoric disorder. Psychoneuroendocrinology 2003;28(Suppl 3):39–53.

50. Sepede G, Sarchione F, Matarazzo I, et al. Premenstrual dysphoric disorder without comorbid psychiatric conditions: a systematic review of therapeutic options. Clin Neuropharmacol 2016;39(5):241–61.

51. Baker FC, Lamarche LJ, Iacovides S, et al. Sleep and menstrual-related disorders. Sleep Med Clin 2008;3:25–35.

52. Gupta R, Lahan V, Bansal S. Subjective sleep problems in young women suffering from premenstrual dysphoric disorder. N Am J Med Sci 2012;4(11): 593–5.

53. Khazaie H, Ghadami MR, Khaledi-Paveh B, et al. Sleep quality in university students with premenstrual dysphoric disorder. Shanghai Arch Psychiatry 2016;28(3):131–8.

54. Kuan AJ, Carter DM, Ott FJ. Premenstrual complaints before and after 40 years of age. Can J Psychiatry 2004;49(3):215.

55. Mauri M. Sleep and the reproductive cycle: a review. Health Care Women Int 1990;11(4):409–21.

56. Lamarche LJ, Driver HS, Wiebe S, et al. Nocturnal sleep, daytime sleepiness, and napping among women with significant emotional/behavioral premenstrual symptoms. J Sleep Res 2007;16(3): 262–8.

57. Baker FC, Colrain IM. Daytime sleepiness, psychomotor performance, waking EEG spectra and evoked potentials in women with severe premenstrual syndrome. J Sleep Res 2010;19(1 Pt 2): 214–27.

58. Parry BL, LeVeau B, Mostofi N, et al. Temperature circadian rhythms during the menstrual cycle and sleep deprivation in premenstrual dysphoric disorder and normal comparison subjects. J Biol Rhythms 1997;12(1):34–46.

59. Parry BL, Martinez LF, Maurer EL, et al. Sleep, rhythms and women's mood. Part I. Menstrual cycle, pregnancy and postpartum. Sleep Med Rev 2006; 10(2):129–44.

60. Shechter A, Lesperance P, Ng Ying Kin NM, et al. Pilot investigation of the circadian plasma melatonin rhythm across the menstrual cycle in a small group of women with premenstrual dysphoric disorder. PLoS One 2012;7(12):e51929.

61. Shechter A, Lesperance P, Ng Ying Kin NM, et al. Nocturnal polysomnographic sleep across the menstrual cycle in premenstrual dysphoric disorder. Sleep Med 2012;13(8):1071–8.

62. Parry BL, Meliska CJ, Sorenson DL, et al. Reduced phase-advance of plasma melatonin after bright morning light in the luteal, but not follicular, menstrual cycle phase in premenstrual dysphoric disorder: an extended study. Chronobiol Int 2011;28(5): 415–24.

63. Parry BL, Berga SL, Mostofi N, et al. Plasma melatonin circadian rhythms during the menstrual cycle and after light therapy in premenstrual dysphoric disorder and normal control subjects. J Biol Rhythms 1997;12(1):47–64.

64. Krasnik C, Montori VM, Guyatt GH, et al. The effect of bright light therapy on depression associated with premenstrual dysphoric disorder. Am J Obstet Gynecol 2005;193(3 Pt 1):658–61.

65. (NSF) NSF. Women and sleep poll. 1998. Available at: www.sleepfoundation.org. Accessed February 24, 2006.

66. Davis S, Mirick DK. Circadian disruption, shift work and the risk of cancer: a summary of the evidence and studies in Seattle. Cancer Causes Control 2006;17(4):539–45.

67. Woosley JA, Lichstein KL. Dysmenorrhea, the menstrual cycle, and sleep. Behav Med 2014;40(1):14–21.

68. Liu X, Chen H, Liu ZZ, et al. Early menarche and menstrual problems are associated with sleep disturbance in a large sample of Chinese adolescent girls. Sleep 2017;40(9).

69. Baker FC, Driver HS, Rogers GG, et al. High nocturnal body temperatures and disturbed sleep in women with primary dysmenorrhea. Am J Physiol 1999;277(6 Pt 1):E1013–21.

70. Iacovides S, Avidon I, Bentley A, et al. Diclofenac potassium restores objective and subjective measures of sleep quality in women with primary dysmenorrhea. Sleep 2009;32(8):1019–26.

71. Iacovides S, George K, Kamerman P, et al. Sleep fragmentation hypersensitizes healthy young women to deep and superficial experimental pain. J Pain 2017;18(7):844–54.

72. Iacovides S, Avidon I, Baker FC. What we know about primary dysmenorrhea today: a critical review. Hum Reprod Update 2015;21(6):762–78.

73. Gogos A, Wu YC, Williams AS, et al. The effects of ethinylestradiol and progestins ("the pill") on cognitive function in pre-menopausal women. Neurochem Res 2014;39(12):2288–300.

74. Cedars MI. Triphasic oral contraceptives: review and comparison of various regimens. Fertil Steril 2002;77(1):1–14.

75. Baker FC, Waner JI, Vieira EF, et al. Sleep and 24 hour body temperatures: a comparison in young men, naturally cycling women and women taking hormonal contraceptives. J Physiol 2001;530(Pt 3):565–74.

76. Baker FC, Mitchell D, Driver HS. Oral contraceptives alter sleep and raise body temperature in young women. Pflugers Arch 2001;442(5): 729–37.

77. Shine-Burdick R, Hoffmann R, Armitage R. Short note: oral contraceptives and sleep in depressed and healthy women. Sleep 2002;25(3):347–9.

78. Plante DT, Goldstein MR. Medroxyprogesterone acetate is associated with increased sleep spindles during non-rapid eye movement sleep in women referred for polysomnography. Psychoneuroendocrinology 2013;38(12):3160–6.

79. Kloss JD, Perlis ML, Zamzow JA, et al. Sleep, sleep disturbance, and fertility in women. Sleep Med Rev 2015;22:78–87.

80. Boyar R, Finkelstein J, Roffwarg H, et al. Synchronization of augmented luteinizing hormone secretion with sleep during puberty. N Engl J Med 1972; 287(12):582–6.

81. Shaw ND, Butler JP, McKinney SM, et al. Insights into puberty: the relationship between sleep stages and pulsatile LH secretion. J Clin Endocrinol Metab 2012;97(11):E2055–62.

82. Hall JE, Sullivan JP, Richardson GS. Brief wake episodes modulate sleep-inhibited luteinizing hormone secretion in the early follicular phase. J Clin Endocrinol Metab 2005;90(4):2050–5.

83. Lim AJ, Huang Z, Chua SE, et al. Sleep duration, exercise, shift work and polycystic ovarian syndrome-related outcomes in a healthy population: a cross-sectional study. PLoS One 2016;11(11):e0167048.

84. Nam GE, Han K, Lee G. Association between sleep duration and menstrual cycle irregularity in Korean female adolescents. Sleep Med 2017;35:62–6.

Impact of Shift Work on the Circadian Timing System and Health in Women

Laura Kervezee, PhD[a], Ari Shechter, PhD[b],
Diane B. Boivin, MD, PhD[a],*

KEYWORDS

- Shift work • Circadian clock • Sleep • Women • Sex differences • Circadian misalignment
- Chronobiology

KEY POINTS

- Shift workers experience circadian misalignment, which leads to acute physiologic effects that may contribute to long-term health problems.
- Sex differences in the circadian timing system are present on molecular, physiologic, behavioral, and cognitive levels, which contribute to sex-specific health and safety concerns related to shift work.
- Recent epidemiologic evidence indicates that women who work night shifts have an increased risk of developing cancer, metabolic syndrome, cardiovascular disease, diabetes, and reproductive disturbances compared with women who work during traditional working hours.
- Night shift workers who have not adapted to their work schedule can experience the lowest alertness and performance during their work period and, importantly, during their commute home in the morning.

INTRODUCTION

Shift work, commonly defined as work that is performed outside the conventional 9-to-5 working day, is a necessary product of the 24-7 society that requires many industries to be operational around the clock. Data from the 2010 National Health Interview Survey in the United States revealed that 29% of the workforce described their work time arrangement as different from a regular day shift.[1] The 2005 General Social Survey in Canada arrived at a similar percentage, with 28% of the workforce working in shifts.[2] In the European Union (EU), 21% of the workers report working in nonstandard shifts and 19% work at night at least once a month.[3] The percentages of men and women involved in shift work are equal in both North America and the EU.[1–3]

Shift work is associated with various adverse health effects[4,5] and is regarded as probably carcinogenic in humans by the International Agency for Research on Cancer (IARC).[6] Although there is

Disclosure Statement: This research was supported by operating grants from the Canadian Institutes of Health Research (CIHR, MOP-137052) and The Institut De Recherche Robert-Sauvé En Santé Et En Sécurité Du Travail (IRSST, operating grant 2013-0046). L. Kervezee received a postdoctoral fellowship from the Fonds de Recherche du Québec–Santé. D.B. Boivin provides conferences and legal expert advices on various cases related to shift work.
a Department of Psychiatry, Centre for Study and Treatment of Circadian Rhythms, Douglas Mental Health University Institute, McGill University, 6875 LaSalle Boulevard, Montreal, Quebec H4H 1R3, Canada; b Department of Medicine, Center for Behavioral Cardiovascular Health, Columbia University, 622 West 168th Street, Room 9-300B, New York, NY 10032, USA
* Corresponding author.
E-mail address: diane.boivin@douglas.mcgill.ca

increasing evidence that sex differences exist on all biological levels (see later discussion of chronobiology), women remain an underrepresented group in biomedical research. Therefore, it is crucial to address the specific challenges faced by female shift workers. This review provides a brief overview of the circadian timing system, the disruption of which is thought to contribute to the adverse health effects associated with shift work. Focusing on scientific literature involving actual shift workers or laboratory-based studies in healthy human subjects, we discuss sex differences in the regulation of the circadian timing system and the sleep–wake cycle that may underlie female-specific susceptibility to adverse effects of shift work. The health concerns for the female shift worker and countermeasures that might aid in the adaptation to the shifted work schedule and, possibly, in the prevention of the adverse health effects are described.

CIRCADIAN TIMING SYSTEM

Daily variations have been found in many physiologic and behavioral processes in humans, such as hormone levels, sleep propensity, alertness, and organ function. These daily rhythms are generated by the circadian system (from the Latin circa dies: approximately 1 day), an endogenous timing system that emerged early in evolutionary history as an adaptation to predictable, cyclic changes in light, temperature, and food availability.[7]

Although sex differences in the period length for circadian rhythms have been identified (see later discussion), the endogenous circadian timing system in humans has an average period of 24.2 hours, and hence requires daily resetting to remain entrained to the 24-hour light–dark cycles on Earth.[8] Light, the most prominent synchronizer in humans and other mammals, is transmitted from the retina to the central clock located in the suprachiasmatic nuclei (SCN) of the anterior hypothalamus.[9] Within the SCN, photic input is integrated and conveyed to peripheral tissues (Fig. 1A). Cells in the SCN show self-sustained circadian rhythms, which are generated by a molecular transcriptional/translational feedback loop that autonomously sustains a rhythm with a period of approximately 24 hours in each neuron (Fig. 1B).[10]

The transcriptional–translational feedback loop is not unique to the cells of the SCN. In fact, most cell types in the body express a similar set of clock genes[11,12] that can oscillate autonomously.[13] In humans, 24-hour rhythms in the expression levels of clock genes have been found in many peripheral tissues, including peripheral blood mononuclear cells,[14] adipose tissue,[15,16] oral mucosa,[17] fibroblasts,[18] bone marrow,[19] and several brain regions.[20,21] The core clock genes not only regulate their own expression but also that of clock-controlled genes. Early microarray studies in mice revealed that up to 10% of genes in the SCN and the liver show circadian expression patterns.[22,23] In humans, genome-wide gene

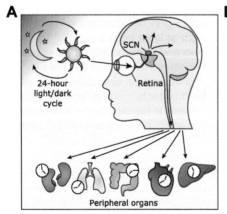
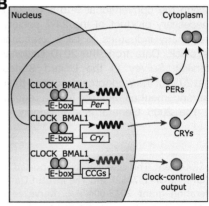

Fig. 1. Organization of the circadian timing system at (A) the level of the organism and (B) of the cell. (A) The biological clock is located in the SCN. Light information from the environment is transmitted from the retina to the SCN in the hypothalamus. Neuronal and humoral signals from the SCN synchronize the circadian oscillators in peripheral organs. (B) At the cellular level, a 24-hour rhythm is generated by a translational or transcriptional feedback loop. The transcription factors CLOCK and BMAL1 bind to E-box elements in the promotor of other clock genes (*period1, 2* and *cryptochrome1, 2*) and of clock-controlled genes (CCGs), thereby activating their transcription. After translation in the cytoplasm, PER and CRY dimerize and translocate to the nucleus, where they inhibit the transcriptional activity of CLOCK and BMAL1. Hereby, the 2 proteins down-regulate their own transcription. This (simplified) process creates oscillations in gene expression with a period of approximately 24 hours.

expression studies in blood,[24–26] brain tissue,[27–29] adipose tissue,[30] and hair follicle cells[31] have revealed that a similar proportion of the human transcriptome shows 24-hour variation.

An important difference between the core clock machinery in the central clock in the SCN and peripheral clocks in other tissues is that SCN neurons can be directly entrained by environmental synchronizers, the most powerful of which is light.[32] Depending on the timing, spectral composition, and intensity of light exposure, the central circadian clock can be rapidly shifted to earlier or later phases,[33] whereas peripheral tissues take longer to synchronize to shifts in the environmental light–dark cycle in rats.[34] However, recently, a laboratory-based shift work protocol in healthy adults was conducted in which sleep periods were delayed by 10 hours.[35] The findings show that, in humans, bright light exposure can synchronize peripheral clock gene expression more rapidly than previously expected based on animal experiments. However, assessment of genome-wide gene expression levels is required to determine to what extent the entire circadian transcriptome adapts to a night-oriented shift work schedule. In addition, it has been shown that feeding cycles can differentially affect the central clock and peripheral clocks, although the exact mechanism remains to be elucidated.[36]

The circadian timing system interacts with the homeostatic drive for sleep to regulate the daily pattern of wakefulness and sleep.[37] The duration of wakefulness increases the need for sleep, while the circadian timing system increasingly promotes wakefulness during the day to counteract the homeostatic need for sleep. These processes interact to maintain wakefulness for approximately 16 hours during the day and consolidated sleep for approximately 8 hours during the night.[38] The timing of sleep relative to the endogenous circadian phase, as measured by core body temperature or melatonin rhythms, was found to depend on the intrinsic circadian period, with a shorter circadian period associated with increased morningness and sleep occurring at a later endogenous circadian phase.[39,40]

SEX DIFFERENCES IN THE CIRCADIAN TIMING SYSTEM

Sex differences in the function of the circadian timing system have been observed on many different levels. In general, the intrinsic circadian period is shorter in women compared with men and a larger percentage of women have period lengths that are shorter than 24 hours.[41] As a result, the phase angle of entrainment; that is, the time between circadian phase markers and habitual wake time, is longer in women than in men.[41–44] Consequently, for similar timing of sleep periods, the circadian phases of many different biological processes are earlier in women compared with men. For example, the phases for several physiologic circadian markers, such as dim light melatonin onset (DLMO) and core body temperature minimum, are also earlier in women compared with men, despite similar habitual sleep times in the study populations.[42–45]

Interestingly, the phases in peak expression levels of the core clock genes *Per2*, *Per3*, and *Arntl1* in the aged human cerebral cortex occur significantly earlier in women compared with men.[21] On the behavioral level, women have an earlier chronotype with a higher preference for morningness compared with men.[46–49] This difference is most pronounced at the end of adolescence and disappears around 50 years of age, the average age of menopause, suggesting the involvement of sex hormones in the regulation of chronotype.[49]

Furthermore, the timing of a wide range of sleep measures shows significant sex differences. For example, in a recent study, an ultradian sleep–wake cycle protocol was used in which participants alternated 1-hour naps with 1-hour wake episodes for 72 hours. The diurnal and circadian variation in vigilance levels and sleep measures, such as sleep efficiency and sleep onset latency, were quantified, as well as the amount of slow wave sleep, rapid eye movement (REM) sleep, and non-REM sleep.[42] These measures varied significantly over the 24-hour period and were phase-advanced by approximately 2 hours relative to habitual bedtimes in women compared with men.[42] This phase advance is explained by the additive effects of earlier timing of the circadian variation of sleep and a longer phase angle of entrainment in women.[42]

Perhaps related to these findings, women also have an increased risk of developing sleep disturbances. For example, women have a 41% higher risk of developing insomnia compared with men[50] and, in general, women report poorer subjective sleep quality, although this is not reflected in objective measures of sleep architecture.[51,52] There is evidence to suggest that sex differences in the circadian timing system may at least partially underlie the increased propensity for developing sleep disturbances. For example, because women have an earlier endogenous circadian phase relative to wake time, the circadian drive for alertness is advanced.[42] It has been suggested that this explains the higher rates of sleep maintenance insomnia and early morning awakenings[53] observed in women compared with men.[41,42]

In terms of performance and alertness, laboratory-based studies have shown that accuracy-related tasks, as well as subjective alertness, display larger circadian variations, with a greater extent of deterioration in these measures during the night in women compared with men.[42,54] These observations may explain the reduced tolerance to shift work[55] and greater risk of work injury associated with shift work[56] reported in women.

Clinical Implications of Sex Differences in Circadian Timing

Sex differences in the circadian timing system have important clinical implications. For example, a specific time-dependent administration of chemotherapeutic drugs significantly improves survival rate in men with metastatic colorectal cancer but had the opposite effect on women compared with the conventional dosing regimen.[57,58] The chronomodulated dosing regimen consisted of a 4-day infusion of fluorouacil and leucovorin at night with peak delivery at 04:00 and oxaliplatin during the day with a peak at 16:00. These phase III clinical trials were based on the rationale that the tolerance and efficacy of drugs depends on the time of day as a result of 24-hour rhythms in drug metabolism, cell division, and DNA repair.[59] However, during determination of the dosing regimen in preclinical and clinical studies, women were underrepresented in the study sample, and the sex-dependent response to the chronomodulated schedule was not specifically addressed.[60] These results emphasize the importance of considering sex differences when studying function of the circadian timing system.

DEREGULATION OF CIRCADIAN TIMING SYSTEM AND SLEEP–WAKE CYCLE IN SHIFT WORK

Shift workers are exposed to atypical or irregular timing of sleep, which leads to misalignment between the endogenous circadian timing system and the sleep–wake cycle. When measured by a circadian marker such as phase of the melatonin rhythm, the exact proportion of night shift workers in which the central clock adapts to the shifted sleep–wake schedule remains controversial, with estimates ranging from as low as 3%[61] up to 41%.[62] Regardless of the exact estimate, the central clock does not seem to adapt to a nightly work schedule in most shift workers.

The acute physiologic consequences of circadian misalignment have been described in laboratory-based studies of healthy subjects. Circadian misalignment is associated with alterations of physiologic processes, such as decreased total daily energy expenditure,[63] reduced glucose tolerance and insulin sensitivity,[64–67] lowered leptin levels,[67] increased blood pressure and cardiac vagal modulation,[62,68] elevated systemic inflammatory markers,[65,68,69] and a desynchrony between rhythmic cytokine release and fluctuating numbers of monocytes and T lymphocytes.[70] Furthermore, a novel hypothesis is that at least some of the physiologic health effects of circadian misalignment are related to disturbances of gut microbiota, which warrants further investigation.[71] The alterations in metabolic, inflammatory, and cardiovascular markers due to short-term circadian misalignment provide insights into the underlying physiologic mechanisms of adverse health effects associated with shift work.

In addition, circadian misalignment has a direct impact on fatigue and performance. Arousal depends both on time awake, which increases the homeostatic sleep drive, and on circadian phase. From a circadian perspective, arousal is lowest near the circadian body temperature minimum at the end of the night and this trough in arousal is aggravated by prolonged wakefulness.[72] Hence, night shift workers who have not adapted to their work schedule can experience the lowest alertness and performance during their work period and, importantly, during their commute home in the morning.[73] As a result, shift work can lead to an increased risk of accidents in the workplace and on the road.[74–76] Therefore, research that contributes to the development of strategies to enhance adaptation among shift workers is crucial for preventing long-term health consequences, as well as improving work safety.

HEALTH EFFECTS OF SHIFT WORK IN WOMEN

The last decade has seen a large number of epidemiologic studies in shift workers that investigate the association between shift work and the risk of developing a variety of adverse health effects, including cancer, type 2 diabetes mellitus (T2DM), cardiovascular disorders, reproductive health issues, and sleep disturbances. The authors review this literature by focusing primarily on meta-analyses and systematic reviews on the association between shift work and negative health effects in women. Recent large-scale epidemiologic studies of female shift workers that have not yet been included in meta-analyses are also discussed.

Sleep Disturbances

Shift work has a major impact on sleep because atypical work schedules often interfere with the biologically optimal time for sleep.[77] A systematic review concluded that, although the evidence is not unequivocal, women generally show reduced tolerance to shift work compared with men; that is, they have more sleep problems, higher levels of fatigue and sleepiness, and higher rates of disability.[55] Shift workers who experience insomnia or excessive sleepiness associated with a work schedule that overlaps with their usual sleep period should be assessed for a specific type of circadian rhythm sleep–wake disorder diagnosed as shift work disorder (SWD).[78,79] The prevalence of SWD among shift workers is currently unknown, with estimates ranging from 10%[80] and 44%[81] in rotating and night shift workers. Despite the higher number of female shift workers who report sleep problems, SWD has been reported more frequently in male shift workers.[81–83]

Injury

The risk for work-related injuries is high in adults who work night shifts, and it has been estimated that 13% of these injuries could be due to sleep problems.[84] A meta-analysis on the association between sleep problems and work injuries concluded that studies with a higher proportion of female participants tended to find a higher risk for occupational injury.[84] In addition, among a sample of Canadian workers, women who did shift work were found to have a higher risk of work injury compared with day workers than men who did shift work.[56] The extent to which sex differences in night shift work-related injuries can be attributable to biological sex differences in circadian variations in performance remains to be investigated. Furthermore, additional nonwork-related obligations potentially faced more frequently by women than men (eg, childcare or other domestic responsibilities) also require consideration in future research and in clinical practice.

Cancer

In 2007, the IARC concluded that shift work involving circadian disruption is probably carcinogenic to humans. This conclusion was based on sufficient mechanistic evidence in animal studies, as well as limited evidence from epidemiologic studies of the association between night shift work and breast cancer.[6] Since the IARC publication, various meta-analyses have evaluated the scientific literature available on this topic. Most meta-analyses reported a significant association between night shift work and the risk of breast cancer,[85–88] although limited evidence was found in 2 other publications.[89,90] Overall, studies that found a significant association indicate that exposure to night shift work increases the risk of breast cancer by 6% to 20% compared with no exposure to night shift work.[85–88]

In a few studies that attempted to find an exposure–effect relationship, the number of years involved in shift work was positively associated with the risk of developing breast cancer.[86–88] However, the quantification of shift work exposure is challenging because it not only entails the number of years involved in shift work but also the intensity and frequency during those years. Future research is warranted to develop a validated measure of shift work exposure that takes into account all of these variables.

Importantly, recent results from the Nurses' Health Study, which involves 2 large cohort studies among almost 200,000 nurses in the United States, revealed that the risk of developing breast cancer increased in women who accumulated years of night shift work early in their career (hazard ratio [HR] 2.15, 95% CI 1.23–3.73) but that the increased risk may wane over time after night shift work has stopped.[91] These observations offer a possible explanation for some of the inconsistent results obtained in the meta-analyses. In addition, it shows that researchers who are investigating exposure–effect relationships should also consider at what age or career stage the exposure occurred.

A recently published report on the risk of breast cancer associated with night shift work included 3 prospective studies involving almost 800,000 women in the United Kingdom; the investigators concluded that there is no evidence for increased risk of breast cancer among shift workers.[92] However, the methodology in this report was subsequently criticized because of the very short follow-up of 3 years and the characteristics of the study population, who were mainly retired women who would have a declining risk associated with shift work accumulated at an earlier point during their career.[93–95]

In addition to breast cancer, endometrial cancer is another female-specific malignancy that was found to be associated with increased exposure to night shift work in the Nurses' Health Study, particularly in obese women.[96] On the other hand, another study found that night shift work was not associated with an increased risk in ovarian cancer.[97]

Mechanistically, circadian disturbances and increased exposure to light at night resulting from night shift work are thought to lead to altered clock gene expression, melatonin suppression, and modulation of sex hormone levels.[98] These physiologic changes may in turn contribute to increased tumorigenesis in breast cancer by disrupting the cell cycle, modulating apoptosis, and altering cellular metabolism.[98]

Metabolic Syndrome, Type 2 Diabetes, and Cardiovascular Disease

Metabolic syndrome is a group of characteristics consisting of increased body weight, elevated lipids, increased blood pressure, and impaired glucose homeostasis. The combination of these characteristics leads to an increased risk of developing T2DM, cardiovascular disease, and all-cause mortality.[99] A recent meta-analysis concluded that night shift work is associated with a 1.57 (95% CI 1.24–1.98) increased relative risk (RR) of metabolic syndrome, with female workers having a higher risk compared with male shift workers (RR 1.61, 95% CI 1.10–2.34 vs RR 1.36, 95% CI 1.03–1.81).[100]

The association between metabolic syndrome and shift work may partly be attributed to changes in diet and physical activity that have been observed in shift workers.[101,102] However, there is increasing evidence that changes in sleep and circadian disruption may also play a role.[103] For example, in a cross-sectional study among female health care workers, the association between shift work and metabolic syndrome was mediated by sleep duration when measured with actigraphy[104] but not with a self-reported sleep duration.[105] A meta-analysis on the association between sleep duration and metabolic syndrome supports the finding that short sleep duration, as commonly experienced by shift workers, is associated with metabolic syndrome.[106] However, there is increasing evidence that circadian disruption per se is also related to the development of metabolic syndrome characteristics.[103] For example, various laboratory-based studies in healthy humans have shown that circadian misalignment reduces glucose tolerance[66,67,107] independent of sleep loss.[65] This finding was recently confirmed in male and female shift workers with at least 1 year of consecutive shift work experience.[108]

In line with the association between metabolic syndrome and shift work, recent epidemiologic evidence in females has linked shift work to the risk of developing T2DM. In a cohort study of 19,873 nurses in Denmark, the risk for diabetes in nurses who worked night shift was significantly increased compared with nurses who worked day shift (HR 1.84, 95% CI 1.46–2.31).[109] Results from the Nurses' Health Study provide evidence for a dose-response relationship, with the duration of shift work exposure associated with a progressive increased risk for T2DM.[110] Women with more than 20 years of shift work exposure had 1.58 (95% CI 1.43–1.74) times the risk of developing T2DM compared with women who never worked night shift.[110] Furthermore, in a study that involved 28,041 African American women, the risk of T2DM was significantly higher for those who worked night shift compared with those who never worked night shift (HR 1.22, 95% CI 1.11–1.34).[111] In all these studies, the risk of developing T2DM associated with shift work was attenuated but still significant, after controlling for body mass index, indicating that the risk of diabetes is partly, though not totally, mediated by body weight in these populations.[109–111] A meta-analysis of 28 independent reports that assessed the association between shift work and T2DM supported these findings, showing that in women shift work has 1.09 (95% CI 1.04–1.14) times the risk of T2DM compared with non-shift work.[112] Interestingly, although female shift workers were reported to have a higher risk of metabolic syndrome than men (see previous discussion), male shift workers were found to have a larger risk of developing T2DM compared with women, namely 1.27 (95% CI 1.20–1.56).[112] Overall, these studies suggest that shift work is associated with an increased risk of T2DM in both women and men.

Metabolic syndrome leads to an increased risk of cardiovascular disease, a major cause of death among women and men.[113] In a meta-analysis investigating the relationship between shift work and cardiovascular events, shift work was significantly associated with risk of myocardial infarction, ischemic stroke, and coronary events but not with cardiovascular events in general or with mortality.[114]

Although sex differences have been observed in other risk factors for cardiovascular disease, and female-specific risk factors for cardiovascular disease do exist (eg, gestational hypertension and polycystic ovary syndrome),[113] the meta-analysis by Vyas and colleagues[114] (2012) did not specify the risk for male and female shift workers separately. A recent report from the Nurses' Health Study on the risk of coronary heart disease among female nurses indicated that longer exposure to rotating night shift work (>5 years) is associated with an increased risk of coronary heart disease and that this effect wanes over time after cessation of shift work.[115] Future research should investigate the potential sex differences in the effect of shift work on the risk of cardiovascular disease.

Reproductive Outcomes

The circadian timing system plays an important role in the regulation of reproductive physiology.[116] For example, animal studies have shown that the surge in luteinizing hormone and subsequent ovulation is gated by the central clock in the SCN[117] and that a mutation in the clock gene disrupts the estrous cycle and maintenance of pregnancy in rodents.[118] Therefore, disruption of the circadian timing system is thought to lead to disturbances of the reproductive axis.[116]

Indeed, shift work has been associated with adverse effects at different stages of the reproductive cycle, although the evidence is not conclusive and effect sizes are uncertain for some outcomes.[119] For example, after adjusting for confounding factors, an association between shift work and menstrual cycle disruption was found in a meta-analysis of 8 studies encompassing 28,479 women, with an odds ratio (OR) of 1.15 (95% CI 1.01–1.31).[120] In the same meta-analysis, an association was found between early spontaneous pregnancy loss and night shift work (OR 1.41, 95% CI 1.22–1.63), but not between infertility and shift work after adjusting for confounding factors.[120] Among a large cohort of nurses, the number of nights worked per month (either on a rotating night schedule or a fixed night schedule) was positively correlated with the prevalence of irregular menstrual cycles.[121] In addition, rotating night work, but not fixed night work, was associated with very short and long cycles, both indicators of reduced fertility.[121] Nevertheless, in the same study, no association was found between current or past shift work exposure and infertility when fertility was measured by duration of current pregnancy attempt among nurses who indicated they were actively trying to get pregnant.[122]

Regarding pregnancy-related outcomes, fixed night shift work, but not rotating night shift work, was associated with risk of miscarriage in a meta-analysis of the available literature (RR 1.51, 95% CI 1.27–1.78).[123] Furthermore, another meta-analysis showed that shift work is associated with preterm delivery (RR 1.14, 95% CI 1.01–1.30) but not with other pregnancy complications such as low birth weight, being small for gestational age, gestational hypertension, or preeclampsia.[124]

COUNTERMEASURES

Countermeasures to prevent the adverse effects of shift work have mainly focused on the short-term consequences, including sleep duration and quality, fatigue, and performance.[125] Various systematic reviews have indicated that scheduled napping, controlled light exposure during the night shift combined with light-blocking glasses during the morning commute, nutrition guidelines, and psychoeducation may be successful in improving sleep quality and reducing fatigue in shift workers.[125–128] The use of melatonin after night shifts is associated with increased sleep duration, although the evidence is of low quality.[125,129] Other pharmacologic interventions, such as the use of hypnotics to improve sleep or stimulants to enhance alertness, show mixed effectiveness and are associated with adverse side effects.[125,129] In general, systematic reviews on strategies for shift workers mention the large degree of heterogeneity between studies and call for high-quality studies with longer follow-up.

Importantly, individual differences, as well as characteristics of the work environment, should be considered when designing strategies to enhance adaptation to shift work. Not only will personal preferences and nonwork-related obligations affect a given countermeasure but sex differences may also play a role. For example, men were found to show increased vigilance and higher frontal slow-wave activity during sleep following exposure to blue-enriched light in the late evening compared non–blue-enriched light, while these effects were not observed in women.[130] Thus, sex differences in light sensitivity need to be considered when designing light interventions to enhance adaptation to shift work.

In addition, chronotype modulates sleep duration in shift workers.[131,132] In 1 study, late chronotype participants had shorter sleep duration on morning shifts, whereas early chronotype participants had shorter sleep duration on night shifts.[131] In a 5-month intervention study among 114 mostly male factory workers, sleep duration, sleep quality, and wellbeing were increased in early and late chronotypes when the exposure to their most strenuous shift was reduced (ie, when early chronotypes only worked morning and evening shifts, and late chronotypes only worked evening and night shifts).[133] Because the average woman has an earlier chronotype than the average man, potential sex differences in the response to an intervention may be confounded by chronotype, although this has not been formally tested.

Overall, these observations highlight the need for strategies tailored to individual needs and working conditions. Future research is warranted to assess the effect of preventive strategies on the long-term health consequences associated with shift work and to determine their applicability to specific populations of women by age group; by reproductive status; such as pregnancy and premenopause or postmenopause; and by chronotype.

SUMMARY

Women who do shift work make up a large part of the workforce.[56] Like their male counterparts, female shift workers experience circadian misalignment and disturbed physiologic rhythms as a result of shifted sleep periods. However, sex differences in the functioning of the circadian timing system are observed at many different biological levels. Emerging evidence indicates that the implications of these sex differences are potentially far-reaching: they may contribute to women's reduced tolerance to shift work and their increased risk of work injury related to shift work.

Recent epidemiologic studies and meta-analyses have started to shed light on women's health risks associated with shift work, both in terms of an altered risk compared with men (cardiometabolic disorders, sleep disturbances) and the risk of female-specific disorders (breast cancer, menstrual cycle disruption, reproductive problems). Although these studies generally point to an increased health risk associated with shift work, many meta-analyses cited in this review note that epidemiologic studies frequently suffer from several limitations, including incomplete exposure measurements, lack of standardized definition of shift work, difficulties quantifying exposure, and inclusion of a limited number of occupational groups.[85–90,100,112,120,123,124]

Future studies need to address these limitations to obtain a more precise risk estimate. Nevertheless, there is a clear need for strategies to improve adaptation to alternative work schedules. No 1-size-fits-all solution exists, and shift work research should focus on strategies that can be tailored to individual needs for women at various reproductive stages.

REFERENCES

1. Alterman T, Luckhaupt SE, Dahlhamer JM, et al. Prevalence rates of work organization characteristics among workers in the U.S.: data from the 2010 national health interview survey. Am J Ind Med 2013;56:647–59.
2. Williams C. Work-life balance of shift workers. Statistics Canada Perspectives 2008;75-001-X. Available at: http://www.statcan.gc.ca/pub/75-001-x/2008108/pdf/10677-eng.pdf. Accessed May 29, 2018.
3. Eurofound. Sixth European Working Conditions Survey 2015. Available at: https://www.eurofound.europa.eu/surveys/european-working-conditions-surveys/sixth-european-working-conditions-survey-2015. Accessed May 29, 2018.
4. Kecklund G, Axelsson J. Health consequences of shift work and insufficient sleep. BMJ 2016;355:i5210.
5. Boivin DB, Boudreau P. Impacts of shift work on sleep and circadian rhythms. Pathologie Biolo (Paris) 2014;62:292–301.
6. Straif K, Baan R, Grosse Y, et al. Carcinogenicity of shift-work, painting, and fire-fighting. Lancet Oncol 2007;8(12):1065–6.
7. Gerhart-Hines Z, Lazar MA. Circadian metabolism in the light of evolution. Endocr Rev 2015;36(3):289–304.
8. Czeisler CA, Duffy JF, Shanahan TL, et al. Stability, precision, and near-24-hour period of the human circadian pacemaker. Science 1999;284(5423):2177–81.
9. Dibner C, Schibler U, Albrecht U. The mammalian circadian timing system: organization and coordination of central and peripheral clocks. Annu Rev Physiol 2010;72:517–49.
10. Takahashi JS. Transcriptional architecture of the mammalian circadian clock. Nat Rev Genet 2017;18(3):164–79.
11. Balsalobre A, Damiola F, Schibler U. A serum shock induces circadian gene expression in mammalian tissue culture cells. Cell 1998;93:929–37.
12. Zylka MJ, Shearman LP, Weaver DR, et al. Three period homologs in mammals: differential light responses in the suprachiasmatic circadian clock and oscillating transcripts outside of brain. Neuron 1998;20:1103–10.
13. Welsh DK, Yoo S-H, Liu AC, et al. Bioluminescence imaging of individual fibroblasts reveals persistent, independently phased circadian rhythms of clock gene expression. Curr Biol 2004;14:2289–95.
14. Boivin DB, James FO, Wu A, et al. Circadian clock genes oscillate in human peripheral blood mononuclear cells. Blood 2003;102:4143–5.
15. Otway DT, Mantele S, Bretschneider S, et al. Rhythmic diurnal gene expression in human adipose tissue from individuals who are lean, overweight, and type 2 diabetic. Diabetes 2011;60(5):1577–81.
16. Wehrens SMT, Christou S, Isherwood C, et al. Meal timing regulates the human circadian system. Curr Biol 2017;27:1–8.
17. Bjarnason GA, Jordan RC, Wood PA, et al. Circadian expression of clock genes in human oral mucosa and skin: association with specific cell-cycle phases. Am J Pathol 2001;158(5):1793–801.

18. Brown SA, Fleury-Olela F, Nagoshi E, et al. The period length of fibroblast circadian gene expression varies widely among human individuals. PLoS Biol 2005;3(10):e338.

19. Tsinkalovsky O, Smaaland R, Rosenlund B, et al. Circadian variations in clock gene expression of human bone marrow CD34+ cells. J Biol Rhythms 2007;22(2):140–50.

20. Cermakian N, Lamont EW, Boudreau P, et al. Circadian clock gene expression in brain regions of Alzheimer's disease patients and control subjects. J Biol Rhythms 2011;26:160–70.

21. Lim AS, Myers AJ, Yu L, et al. Sex difference in daily rhythms of clock gene expression in the aged human cerebral cortex. J Biol Rhythms 2013;28(2):117–29.

22. Panda S, Antoch MP, Miller BH, et al. Coordinated transcription of key pathways in the mouse by the circadian clock. Cell 2002;109:307–20.

23. Storch K-F, Lipan O, Leykin I, et al. Extensive and divergent circadian gene expression in liver and heart. Nature 2002;417:78–83.

24. Archer SN, Laing EE, Möller-Levet CS, et al. Mistimed sleep disrupts circadian regulation of the human transcriptome. Proc Natl Acad Sci U S A 2014; 111:E682–91.

25. Kervezee L, Cuesta M, Cermakian N, et al. Simulated night shift work induces circadian misalignment of the human peripheral blood mononuclear cell transcriptome. Proc Natl Acad Sci U S A 2018; 115(21):5540–5.

26. Arnardottir ES, Nikonova EV, Shockley KR, et al. Blood-gene expression reveals reduced circadian rhythmicity in individuals resistant to sleep deprivation. Sleep 2014;37:1589–600.

27. Li JZ, Bunney BG, Meng F, et al. Circadian patterns of gene expression in the human brain and disruption in major depressive disorder. Proc Natl Acad Sci U S A 2013;110:9950–5.

28. Chen C-Y, Logan RW, Ma T, et al. Effects of aging on circadian patterns of gene expression in the human prefrontal cortex. Proc Natl Acad Sci U S A 2016;113:206–11.

29. Lim ASP, Klein H-U, Yu L, et al. Diurnal and seasonal molecular rhythms in human neocortex and their relation to Alzheimer's disease. Nat Commun 2017;8:14931.

30. Loboda A, Kraft WK, Fine B, et al. Diurnal variation of the human adipose transcriptome and the link to metabolic disease. BMC Med Genomics 2009;2:7.

31. Akashi M, Soma H, Yamamoto T, et al. Noninvasive method for assessing the human circadian clock using hair follicle cells. Proc Natl Acad Sci U S A 2010;107:15643–8.

32. Welsh DK, Takahashi JS, Kay SA. Suprachiasmatic nucleus: cell autonomy and network properties. Annu Rev Physiol 2010;72:551–77.

33. Duffy JF, Czeisler CA. Effect of light on human circadian physiology. Sleep Med Clin 2009;4(2): 165–77.

34. Yamazaki S, Numano R, Abe M, et al. Resetting central and peripheral circadian oscillators in transgenic rats. Science 2000;288(5466):682–5.

35. Cuesta M, Boudreau P, Cermakian N, et al. Rapid resetting of human peripheral clocks by phototherapy during simulated night shift work. Sci Rep 2017;7(1):16310.

36. Zarrinpar A, Chaix A, Panda S. Daily eating patterns and their impact on health and disease. Trends Endocrinol Metab 2016;27(2):69–83.

37. Borbely AA, Daan S, Wirz-Justice A, et al. The two-process model of sleep regulation: a reappraisal. J Sleep Res 2016;25(2):131–43.

38. Daan S, Beersma DG, Borbely AA. Timing of human sleep: recovery process gated by a circadian pacemaker. Am J Physiol 1984;246(2 Pt 2): R161–83.

39. Duffy JF, Rimmer DW, Czeisler CA. Association of intrinsic circadian period with morningness-eveningness, usual wake time, and circadian phase. Behav Neurosci 2001;115(4):895–9.

40. Wright KP Jr, Gronfier C, Duffy JF, et al. Intrinsic period and light intensity determine the phase relationship between melatonin and sleep in humans. J Biol Rhythms 2005;20(2):168–77.

41. Duffy JF, Cain SW, Chang A-M, et al. Sex difference in the near-24-hour intrinsic period of the human circadian timing system. Proc Natl Acad Sci U S A 2011;108(Suppl):15602–8.

42. Boivin DB, Shechter A, Boudreau P, et al. Diurnal and circadian variation of sleep and alertness in men vs. naturally cycling women. Proc Natl Acad Sci U S A 2016;113:10980–5.

43. Cain SW, Dennison CF, Zeitzer JM, et al. Sex differences in phase angle of entrainment and melatonin amplitude in humans. J Biol Rhythms 2010;25:288–96.

44. Mongrain V, Lavoie S, Selmaoui B, et al. Phase relationships between sleep-wake cycle and underlying circadian rhythms in morningness-eveningness. J Biol Rhythms 2004;19(3):248–57.

45. Baehr EK, Revelle W, Eastman CI. Individual differences in the phase and amplitude of the human circadian temperature rhythm: with an emphasis on morningness-eveningness. J Sleep Res 2000; 9(2):117–27.

46. Adan A, Natale V. Gender differences in morningness-eveningness preference. Chronobiol Int 2002;19(4):709–20.

47. Tonetti L, Fabbri M, Natale V. Sex difference in sleep-time preference and sleep need: a cross-sectional survey among Italian pre-adolescents, adolescents, and adults. Chronobiology Int 2008; 25:745–59.

48. Fischer D, Lombardi DA, Marucci-Wellman H, et al. Chronotypes in the US – influence of age and sex. Plos One 2017;12:e0178782.

49. Roenneberg T, Kuehnle T, Pramstaller PP, et al. A marker for the end of adolescence. Curr Biol 2004;14(24):R1038–9.

50. Zhang B, Wing YK. Sex differences in insomnia: a meta-analysis. Sleep 2006;29(1):85–93.

51. Mong JA, Baker FC, Mahoney MM, et al. Sleep, rhythms, and the endocrine brain: influence of sex and gonadal hormones. J Neurosci 2011;31:16107–16.

52. van den Berg JF, Miedema HME, Tulen JHM, et al. Sex differences in subjective and actigraphic sleep measures: a population-based study of elderly persons. Sleep 2009;32:1367–75.

53. Li RH, Wing YK, Ho SC, et al. Gender differences in insomnia–a study in the Hong Kong Chinese population. J Psychosom Res 2002;53(1):601–9.

54. Santhi N, Lazar AS, McCabe PJ, et al. Sex differences in the circadian regulation of sleep and waking cognition in humans. Proc Natl Acad Sci U S A 2016;113:E2730–9.

55. Saksvik IB, Bjorvatn B, Hetland H, et al. Individual differences in tolerance to shift work–a systematic review. Sleep Med Rev 2011;15(4):221–35.

56. Wong IS, McLeod CB, Demers PA. Shift work trends and risk of work injury among Canadian workers. Scand J Work Environ Health 2011;37(1):54–61.

57. Giacchetti S, Bjarnason G, Garufi C, et al. Phase III trial comparing 4-day chronomodulated therapy versus 2-day conventional delivery of fluorouracil, leucovorin, and oxaliplatin as first-line chemotherapy of metastatic colorectal cancer: the European Organisation for Research and Treatment of Cancer Chronotherapy Group. J Clin Oncol 2006;24(22):3562–9.

58. Giacchetti S, Dugue PA, Innominato PF, et al. Sex moderates circadian chemotherapy effects on survival of patients with metastatic colorectal cancer: a meta-analysis. Ann Oncol 2012;23(12):3110–6.

59. Lévi F, Okyar A, Dulong S, et al. Circadian timing in cancer treatments. Annu Rev Pharmacol Toxicol 2010;50:377–421.

60. Li XM, Mohammad-Djafari A, Dumitru M, et al. A circadian clock transcription model for the personalization of cancer chronotherapy. Cancer Res 2013;73(24):7176–88.

61. Folkard S. Do permanent night workers show circadian adjustment? A review based on the endogenous melatonin rhythm. Chronobiol Int 2008;25(2):215–24.

62. Boudreau P, Dumont GA, Boivin DB. Circadian adaptation to night shift work influences sleep, performance, mood and the autonomic modulation of the heart. PloS One 2013;8:e70813.

63. McHill AW, Melanson EL, Higgins J, et al. Impact of circadian misalignment on energy metabolism during simulated nightshift work. Proc Natl Acad Sci U S A 2014;111:17302–7.

64. Morris CJ, Yang JN, Garcia JI, et al. Endogenous circadian system and circadian misalignment impact glucose tolerance via separate mechanisms in humans. Proc Natl Acad Sci U S A 2015;112(17):E2225–34.

65. Leproult R, Holmback U, Van Cauter E. Circadian misalignment augments markers of insulin resistance and inflammation, independently of sleep loss. Diabetes 2014;63(6):1860–9.

66. Buxton OM, Cain SW, O'Connor SP, et al. Adverse metabolic consequences in humans of prolonged sleep restriction combined with circadian disruption. Sci Transl Med 2012;4(129):129ra43.

67. Scheer FAJL, Hilton MF, Mantzoros CS, et al. Adverse metabolic and cardiovascular consequences of circadian misalignment. Proc Natl Acad Sci U S A 2009;106:4453–8.

68. Morris CJ, Purvis TE, Hu K, et al. Circadian misalignment increases cardiovascular disease risk factors in humans. Proc Natl Acad Sci 2016;113:E1402–11.

69. Wright KP Jr, Drake AL, Frey DJ, et al. Influence of sleep deprivation and circadian misalignment on cortisol, inflammatory markers, and cytokine balance. Brain Behav Immun 2015;47:24–34.

70. Cuesta M, Boudreau P, Dubeau-Laramée G, et al. Simulated night shift disrupts circadian rhythms of immune functions in humans. J Immunol 2016;196:2466–75.

71. Reynolds AC, Paterson JL, Ferguson SA, et al. The shift work and health research agenda: considering changes in gut microbiota as a pathway linking shift work, sleep loss and circadian misalignment, and metabolic disease. Sleep Med Rev 2017;34:3–9.

72. Wright KP, Lowry CA, Lebourgeois MK. Circadian and wakefulness-sleep modulation of cognition in humans. Front Mol Neurosci 2012;5:50.

73. Lee ML, Howard ME, Horrey WJ, et al. High risk of near-crash driving events following night-shift work. Proc Natl Acad Sci U S A 2016;113(1):176–81.

74. Ayas NT, Barger LK, Cade BE, et al. Extended work duration and the risk of self-reported percutaneous injuries in interns. JAMA 2006;296(9):1055–62.

75. Crummy F, Cameron PA, Swann P, et al. Prevalence of sleepiness in surviving drivers of motor vehicle collisions. Intern Med J 2008;38(10):769–75.

76. Philip P, Akerstedt T. Transport and industrial safety, how are they affected by sleepiness and sleep restriction? Sleep Med Rev 2006;10(5):347–56.

77. Akerstedt T, Wright KP Jr. Sleep loss and fatigue in shift work and shift work disorder. Sleep Med Clin 2009;4(2):257–71.
78. Wright KP Jr, Bogan RK, Wyatt JK. Shift work and the assessment and management of shift work disorder (SWD). Sleep Med Rev 2013; 17(1):41–54.
79. American Academy of Sleep Medicine. International classification of sleep disorders. 3rd edition. Darien (IL): American Academy of Sleep Medicine; 2014.
80. Drake CL, Roehrs T, Richardson G, et al. Shift work sleep disorder: prevalence and consequences beyond that of symptomatic day workers. Sleep 2004;27(8):1453–62.
81. Flo E, Pallesen S, Mageroy N, et al. Shift work disorder in nurses–assessment, prevalence and related health problems. PLoS One 2012;7(4): e33981.
82. Waage S, Pallesen S, Moen BE, et al. Predictors of shift work disorder among nurses: a longitudinal study. Sleep Med 2014;15(12):1449–55.
83. Di Milia L, Waage S, Pallesen S, et al. Shift work disorder in a random population sample– prevalence and comorbidities. PLoS One 2013; 8(1):e55306.
84. Uehli K, Mehta AJ, Miedinger D, et al. Sleep problems and work injuries: a systematic review and meta-analysis. Sleep Med Rev 2014;18(1): 61–73.
85. Jia Y, Lu Y, Wu K, et al. Does night work increase the risk of breast cancer? A systematic review and meta-analysis of epidemiological studies. Cancer Epidemiol 2013;37(3):197–206.
86. Wang F, Yeung KL, Chan WC, et al. A meta-analysis on dose-response relationship between night shift work and the risk of breast cancer. Ann Oncol 2013;24(11):2724–32.
87. Lin X, Chen W, Wei F, et al. Night-shift work increases morbidity of breast cancer and all-cause mortality: a meta-analysis of 16 prospective cohort studies. Sleep Med 2015;16(11):1381–7.
88. He C, Anand ST, Ebell MH, et al. Circadian disrupting exposures and breast cancer risk: a meta-analysis. Int Arch Occup Environ Health 2015;88(5): 533–47.
89. Kamdar BB, Tergas AI, Mateen FJ, et al. Night-shift work and risk of breast cancer: a systematic review and meta-analysis. Breast Cancer Res Treat 2013; 138(1):291–301.
90. Ijaz S, Verbeek J, Seidler A, et al. Night-shift work and breast cancer–a systematic review and meta-analysis. Scand J Work Environ Health 2013; 39(5):431–47.
91. Wegrzyn LR, Tamimi RM, Rosner BA, et al. Rotating night shift work and risk of breast cancer in the nurses' health studies. Am J Epidemiol 2017; 186(5):532–40.
92. Travis RC, Balkwill A, Fensom GK, et al. Night shift work and breast cancer incidence: three prospective studies and meta-analysis of published studies. J Natl Cancer Inst 2016;108(12).
93. Hansen J. RE: night shift work and breast cancer incidence: three prospective studies and meta-analysis of published studies. J Natl Cancer Inst 2017;109(4):344.
94. Schernhammer ES. RE: night shift work and breast cancer incidence: three prospective studies and meta-analysis of published studies. J Natl Cancer Inst 2017;109(4):2.
95. Stevens RG. RE: night shift work and breast cancer incidence: three prospective studies and meta-analysis of published studies. J Natl Cancer Inst 2017;109(4):342.
96. Viswanathan AN, Hankinson SE, Schernhammer ES. Night shift work and the risk of endometrial cancer. Cancer Res 2007;67(21):10618–22.
97. Poole EM, Schernhammer ES, Tworoger SS. Rotating night shift work and risk of ovarian cancer. Cancer Epidemiol Biomarkers Prev 2011;20(5): 934–8.
98. Blakeman V, Williams JL, Meng QJ, et al. Circadian clocks and breast cancer. Breast Cancer Res 2016;18(1):89.
99. Kaur J. A comprehensive review on metabolic syndrome. Cardiol Res Pract 2014;2014:943162.
100. Wang F, Zhang L, Zhang Y, et al. Meta-analysis on night shift work and risk of metabolic syndrome. Obes Rev 2014;15(9):709–20.
101. Lowden A, Moreno C, Holmback U, et al. Eating and shift work - effects on habits, metabolism and performance. Scand J Work Environ Health 2010; 36(2):150–62.
102. Atkinson G, Fullick S, Grindey C, et al. Exercise, energy balance and the shift worker. Sports Med 2008;38(8):671–85.
103. Qian J, Scheer FA. Circadian system and glucose metabolism: implications for physiology and disease. Trends Endocrinol Metab 2016; 27(5):282–93.
104. Korsiak J, Tranmer J, Day A, et al. Sleep duration as a mediator between an alternating day and night shift work schedule and metabolic syndrome among female hospital employees. Occup Environ Med 2017;75(2):132–8.
105. Lajoie P, Aronson KJ, Day A, et al. A cross-sectional study of shift work, sleep quality and cardiometabolic risk in female hospital employees. BMJ Open 2015;5(3):e007327.
106. Iftikhar IH, Donley MA, Mindel J, et al. Sleep duration and metabolic syndrome. An updated dose-risk metaanalysis. Ann Am Thorac Soc 2015; 12(9):1364–72.
107. Eckel RH, Depner CM, Perreault L, et al. Morning circadian misalignment during short sleep duration

impacts insulin sensitivity. Curr Biol 2015;25(22): 3004–10.

108. Morris CJ, Purvis TE, Mistretta J, et al. Effects of the internal circadian system and circadian misalignment on glucose tolerance in chronic shift workers. J Clin Endocrinol Metab 2016;101(3): 1066–74.

109. Hansen AB, Stayner L, Hansen J, et al. Night shift work and incidence of diabetes in the Danish Nurse Cohort. Occup Environ Med 2016;73(4): 262–8.

110. Pan A, Schernhammer ES, Sun Q, et al. Rotating night shift work and risk of type 2 diabetes: two prospective cohort studies in women. PLoS Med 2011;8(12):e1001141.

111. Vimalananda VG, Palmer JR, Gerlovin H, et al. Night-shift work and incident diabetes among African-American women. Diabetologia 2015; 58(4):699–706.

112. Gan Y, Yang C, Tong X, et al. Shift work and diabetes mellitus: a meta-analysis of observational studies. Occup Environ Med 2015;72(1):72–8.

113. Appelman Y, van Rijn BB, Ten Haaf ME, et al. Sex differences in cardiovascular risk factors and disease prevention. Atherosclerosis 2015;241(1): 211–8.

114. Vyas MV, Garg AX, Iansavichus AV, et al. Shift work and vascular events: systematic review and meta-analysis. BMJ 2012;345:e4800.

115. Vetter C, Devore EE, Wegrzyn LR, et al. Association between rotating night shift work and risk of coronary heart disease among women. JAMA 2016; 315:1726.

116. Gamble KL, Resuehr D, Johnson CH. Shift work and circadian dysregulation of reproduction. Front Endocrinol (Lausanne) 2013;4:92.

117. Levine JE. New concepts of the neuroendocrine regulation of gonadotropin surges in rats. Biol Reprod 1997;56(2):293–302.

118. Miller BH, Olson SL, Turek FW, et al. Circadian clock mutation disrupts estrous cyclicity and maintenance of pregnancy. Curr Biol 2004;14(15): 1367–73.

119. Fernandez RC, Marino JL, Varcoe TJ, et al. Fixed or rotating night shift work undertaken by women: implications for fertility and miscarriage. Semin Reprod Med 2016;34(2):74–82.

120. Stocker LJ, Macklon NS, Cheong YC, et al. Influence of shift work on early reproductive outcomes: a systematic review and meta-analysis. Obstet Gynecol 2014;124(1):99–110.

121. Lawson CC, Johnson CY, Chavarro JE, et al. Work schedule and physically demanding work in relation to menstrual function: the Nurses' Health Study 3. Scand J Work Environ Health 2015; 41(2):194–203.

122. Gaskins AJ, Rich-Edwards JW, Lawson CC, et al. Work schedule and physical factors in relation to fecundity in nurses. Occup Environ Med 2015; 72(11):777–83.

123. Bonde JP, Jorgensen KT, Bonzini M, et al. Miscarriage and occupational activity: a systematic review and meta-analysis regarding shift work, working hours, lifting, standing, and physical workload. Scand J Work Environ Health 2013;39(4): 325–34.

124. Palmer KT, Bonzini M, Harris EC, et al. Work activities and risk of prematurity, low birth weight and pre-eclampsia: an updated review with meta-analysis. Occup Environ Med 2013;70(4):213–22.

125. Neil-Sztramko SE, Pahwa M, Demers PA, et al. Health-related interventions among night shift workers: a critical review of the literature. Scand J Work Environ Health 2014;40(6):543–56.

126. Richter K, Acker J, Adam S, et al. Prevention of fatigue and insomnia in shift workers-a review of non-pharmacological measures. EPMA J 2016;7:16.

127. Ruggiero JS, Redeker NS. Effects of napping on sleepiness and sleep-related performance deficits in night-shift workers: a systematic review. Biol Res Nurs 2014;16(2):134–42.

128. Boivin DB, Boudreau P, James FO, et al. Photic resetting in night-shift work: impact on nurses' sleep. Chronobiol Int 2012;29:619–28.

129. Liira J, Verbeek J, Ruotsalainen J. Pharmacological interventions for sleepiness and sleep disturbances caused by shift work. JAMA 2015;313(9): 961–2.

130. Chellappa SL, Steiner R, Oelhafen P, et al. Sex differences in light sensitivity impact on brightness perception, vigilant attention and sleep in humans. Sci Rep 2017;7(1):14215.

131. Juda M, Vetter C, Roenneberg T. Chronotype modulates sleep duration, sleep quality, and social jet lag in shift-workers. J Biol Rhythms 2013;28(2): 141–51.

132. Korsiak J, Tranmer J, Leung M, et al. Actigraph measures of sleep among female hospital employees working day or alternating day and night shifts. J Sleep Res 2017. [Epub ahead of print].

133. Vetter C, Fischer D, Matera JL, et al. Aligning work and circadian time in shift workers improves sleep and reduces circadian disruption. Curr Biol 2015; 25(7):907–11.

Sleep Health in Pregnancy
A Scoping Review

Clare Ladyman, BSc, PGDip, T. Leigh Signal, PhD*

KEYWORDS

- Pregnancy • Trimester • Sleep health • Sleep duration • Sleep efficiency or continuity
- Sleep timing • Sleepiness or alertness • Perceptions of sleep quality

KEY POINTS

- Information on sleep health in pregnancy focuses primarily on sleep duration and sleep continuity/efficiency with limited data available on changes in sleep timing, perceived sleep quality and alertness/sleepiness across pregnancy.
- Sleep is highly variable between pregnant women but healthy sleep does not seem to change markedly across pregnancy. There may be an increase in sleep disturbances in the third trimester.
- Sleep positioning should be considered an aspect of sleep health in pregnancy.
- Research on sleep health across pregnancy is needed, with sample screening criteria clearly specified and women screened for complications throughout data collection not just at recruitment.

INTRODUCTION

For most women, altered sleep is among a multitude of physiologic changes occurring during pregnancy. It is also among the most noticed changes[1] and is a topic women regularly seek information on, yet there is still limited empirical information available on what constitutes healthy sleep in each trimester of pregnancy. This makes it difficult for maternal health care providers to advise women on what changes are within the range of normal.

Previous literature suggests there are alterations to sleep duration, the architecture of sleep, and perceptions of sleep quality, with clear changes occurring between trimesters.[2–4] Many studies in this area have focused on the possible consequences of altered or disturbed sleep for the health of pregnant women and the health of their growing babies. These have revealed important findings, showing, for example, that short and/or long sleep duration and/or disturbed sleep are risk factors for preterm birth,[5,6] gestational diabetes,[7,8] hypertension,[9] preeclampsia,[10] increased labor duration, and a greater likelihood of cesarean delivery.[11] Poorer antenatal mood and depression[12–14] and poorer postnatal mood[15] have also been associated with disturbed sleep in pregnancy. These health outcomes have consequences for women and children both in the short term and across the lifespan.

Like the studies that have investigated sleep during pregnancy, sleep science and sleep medicine focus more generally on what can go wrong with sleep. This approach has been important in advancing the understanding of the role of sleep in the development of ill health and disease.[16–18] However, there is growing recognition that healthy sleep is more than just an absence of sleep problems or a sleep disorder. A sufficient amount of good quality sleep is being acknowledged as among the fundamental components of good health, along with diet and physical activity.[19,20]

Disclosure Statement: The authors have nothing to disclose.
Sleep/Wake Research Centre, College of Health, Massey University, PO Box 756, Wellington 6140, New Zealand
* Corresponding author.
E-mail address: T.L.Signal@massey.ac.nz

Sleep Med Clin 13 (2018) 307–333
https://doi.org/10.1016/j.jsmc.2018.04.004

Recently there has been an effort to frame sleep positively and to look at the potential benefits of good sleep. Buysse[21] has defined sleep health as "...a multidimensional pattern of sleep-wake-fulness, adapted to individual, social, and environmental demands, that promotes physical and mental well-being." He proposes 5 dimensions of good sleep health: "subjective satisfaction, appropriate timing, adequate duration, high efficiency, and sustained alertness during waking hours."

This shift in focus is highly relevant during pregnancy, a time when women have greater awareness of their own health and are concerned about the consequences for their child. Women also have more frequent interactions with health professionals and are receptive to information on maintaining or improving their health. Pregnancy is normally viewed as a positive time for most women and it is, therefore, relevant to focus on sleep health as a positive component of pregnancy. To do so, women and health professionals need practical, evidence-based information about different aspects of sleep and what constitutes normal healthy ranges. Such information would also allow health professionals to know when women need further assessment and possibly referral for sleep problems.

To the authors' knowledge, there has been no previous attempt to define sleep health in pregnancy. This review summarizes the available research evidence on healthy sleep in each trimester of pregnancy, using a scoping review underpinned by Buysse's[21] definition of sleep health.

METHODS

The methodology outlined by Arksey and O'Malley[22] is the basis for this scoping review. The following key steps were followed: (1) consultation; (2) identifying the research question; (3) identifying the relevant studies; (4) study selection; (5) charting the data, and (6) collating, summarizing, and reporting the results.

Identifying the Research Question

To ensure the topic addressed by the review was relevant and the findings practically useful, potential end users were consulted. These were health care providers working with pregnant women and included an obstetrician, community-based midwife, an antenatal information coordinator at a large regional hospital, and a pregnancy and childbirth education manager of a community-based service. All agreed that information on healthy sleep in pregnancy is sparse,

at best, and that information on this topic would be useful in their clinical environment. This consultation formed the rationale for this scoping review.

Based on the multidimensional definition of sleep health by Buysse,[21] this review examines the extent of knowledge on sleep duration, sleep continuity/efficiency, sleep timing, daytime alertness/sleepiness, and perceived satisfaction/quality of sleep. It is proposed that healthy sleep is most likely to occur in a healthy, uncomplicated pregnancy; therefore, studies included in this review needed to clearly specify the criteria used to assure that the participating women were healthy. Thus, the research question was: What is known about sleep health in each trimester of pregnancy?

Identifying Relevant Studies

The initial literature search was conducted in the Cochrane Library, PubMed, Medline, psycINFO, Web of Science, CINAHL Complete, and Scopus databases. These databases were systematically searched using key terms for sleep and pregnancy to form a Boolean string. The final string was as follows: (pregnan* OR gestat*) AND (sleep*) AND (quality OR duration OR timing) AND (week* OR trimester* OR early OR mid OR late).

Inclusion or Exclusion Criteria

To ensure broad coverage, studies published in the English language from January 1975 to December 2017 were considered eligible. Only studies that reported sleep in a healthy sample or subsample of pregnant women were included. Data from control groups or subsamples that sufficiently screened participating women were eligible for consideration. For a study to be included in the review, sleep data needed to be presented in sufficient detail; to report means, standard deviations (SDs), or proportions higher or lower than specified cut-offs; and to specify the trimester or gestational week.

Due to an established relationship with altered sleep, the exclusion criteria in each study had to stipulate that participating women self-reported or were screened for current mood disorders and sleep problems. At a minimum, each sample also had to be screened for pregnancy complications or pregnancy-related health issues, which were assumed (if not specifically stated) to include gestational diabetes, hypertensive disorders (eg, hypertension and/or preeclampsia or eclampsia), and other health concerns associated with small for gestational age infants and preterm birth.

Study Selection

Endnote reference management software was used to import and manage references. The initial search produced 1946 articles, of which 1218 were duplicates, leaving 728 for initial screening. The titles, abstracts, and keywords of the 728 identified articles were reviewed by 2 researchers and 503 records were excluded as not relevant to the topic. Full text of the remaining 225 articles were read by both researchers to assess topic relevance, and a further 57 articles were excluded. Thirty-nine articles were considered central to the topic and 8 articles were identified as review papers. The reference lists of these review papers and key articles were reviewed and yielded a further 88 studies, 14 of these were additional review papers and their reference lists were also screened.

Careful screening of the participant inclusion or exclusion criteria was completed for 248 articles and 224 records were excluded. This resulted in 24 studies being included in the review. **Fig. 1** outlines the study selection pathway. Throughout the entire process, a conservative approach was taken; if there was uncertainty about the inclusion or exclusions criteria, both researchers discussed the study and reached consensus.

Charting the Data

Data were extracted from the final 24 studies and charted in Excel. The following information was recorded: investigator, year of publication, geographic location, sample size, gestational age, participant characteristics, sleep measurement tools, sleep parameters reported, aims, and conclusions. **Table 1** summarizes

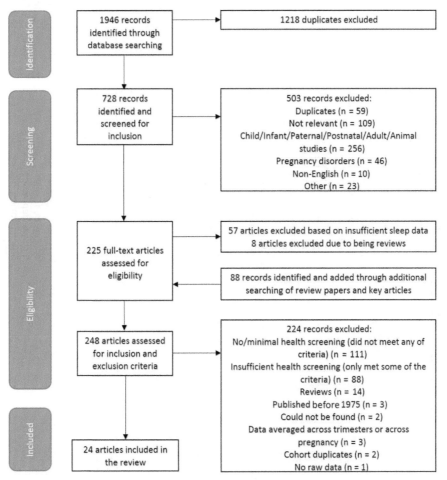

Fig. 1. Flow diagram of the study selection process. 1946 publications were identified from the initial search. After the assessment and exclusion process 24 research papers were included in this scoping review.

Table 1
Summary of characteristics of 24 studies (alphabetically by investigators)

Investigator, Year, Country	Number of Subjects	Trimester (Gestational Week)	Participant Characteristics	Sleep Measure	Sleep Parameters Reported	Aim or Overview	Conclusions
Baker et al,[47] 2016; United States	172	1st trimester (10–12 wk) 2nd trimester (14–16 wk and 18–20 wk)	Parity: does not specify Mean age: 29.3 ± 4.9 y Recruitment setting: self-referral, physician referrals, local advertisements, or university research registries Other characteristics reported: BMI, marital status, household annual income, education, ethnicity	Objective: actigraphy (acti) Subjective: diary (diary), PSQI	Objective Duration: TST (min)$_{acti}$ Continuity/Efficiency: WASO (min)$_{acti}$ SE (%)$_{acti}$ SOL (min)$_{acti}$ Subjective Duration: TST (min)$_{diary}$ Continuity/Efficiency: WASO (min)$_{diary}$ SE (%)$_{diary}$ SOL (min)$_{diary}$ Satisfaction/Quality: PSQI (global)	To examine whether varying degrees of exercise were associated with better nocturnal sleep among pregnant women during early gestation	Some level of exercise among pregnant women seems to be more advantageous than no exercise at all
Brunner et al,[2] 1994; Switzerland	9	1st trimester (9–14 wk) 2nd trimester (18–23 wk) 3rd trimester (32–35 wk)	Parity: 5 primiparous, 4 multiparous Mean age: 30.6 ± 2.9 y Recruitment setting: university obstetrics clinic Other characteristics reported: nil	Objective: in-laboratory PSG Subjective: nil	Objective Duration: TST (min)$_{psg}$ Continuity/Efficiency: SE (%)$_{psg}$ SOL (min)$_{psg}$ WASO (min)$_{psg}$ Other: REM latency (min)$_{psg}$ NREM1 (min)$_{psg}$ NREM2 (min)$_{psg}$ NREM3 (min)$_{psg}$ NREM4 (min)$_{psg}$ REM (min)$_{psg}$ SWS sleep (min)$_{psg}$ Movement time (min)$_{psg}$	To investigate changes in sleep in the course of pregnancy, PSG was recorded and analyzed in 9 healthy women on 2 consecutive nights during each trimester	Documents alterations in electroencephalogram spectral power that may be associated with hormonal changes during pregnancy
Crowley et al,[28] 2016; United States	14	2nd trimester (21.0 ± 1.0 wk)	Parity: All primiparous Mean age: 29.9 ± 4.7 y Recruitment setting: community Other characteristics reported: ethnicity, education, family income, depression history, anxiety history, EPDS, STAI	Objective: actigraphy Subjective: diary, PSQI	Objective Continuity/Efficiency: WASO (min)$_{acti}$ fragmentation index$_{acti}$ SOL (min)$_{acti}$ Subjective Continuity/Efficiency: SOL (min)$_{diary}$ Satisfaction/Quality: PSQI (global)	Pilot study to examine associations among stress-related physiologic factors (including GABA-ergic neurosteroids) and stress-related behavioral indices of anxiety during pregnancy	Data suggest that cortisol, progesterone, and ALLO + pregnanolone levels in 2nd trimester are inversely related to negative emotional symptoms and the negative impact of acute stress challenge seems to exert its effects by reducing these steroids to further promote negative emotional responses

	n	Timepoint	Sample	Measures	Sleep variables	Aim	Findings
Ebert et al,[39] 2015; United States	161	1st trimester (10–12 wk) 2nd trimester (14–16 wk and 18–20 wk)	Parity: 83 primiparous, 78 multiparous Mean age: 29.3 ± 4.9 y Recruitment setting: self-referral, physician referrals, local advertisements, or university research registries Other characteristics reported: education, ethnicity, marital status, income, children at home, prepregnancy weight, BMI at week 10, BP at week 10, caffeine, exercise, IDS, PSS	Objective: actigraphy Subjective: diary	Objective Duration: TST (nighttime) $(min)_{acti}$ Continuity/Efficiency: WASO $(min)_{acti}$ SOL $(min)_{acti}$, SE_{acti} Subjective Duration: TST (nighttime) $(min)_{diary}$ Continuity/Efficiency: WASO $(min)_{diary}$ SE $(\%)_{diary}$ SOL $(min)_{diary}$ Other: naps taken	To assess whether daytime naps negatively affect nocturnal sleep	The number of daytime naps have minimal impact on nocturnal sleep parameters; however, long nappers did exhibit modestly impaired sleep continuity and sleep quality Overall, daytime naps were a beneficial countermeasure to sleep disruption commonly reported by pregnant women
Elek et al,[44] 1997; United States	24	3rd trimester 7th mo (26.0 ± 0.8 wk) 8th mo (31.3 ± 1.0 wk) 9th mo (36.4 ± 1.1 wk)	Parity: all primiparous Mean age: 25.3 y (range 21–32 y) Recruitment setting: private physician offices Other characteristics reported: ethnicity, marital status, minimum education, employment status, income (per couple)	Objective: actigraphy Subjective: diary, VAS-F (13-item)	Objective Duration: TST_{diary} Continuity/Efficiency: number of undisturbed 90-min sleep cycles Subjective Other: morning and evening fatigue	This pilot study examined parents' levels of morning or evening fatigue, number of uninterrupted sleep periods, and length of sleep during 3rd trimester; and relationship of sleep to parents' reports of fatigue	The findings support the multidimensional nature of fatigue and indicate need for perinatal health caregivers to develop individualized interventions for mothers during the 3rd trimester Fathers should also participate in future research on factors influencing prenatal and postpartum experience

(continued on next page)

Table 1
(continued)

Investigator, Year, Country	Number of Subjects	Trimester (Gestational Week)	Participant Characteristics	Sleep Measure	Sleep Parameters Reported	Aim or Overview	Conclusions
Haney et al,[38] 2014; United States	161	1st trimester (10–12 wk) 2nd trimester (14–16 wk and 18–20 wk)	Parity: does not describe (37% with at least 1 child <18 y living at home) Mean age: 29.0 ± 5.0 y Recruitment setting: community Other characteristics reported: prepregnancy weight, weight at 1st trimester, BMI at 1st trimester, BP at 1st trimester, PSS, IDS, ethnicity, marital status, number of children	Objective: actigraphy Subjective: diary	Objective Duration: TST (nighttime) $(min)_{acti}$ Continuity/Efficiency: WASO $(min)_{acti}$ SOL $(min)_{acti}$ Subjective Duration: TST (nighttime) $(min)_{diary}$ Continuity/Efficiency: WASO $(min)_{diary}$ SOL $(min)_{diary}$	To examine whether women with poor sleep (defined as short sleep duration, longer WASO or longer SOL at 10–12 wk, measured by sleep diary and actigraphy) would have higher BP or higher BMI across early pregnancy (10–20 wk) and whether women with sleep disturbance (ie, poor sleep between 10 and 20 wk) would have greater increases in BP or BMI	A subset of women report substantial difficulty initiating and maintaining sleep during early pregnancy and this may augment risk of higher BP and BMI Assessing sleep in early pregnancy is important to allow time for appropriate intervention
Hertz et al,[30] 1992; United States	12	3rd trimester (30–38 wk)	Parity: 7 primiparous, 5 multiparous Mean age: 30.5 ± 5.1 y Recruitment setting: hospital obstetrics department Other characteristics reported: nil	Objective: in-laboratory PSG Subjective: SSS	Objective Duration: TIB $(min)_{psg}$, TST (nighttime) $(min)_{psg}$ Continuity/Efficiency: SE $(\%)_{psg}$, SOL $(min)_{psg}$, WASO $(min)_{psg}$, number of $awakenings_{psg}$ Other: REM latency $(min)_{psg}$, NREM1 $(min)_{psg}$, NREM2 $(min)_{psg}$, NREM3-4 $(min)_{psg}$, REM $(min)_{psg}$ Subjective Alertness/Sleepiness: SSS Satisfaction/Quality: restless sleep Other: snoring, bad dreams	To present a detailed investigation of sleep patterns, respiration, and leg muscle electromyography of 12 women in 3rd trimester	In accordance with subjective reports, women in 3rd trimester demonstrated PSG patterns of sleep maintenance insomnia

Source; Year; Country	N	Gestational Age	Sample Characteristics	Sleep Assessment	Study Aim	Sleep Measures	Key Findings
Hux et al,[48] 2017; United States	103	1st trimester (12.2 ± 1.1 wk)	Parity: 63 primiparous, 40 multiparous Mean age: 29.8 ± 5.0 y Recruitment setting: self-referral, physician referrals, local advertisements, or university research registries Other characteristics reported: ethnicity, income, education, socioeconomic score, mean gestational age at delivery, preterm birth, preeclampsia, gestational diabetes	Objective: nil Subjective: PSQI	To validate previously developed novel model of AL in early pregnancy by evaluating associations between AL scores and subjective measures of stress and proxies of chronic stress, including race or ethnicity, sleep quality, and socioeconomic status	Subjective Satisfaction/Quality: PSQI (global)	Higher AL, measured by the pregnancy-specific model, was associated with poorer sleep quality and lower educational attainment, both considered chronic stressors These relationships were consistent with previous findings in nonpregnant populations, and suggest that AL may be useful for capturing the physiologic impact of chronic stress in early pregnancy
Lee et al,[41] 2000; United States	31	3rd trimester (35–36 wk)	Parity: does not specify Mean age: 31.6 ± 4.5 y Recruitment setting: media advertisements, flyers on university campus Other characteristics reported: annual income, employment status, marital satisfaction	Objective: in-home PSG Subjective: diary, POMS	To test the hypothesis that increases in endogenous progesterone levels during luteal phase of menstrual cycle will alter REM sleep and mood state, and that decrease in endogenous progesterone levels postpartum will also alter REM sleep and mood state	Objective Duration: TST (nighttime) (min)$_{psg}$ Continuity/Efficiency: SE (%)$_{psg}$, wake (%)$_{psg}$ Other: REM latency (min)$_{psg}$, NREM1 (%)$_{psg}$, NREM2 (%)$_{psg}$, SWS (%)$_{psg}$, REM (%)$_{psg}$ Subjective Other: fatigue (POMS)	REM sleep and mood state were related to low progesterone levels during menstrual cycle but postpartum REM sleep and mood state were related to increased wake time rather than changes in progesterone levels
Lee et al,[3] 2000; United States	33	1st trimester (11–12 wk) 3rd trimester (35–36 wk)	Parity: 16 primiparous, 17 multiparous Mean age: 30.5 ± 3.7 y (primiparas), 31.5 ± 3.0 y (multiparas) Recruitment setting: advertisements on university campus Other characteristics reported: ethnicity, annual income, employment status, education, marital satisfaction	Objective: In-home PSG Subjective: diary	To describe changes in women's sleep patterns from prepregnancy to postpartum	Objective Duration: TST (nighttime) (min)$_{psg}$ Continuity/Efficiency: SE (%)$_{psg}$, SOL (min)$_{psg}$, wake (%)$_{psg}$ Other: REM latency (min)$_{psg}$, NREM1 (min)$_{psg}$, NREM2 (min)$_{psg}$, NREM3-4 (min)$_{psg}$, REM (min)$_{psg}$	Sleep disturbance was greatest during the first postpartum month, particularly for 1st-time mothers

(continued on next page)

Table 1
(continued)

Investigator, Year, Country	Number of Subjects	Trimester (Gestational Week)	Participant Characteristics	Sleep Measure	Sleep Parameters Reported	Aim or Overview	Conclusions
Okun et al,[40] 2015; United States	143	1st trimester (10–12 wk) 2nd trimester (14–16 wk and 18–20 wk)	Parity: 85 primiparous, 54 multiparous Mean age: 30.4 ± 5.8 y (with insomnia), 29.1 ± 4.6 y (no insomnia) Recruitment setting: self-referral, physician referrals, local advertisements, or university research registries Other characteristics reported: education, ethnicity, marital status, employment status, income	Objective: actigraphy Subjective: diary, ISQ, PSQI	Objective Duration: TST (min)$_{acti}$, TIB (min)$_{acti}$ Continuity/Efficiency: WASO (min)$_{acti}$, SOL (min)$_{acti}$, SE (%)$_{acti}$ Timing: bedtime$_{acti}$ Subjective Duration: TST (min)$_{diary}$, TIB (min)$_{diary}$ Continuity/Efficiency: WASO (min)$_{diary}$, SOL (min)$_{diary}$, SE (%)$_{diary}$ Timing: bedtime$_{diary}$ Satisfaction/Quality: PSQI (global)	To provide additional psychometric evaluation and validation of ISQ and to establish prevalence rates of insomnia among a women during early gestation	Insomnia is a health problem for many pregnant women at all stages in pregnancy These data support validity and reliability of the ISQ to identify insomnia in pregnant women The ISQ is a short and cost-effective tool that can be quickly used in large observational studies or in clinical practice with perinatal women
Strange et al,[29] 2009; United States	220	2nd trimester (20–29 wk)	Parity: does not specify Mean age: does not specify Recruitment setting: obstetric practices Other characteristics reported: nil	Objective: nil Subjective: PSQI, ESS	Subjective Duration: TST$_{psqi}$ Continuity/Efficiency: SE (%)$_{psqi}$, SE (score)$_{psqi}$, SOL (min)$_{psqi}$, SOL (score)$_{psqi}$, disturbances$_{psqi}$ Alertness/Sleepiness: ESS, dysfunction$_{psqi}$ Satisfaction/Quality: PSQI (global), quality$_{psqi}$ Other: use of sleep medications	This study examined subjective sleep quality and daytime sleepiness in relation to preterm birth	Disturbed sleep in pregnancy may be associated with preterm birth Future studies should examine specific physiologic factors that underlie this increased vulnerability

Study	N	Gestational age	Sample characteristics	Methods	Sleep measures	Aim	Conclusions
Tsai et al,[24] 2017; Taiwan	204	1st trimester (11.8 ± 2.30 wk) 2nd trimester (16–28 wk) 3rd trimester (>29 wk)	Parity: 107 primiparous, 97 multiparous Mean age: 32.5 ± 4.0 y Recruitment setting: medical center outpatient obstetric clinic Other characteristics reported: marital status, education, weekly working hours, BMI, CES-D	Objective: actigraphy Subjective: diary, PSQI, ESS	Objective Duration: TST (nighttime) (min)$_{acti}$, TST (daytime) (min)$_{acti}$ Continuity/Efficiency: WASO (%)$_{acti}$ Other: daytime sleep$_{acti}$ Subjective Alertness/Sleepiness: ESS (global), ESS (global ≥10) Satisfaction/Quality: PSQI (global), PSQI (global >5) Other: snoring (n, %)	To examine 1st trimester maternal characteristics associated with persistent and new onset daytime sleepiness in pregnancy	Snoring in the 1st trimester is involved in both persistent and new-onset daytime sleepiness with elevated depressive symptoms related to new-onset daytime sleepiness Intervention strategies for alleviating daytime sleepiness in pregnant women should focus on managing snoring and symptoms of depression in early pregnancy with special attention to primiparous and employed women
Tsai et al,[42] 2016; Taiwan	274	3rd trimester (33.2 ± 2.6 wk)	Parity: all primiparous Mean age: 31.9 ± 4.1 y Recruitment setting: university-affiliated obstetrics and gynecology clinics Other characteristics reported: marital status, employment status, BMI, caffeine intake, smoking and alcohol consumption, education, CES-D scores	Objective: actigraphy Subjective: diary, PSQI, ESS	Objective Duration: TST (nighttime) (min)$_{acti}$ TST (nighttime <6 h)$_{acti}$ TST (daytime) (min)$_{acti}$ TST (24 h) (min)$_{acti}$ TST (24 h <7 h)$_{acti}$ Continuity/Efficiency: SOL (min)$_{acti}$ SOL (>30 min)$_{acti}$ SE (%)$_{acti}$, SE (<85%) (%)$_{acti}$ Subjective Alertness/Sleepiness: ESS (global), ESS (global >10) Satisfaction/Quality: PSQI (global), PSQI (global >5) Other: napping	To examine objective and self-reported sleep disturbances and symptoms of depression and daytime sleepiness in a group of healthy pregnant women	Both objective nighttime sleep <6 h and self-reported poor sleep quality in healthy 3rd trimester pregnant women is associated with significant risks for clinical depression Improving sleep may reduce depression symptom severity and attenuate prevalence of depression in pregnant women

(continued on next page)

Table 1
(continued)

Investigator, Year, Country	Number of Subjects	Trimester (Gestational Week)	Participant Characteristics	Sleep Measure	Sleep Parameters Reported	Aim or Overview	Conclusions
Tsai et al,[4] 2016; Taiwan	164	1st trimester (11.7 ± 2.4 wk) 2nd trimester (22.3 ± 2.3 wk) 3rd trimester (33.7 ± 2.3 wk)	Parity: 85 primiparous, 79 multiparous Mean age: 32.7 ± 4.0 y Recruitment setting: university-affiliated hospital Other characteristics reported: education, employment status, prepregnancy BMI	Objective: actigraphy Subjective: diary, PSQI	Objective Duration: TST (nighttime) (h)$_{acti}$, TST (daytime) (min)$_{acti}$ Continuity/Efficiency: WASO (min)$_{acti}$, SE (%)$_{acti}$ Subjective Satisfaction/Quality: PSQI (global), PSQI (global >5)	To examine cross-sectional and longitudinal association between sleep and health-related quality of life in pregnant women	Sleep disturbances are highly prevalent and a persistent problem in pregnant women Adequate sleep is essential at all pregnancy stages and improving nocturnal sleep quantity and quality in early gestation is important for health-related quality of life later in pregnancy
Tsai et al,[26] 2012; Taiwan	38	3rd trimester (32.6 ± 2.8 wk)	Parity: 38 primiparous Mean age: 32.1 ± 5.1 y Recruitment setting: university-affiliated hospital Other characteristics reported: BMI, education, working hours per week, CES-D	Objective: actigraphy Subjective: diary, PSQI, VAS-F	Objective Duration: TST (nighttime) (min)$_{acti}$ Continuity/Efficiency: WASO (min)$_{acti}$ Subjective Duration: TST (min)$_{psqi}$ Continuity/Efficiency: SOL (min)$_{psqi}$ Timing: bedtime$_{acti}$, risetime$_{acti}$ Alertness/Sleepiness: morning fatigue, midday fatigue, afternoon fatigue, evening fatigue Satisfaction/Quality: PSQI (global), PSQI (global >5) Other: number days napped$_{psqi}$, number naps on a given day$_{psqi}$	To examine association among nighttime sleep and daytime napping behaviors, depressive symptoms, and perception of fatigue in pregnant women	Interventions designed to increase sleep duration and decrease depressive symptoms have the potential to prevent, ameliorate, or reduce fatigue in pregnant women Depressive symptoms during pregnancy likely share some psychological and behavioral tendencies with fatigue or sleep disturbance, which may complicate evaluation of intervention effect

Source	n	GA	Sample characteristics	Sleep measures	Sleep variables	Aim	Key findings
Tsai et al,[27] 2011; Taiwan	30	3rd trimester (32.9 ± 2.7 wk)	Parity: 30 primiparous Mean age: 30.8 ± 4.8 y Recruitment setting: university-associated hospital prenatal clinics Other characteristics reported: BMI, education, daily work hours, CES-D	Objective: actigraphy Subjective: diary, PSQI	Objective Duration: TST (min)$_{acti}$, TST (wkend) (min)$_{acti}$, TST (wkday) (min)$_{acti}$ Continuity/Efficiency: WASO (min)$_{acti}$, WASO (wkend) (min)$_{acti}$, WASO (wkday) (min)$_{acti}$, SE (%)$_{acti}$, SE (wkend) (%)$_{acti}$, SE (wkday) (%)$_{acti}$, SOL (min)$_{acti}$, SOL (wkend) (%)$_{acti}$, SOL (wkday) (%)$_{acti}$ Timing: bedtime$_{acti}$, bedtime (wkend)$_{acti}$, bedtime (wkday)$_{acti}$, risetime$_{acti}$, risetime (wkend)$_{acti}$, risetime (wkday)$_{acti}$ Subjective Duration: bedtime$_{psqi}$, risetime$_{psqi}$, TIB (h)$_{psqi}$, TST (h)$_{psqi}$ Continuity/Efficiency: SE (%)$_{psqi}$, SOL (min)$_{psqi}$ Satisfaction/Quality: PSQI (global), PSQI (global >5)	To identify sociodemographic, lifestyle, and health-related factors associated with poor sleep quality in women during 3rd trimester	Primiparous women experience both objective and subjective sleep disturbances, and their sleep patterns differ between weekdays and weekends during 3rd trimester Maternal sleep patterns may be improved by maintaining a regular and earlier bedtime so women have more opportunity to obtain sufficient nocturnal sleep and improve sleep quality
Tsai et al,[31] 2013; Taiwan	80	3rd trimester (32.8 ± 2.7 wk)	Parity: 80 primiparous Mean age: 31.7 ± 4.6 y Recruitment setting: university hospital obstetric clinics Other characteristics reported: education years, employment	Objective: actigraphy Subjective: diary, PSQI, VAS-F (7-item)	Other: number naps/d, number naps/wk, number naps on weekdays, number naps on weekends, use of sleep-enhancement strategies Objective Duration: TST (nighttime) (min)$_{acti}$, TST (daytime) (min)$_{acti}$, TST (in 24 h) (min)$_{acti}$ Continuity/Efficiency: WASO (min)$_{acti}$, SE (%)$_{acti}$, fragmentation index$_{acti}$	To examine temporal association of nighttime sleep quality and quantity with subsequent daytime naps and temporal association of daytime naps with sleep quality	Naps during pregnancy might indicate insufficient nighttime sleep, and longer daytime naps could compromise subsequent nighttime sleep Further research is needed

(continued on next page)

Table 1
(continued)

Investigator, Year, Country	Number of Subjects	Trimester (Gestational Week)	Participant Characteristics	Sleep Measure	Sleep Parameters Reported	Aim or Overview	Conclusions
			status, weekly working hours, BMI, CES-D		Subjective Duration: TST (nighttime) (min)$_{diary}$ Continuity/Efficiency: awakening$_{diary}$ Satisfaction/Quality: PSQI (global), PSQI (global >5) Other: total naps over 7 day$_{diary}$ number of women taking >1 nap on a given day$_{diary}$	and quantity the following night in 3rd trimester	to determine if short sleep duration and longer daytime naps are associated with negative pregnancy outcomes
Tsai et al,[25] 2013; Taiwan	120	3rd trimester (33.7 ± 2.7 wk)	Parity: 120 primiparous Mean Age: 31.3 ± 4.2 y Recruitment setting: university-affiliated hospital Other characteristics reported: gestational age at delivery, prepregnancy BMI, CES-D, infant birth weight, marital status, education, working hours per week, gender of infant, labor duration	Objective: actigraphy Subjective: diary, PSQI	Objective Duration: TST (nighttime) (h)$_{acti}$, TST (nighttime<6) (%)$_{acti}$, TST (daytime) (min)$_{acti}$, TST (in 24 h)$_{acti}$ Continuity/Efficiency: SE (%)$_{acti}$, SE (<85%) (%)$_{acti}$ Other: prevalence daytime napping (%) Subjective Duration: TST (nighttime) (h)$_{psqi}$ Continuity/Efficiency: SE (%)$_{psqi}$ Satisfaction/Quality: PSQI (global), PSQI (global >5)	To examine associations of nighttime and daytime sleep during 3rd trimester with labor duration and risk of cesarean deliveries	There was a beneficial effect of sleep on labor duration, suggesting that studies of sleep duration effects on labor and pregnancy outcomes should consider amount of both daytime and nighttime sleep

Study	N	Timing	Other characteristics	Measures	Sleep outcomes	Aim/Design	Findings
Tsai et al,[43] 2016; Taiwan	197	3rd trimester (33.2 ± 2.7 wk)	Parity: all primiparous Mean age: 32.0 ± 4.2 y Recruitment setting: medical center Other characteristics reported: education, employment hours, BMI, CES-D	Objective: actigraphy Subjective: diary, PSQI, SHPS	Objective Duration: TST (nighttime) (min)$_{acti}$, TST variability (nighttime) (min)$_{acti}$ TST (daytime) (min)$_{acti}$, TST variability (daytime) (min)$_{acti}$ Continuity/Efficiency: SOL (min)$_{acti}$, SOL variability (min)$_{acti}$, WASO (min)$_{acti}$, WASO variability (min)$_{acti}$ Subjective Other: SHPS score	A descriptive study examining associations of sleep hygiene and actigraph measures of sleep with self-reported sleep quality in pregnant women	Findings support avoiding physically, physiologically, emotionally, or cognitively arousing activities before bedtime as a target for sleep-hygiene intervention in pregnant women
Tzeng et al,[45] 2015; Taiwan	139	3rd trimester (36 wk)	Parity: 53 primiparous, 86 multiparous Mean age: 33.6 ± 3.8 y Recruitment setting: antenatal clinics Other characteristics reported: education, employment status, prenatal exercise, planned pregnancy, anemia, use of patient-controlled analgesia, use of pain medication, prepregnancy BMI, EPDS	Objective: nil Subjective: PSQI, FCF	Subjective Duration: TST$_{psqi}$, duration (subscale)$_{psqi}$ Continuity/Efficiency: SOL (subscale)$_{psqi}$, SOL (min)$_{psqi}$, SE (subscale)$_{psqi}$, SE (%)$_{psqi}$ disturbances (subscale)$_{psqi}$ Alertness/Sleepiness: daytime function (subscale)$_{psqi}$ Satisfaction/Quality: PSQI (global), quality (subscale)$_{psqi}$ Other: fatigue (FCF), sleep medication$_{psqi}$, insomnia (%)$_{psqi}$	To identify distinct classes of sleep-disturbance trajectories in women considering elective cesarean from 3rd trimester pregnancy to 6 months postpartum and examine associations of sleep trajectories with BMI, depressive symptoms, and fatigue scores.	Women had 3 distinct sleep-disturbance trajectories before and after elective Cesarean These poor-sleep courses were associated with BMI and psychological well-being Findings suggest need to continuously assess sleep quality in women considering elective Cesarean and up to 6 mo post-Cesarean

(continued on next page)

Table 1
(continued)

Investigator, Year, Country	Number of Subjects	Trimester (Gestational Week)	Participant Characteristics	Sleep Measure	Sleep Parameters Reported	Aim or Overview	Conclusions
Waters et al,[46] 1996; United States	31	3rd trimester (35–36 wk)	Parity: 12 primigravida, 19 multigravida Mean age: 31.3 ± 3.3 y (primiparas), 32.4 ± 5.1 y (multiparas) Recruitment setting: advertisements in obstetric offices and newspapers Other characteristics reported: ethnicity, marital status, number of months married, education, employment status	Objective: PSG (location not specified) Subjective: VAS-F (18-item)	Objective Continuity/Efficiency: SE (%)$_{psg}$ Subjective Other: fatigue (VAS-F), vitality (VAS-F)	To describe differences between primigravidae and multigravidae in their experience of SE, fatigue and vitality, and level of functioning in 3rd trimester of pregnancy and 1st mo postpartum	Maternal role acquisition, experienced by primigravidae results in more fatigue and sleep disruption than maternal role expansion The significant decrease in SE and increase in fatigue in primigravidae after delivery indicates that health care professionals need to provide anticipatory guidance to primigravidae to help smooth the transition from pregnancy to motherhood

| Wilson et al,[23] 2011; Australia | 1st trimester (9–14 wk) 3rd trimester (30–38 wk) | Parity: 9 primiparous and 12 multiparous (1st trimester), 15 primiparous and 12 multiparous (3rd trimester) Mean age: 29.6 ± 3.4 y (1st trimester), 32.3 ± 3.5 y (3rd trimester) Recruitment setting: hospital outpatient obstetrics clinic Other characteristics reported: prepregnancy BMI, marital status, education, employment status | Objective: in-laboratory PSG Subjective: study-specific questionnaire | Objective Continuity/Efficiency: SOL (min)$_{psg}$, WASO (min)$_{psg}$, Arousals/h$_{psg}$, Awakenings$_{psg}$, SE (%)$_{psg}$ Other: REM latency (min)$_{psg}$, respiratory arousals$_{psg}$, limb arousals$_{psg}$, spontaneous arousals$_{psg}$, NREM1 (min)$_{psg}$, NREM2 (min)$_{psg}$, NREM3 (min)$_{psg}$, NREM4 (min)$_{psg}$, REM (min)$_{psg}$, %TST supine$_{psg}$ Subjective Duration: TST (<8 h/night) (%) Continuity/Efficiency: SOL (>20 min) (%), Difficulty falling asleep (%), number of awakenings Satisfaction/Quality: quality and tiredness (study-specific questionnaire) Other: reasons for overnight awakenings | To objectively measure sleep architecture and investigate subjective sleep quality in 1st and 3rd trimester, when compared with nonpregnant state | Sleep during pregnancy is compromised by higher amounts of wake and cortical arousals leading to sleep fragmentation, with greater amounts of light sleep and less deep sleep Mood state did not have an effect on sleep Findings may help health care providers recognize when severe sleep disruption may warrant referral to specialist for appropriate diagnosis and treatment |

(continued on next page)

Table 1
(continued)

Investigator, Year, Country	Number of Subjects	Trimester (Gestational Week)	Participant Characteristics	Sleep Measure	Sleep Parameters Reported	Aim or Overview	Conclusions
Wolfson et al,[15] 2003; United States	38	3rd trimester (34.5 ± 2.3 wk)	Parity: all primiparous Mean age: 30.0 ± 3.8 y Recruitment setting: antenatal classes Other characteristics reported: ethnicity, marital status, education	Objective: nil Subjective: diary (mother's sleep-wake diary)	Subjective Duration: TST (nighttime) $(min)_{diary}$, TST (daytime) $(min)_{diary}$ Continuity/Efficiency: SOL $(min)_{diary}$, disruptions $(min)_{diary}$ Timing: $bedtime_{diary}$, $risetime_{diary}$	To describe and compare diary-reported sleep-wake variables and depressive symptoms during last weeks of pregnancy, at 2–4 wk postpartum, 12–16 wk postpartum, and at 12–15 mo postpartum; and compare sleep-wake variables between depressed and nondepressed mothers at 2–4 wk postpartum	Mothers who developed clinically elevated depressive symptoms (CES–D ≥16) at 2–4 wk postpartum reported more TST risetimes, and more time napping at end of pregnancy compared with mothers who reported fewer symptoms (CES–D <16) at 2–4 wk postpartum

Abbreviations: AL, allostatic load; ALLO, allopregnanolone; BMI, body mass index; BP, blood pressure; CES–D, Center for Epidemiological Studies - Depression; EPDS, Edinburgh Postnatal Depression Scale; ESS, Epworth Sleepiness Scale; FCF, Fatigue Continuum Form; GABA, gamma-aminobutyric acid; IDS, inventory of depressive symptoms; ISQ, insomnia symptom questionnaire; NREM, non-rapid eye movement; POMS, profile of mood states; PSG, polysomnography; PSQI, Pittsburgh Sleep Quality Index; PSS, Perceived Stress Scale; REM, rapid eye movement; SE, sleep efficiency; SHPS, Sleep Hygiene Practice Scale; SOL, sleep onset latency; SSS, Stanford Sleepiness Scale; STAI, Spielberger State-Trait Anxiety; SWS, slow wave sleep; TST, total sleep time; TIB, time in bed; VAS-F, visual analog scale for fatigue; WASO, wake after sleep onset; wkday, weekday; wkend, weekend.

descriptive characteristics of the included studies.

RESULTS

Studies identified in the scoping review are predominantly from Taiwan (38%) and the United States (54%), with only 1 study from Australia[2] and 1 from Switzerland.[23] In reviewing studies from the same investigators or groups of investigators, it became evident that different studies potentially used the same sample of participating women, although this was not always explicitly stated in any publication. To ensure that data from the same cohort of participants was not included in the review multiple times, sample sizes and data collection time frames (when given) were carefully considered. In the first instance, data are presented from studies with the largest number of participants and the widest timeframe. Data from additional studies, thought to use the same sample of women, are included if different sleep variables are provided or if data are presented by subgroups of women (eg, those with and without insomnia symptoms).

Most studies used well-validated and widely accepted sleep measurement tools. Polysomnography (PSG) was used in 6 studies, actigraphy in 14 studies, and sleep diaries in 17 studies. Subjective sleep scales were used in most of the studies, with the Pittsburgh Sleep Quality Index (PSQI) being the most common (n = 14). The Epworth Sleepiness Scale (ESS) and various forms (18-item, 13-item, and 7-item) of the Visual Analog Scale for Fatigue (VAS-F) were used in a limited number of studies. The Fatigue Continuum Form, the Profile of Mood States fatigue subscale, Insomnia Symptom Questionnaire, Stanford Sleepiness Scale, and the Sleep Hygiene Practice Scale were each reported once. Notably, although

studies may have indicated they used these tools, investigators may have chosen not to present data on all measures.

Fig. 2 is an overview of publication dates of the included studies. Recent publications dominate the review, with 71% of the studies published after 2009. However, current literature using PSG measures of sleep is limited, with 5 of the 6 studies published before 2000 and the sixth study published in 2011. The 14 actigraphy studies are more current, with 13 studies published between 2011–2017, and one in 1997.

Sleep data were centered on the third trimester, with 17 articles providing data from this gestational period. Ten articles reported on the first trimester, whereas only 8 articles reported on the second trimester. Five studies spanned 2 trimesters, whereas only 3 studies provided data from all 3 trimesters.[2,4,24]

As seen in **Fig. 3**, most articles reported on continuity/efficiency (42%) and sleep duration (24%). Data were limited for other dimensions of sleep, including satisfaction/quality, timing, and alertness/sleepiness. More than 50% of the data comes from 5 measures of sleep: nighttime total sleep time (TST), sleep efficiency (SE), sleep onset latency (SOL), wake after sleep onset (WASO), and PSQI self-report scores.

Sleep Duration

There are PSG, actigraphy, and self-report data available on the duration of nighttime sleep in each trimester of pregnancy (**Table 2**). Mean PSG and actigraphic nighttime TST values are on average less than 7 hours, with SDs of approximately 1 hour. At each trimester, self-reported TST is longer than PSG and actigraphic TST, with women reporting sleep durations longer than 7 hours on average, particularly in the first and second trimesters. In the third trimester, self-reported TST is similar to PSG and

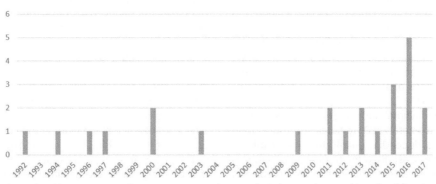

Fig. 2. Number of publications over the past 25 years. This graph indicates the number of publications each year (*Y* axis) over time (*X* axis) between 1992 and 2017.

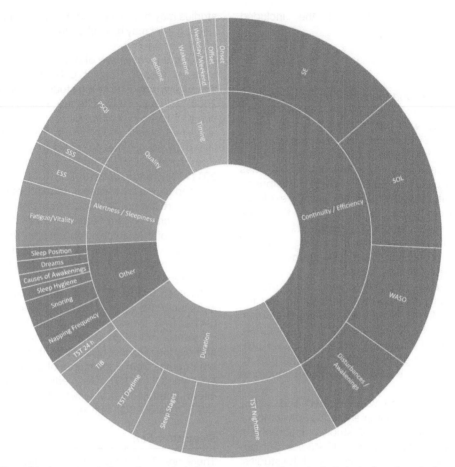

Fig. 3. Hierarchical representation of reported sleep parameters from included studies. A majority of articles report on sleep continuity/efficiency (42%) and sleep duration (24%). Data is limited for other dimensions of sleep including quality, timing and alertness/sleepiness. Over 50% of the data comes from five measures of sleep; nighttime TST, SE, SOL, WASO and PSQI scores. ESS, epworth sleepiness scale; PSQI, pittsburgh sleep quality index; SE, sleep efficiency; SOL, sleep onset latency; SSS, stanford sleepiness scale; TIB, time in bed; TST, total sleep time; WASO, wake after sleep onset.

actigraphic-measured sleep duration. There were limited actigraphic and subjective data on the amount of time pregnant women spend in bed at night, which on average is longer than 8 hours.

Details on the percentage of time and number of minutes spent in the different stages of sleep and wake, rapid eye movement (REM) latency, and movement time is found in **Table 3**. With the exception of non-rapid eye movement (NREM)1 light sleep, the amount of time spent in the different stages of sleep is markedly different between studies.

Average daytime nap durations range widely from approximately 20 minutes to more than 100 minutes, depending on the study (see **Table 2**). Three studies described the frequency of napping in the third trimester.[25–27] The first study reported the prevalence of daytime napping as 97.5%,[25] whereas a second study described 50% of their

cohort napping on 4 days or more (21% on 4–5 days and 29% napping on 6–7 days).[26] The third study reported that the average number of naps per week was 4 plus or minus 3, with 0.64 plus or minus 0.45 naps on weekdays and 0.53 plus or minus 0.45 naps on weekends.[27] There is a small amount of data on TST in 24 hours but only in the third trimester, and values averaged 7 hours (see **Table 2**). Some studies also reported proportions of women obtaining less than 8, less than 7, and less than 6 hours sleep per night (see **Table 2**), and a single study reported on the percentage of time spent in the supine position, dropping from nearly half the night in the first trimester to 20% of the night in the third trimester.[23]

Taken together, this information demonstrates that both nighttime and daytime sleep duration is highly variable among women during a healthy pregnancy.

Table 2
Sleep duration in each trimester as reported for nighttime and daytime periods in studies

Measure	1st Trimester Mean ± SD	2nd Trimester Mean ± SD	3rd Trimester Mean ± SD
PSG TIB (min)	No data	No data	462 ± 52
Actigraphy TIB (min)	478 ± 43 (with insomnia) 483 ± 49 (no insomnia)	No data	No data
Self-Report TIB (min)	509 ± 39 (with insomnia) 508 ± 53 (no insomnia)	No data	493 ± 70
PSG TST (min)	389 ± 10[a] 446 ± 66	401 ± 15	370–415 ± 59–65 430 ± 33 (negative postpartum affect) 412 ± 69 (positive postpartum affect)
Actigraphy TST (min)	390–412 ± 54–64 380 ± 64 (frequent nappers) 439 ± 45 (nonnappers) 400 ± 60 (short nappers) 372 ± 66 (long nappers) 394 ± 65 (with insomnia) 365 ± 69 (no insomnia)	396–398 ± 50–51 383 ± 53 (frequent nappers) 422 ± 51 (nonnappers) 405 ± 47 (short nappers) 381 ± 56 (long nappers)	386–394 ± 52–61 441 ± 61 (frequent nappers) 476 ± 55 (nonnappers) 388 ± 52 (good sleepers) 390 ± 47 (poor sleepers) 388 ± 45 (vaginal delivery) 406 ± 58 (cesarean delivery) 376 ± 54 (frequent nappers) 411 ± 54 (infrequent nappers)
Self-Report TST (min)	461 ± 52 450 ± 49 (frequent nappers) 474 ± 46 (nonnappers) 464 ± 49 (short nappers) 455 ± 57 (long nappers) 444 ± 55 (with insomnia) 466 ± 52 (no insomnia)	454 ± 54 441 ± 61 (frequent nappers) 476 ± 55 (nonnappers) 462 ± 48 (short nappers) 439 ± 65 (long nappers)	408–454 ± 56–92 375 ± 63 (weekdays) 414 ± 72 (weekends) 417 ± 74 (vaginal delivery) 398 ± 80 (cesarean delivery)
Actigraphy Daytime TST (min)	42 ± 33 97 ± 60 (moderate nappers) 82 ± 29 (frequent nappers)	34 ± 26 83 ± 36 (moderate nappers) 91 ± 37 (frequent nappers)	49–84 ± 51–52 46 ± 46 (good sleepers) 38 ± 34 (poor sleepers) 42 ± 36 (vaginal delivery) 41 ± 57 (cesarean delivery) 75 ± 60 (frequent nappers) 22 ± 15 (infrequent nappers)
Self-Report Daytime TST (min)	83 ± 46 (moderate nappers) 93 ± 48 (frequent nappers)	78 ± 41 (moderate nappers) 104 ± 59 (frequent nappers)	18 ± 5[a]
Actigraphy 24-h TST (min)	No data	No data	435–442 ± 57–58 430 ± 51 (vaginal delivery) 448 ± 64 (cesarean delivery) 451 ± 58 (frequent nappers) 433 ± 58 (infrequent nappers)

(continued on next page)

Table 2
(continued)

Measure	1st Trimester Mean ± SD	2nd Trimester Mean ± SD	3rd Trimester Mean ± SD
TST <8 h	71% (PSG, nighttime TST)	No data	74% (PSG, nighttime TST)
TST <7 h	38% (Actigraphy, nighttime TST) 24% (diary, nighttime TST)	25% (actigraphy, nighttime TST) 26% (diary, nighttime TST)	42% (actigraphy, 24 h TST)
TST <6 h	No data	No data	26% (actigraphy, nighttime TST)
PSG %TST in Supine	41 ± 24	No data	19 ± 15

Measured with PSG, actigraphy and self-reports.
[a] SEM rather than SD.
Data from Refs.[2–4,15,23–27,30,31,38–45]

Sleep Continuity/Efficiency

Compared with other dimensions of sleep, there are numerous data available on continuity/efficiency (**Table 4**). Objective SE measured using both PSG and actigraphy range from 71% to 91%, whereas subjective values of SE have a narrower range (83%–91%). PSG WASO values (in minutes) are highest in the third trimester; however, 1 study that reported WASO (percent of sleep) showed little difference between the first and third trimesters.[3] WASO (in minutes) is generally lowest in the third trimester when measured by actigraphy. When measured by self-report, WASO values (in minutes) are lower than either PSG or actigraph-determined WASO. Objective and subjective reports of SOL were similar, ranging from 10 to 27 minutes with an SD of up to 23 minutes. As with sleep duration, the data indicate how variable sleep is between studies and between women.

Table 3
Sleep stages, rapid eye movement latency, and movement time in each trimester

	1st Trimester Mean ± SD	Sleep (%)	2nd Trimester Mean ± SD	Sleep (%)	3rd Trimester Mean ± SD	Sleep (%)
NREM1 (min)	34 ± 4[a] 30 ± 16	3 ± 1	31 ± 4[a]	No data	36 ± 5[a] 35 ± 15	4 ± 1 19 ± 13
NREM2 (min)	215 ± 14[a] 166 ± 44	54 ± 6	234 ± 17[a]	No data	221 ± 14[a] 162 ± 41	56 ± 6 55 ± 14
NREM3 (min)	40 ± 4[a] 85 ± 38	9 ± 3[b]	39 ± 3[a]	No data	36 ± 3[a] 67 ± 28	8 ± 4[b] 12 ± 3[b]
NREM4 (min)	20 ± 4[a] 62 ± 27	No data	24 ± 5[a]	No data	18 ± 6[a] 55 ± 24	No data
REM (min)	80 ± 2[a] 64 ± 16	24 ± 5	73 ± 43[a]	No data	71 ± 6[a] 60 ± 23	21 ± 5 14 ± 4
REM Latency (min)	79 ± 8[a] 118 ± 61 74 ± 26	No data	70 ± 43[a]	No data	65 ± 3[a] 125 ± 51 126 ± 55	No data
Wake (min)	No data	9 ± 6	No data	No data	No data	11 ± 6
Movement Time (min)	10 ± 1[a]	No data	11 ± 41[a]	No data	11 ± 1[a]	No data

Measured with PSG.
[a] SEM rather than SD.
[b] Combined NREM3 and NREM4.
Data from Refs.[2,3,23,30]

Table 4
Sleep continuity/efficiency in each trimester

Measure	1st Trimester Mean ± SD	2nd Trimester Mean ± SD	3rd Trimester Mean ± SD
PSG SE (%)	85–91 ± 6–8 87 ± 2[a] 84 ± 7 (primiparous) 86 ± 9 (multiparous)	88 ± 3[a]	78–89 ± 6–14 75 ± 15 (primiparous) 86 ± 8 (multiparous) 90 ± 4 (primigravidae) 87 ± 7 (multigravidae) 90 ± 6 (negative postpartum affect) 89 ± 6 (positive postpartum affect)
Actigraphy SE (%)	82 ± 7 74 ± 13 (inactive) 76 ± 12 (insufficiently active) 76 ± 12 (sufficiently active) 76 ± 12 (frequent nappers) 82 ± 7 (nonnappers) 78 ± 10 (short nappers) 74 ± 11 (long nappers) 71 ± 13 (with insomnia) 77 ± 11 (no insomnia)	83 ± 6 78 ± 9 (inactive) 81 ± 8 (insufficiently active) 79 ± 8 (sufficiently active) 80 ± 9 (frequent nappers) 80 ± 6 (nonnappers) 80 ± 7 (short nappers) 78 ± 9 (long nappers)	80–81 ± 6–7 81 ± 6 (vaginal delivery) 82 ± 5 (cesarean delivery) 80 ± 6 (frequent nappers) 82 ± 6 (infrequent nappers) 80 ± 7 (weekdays) 80 ± 8 (weekends)
Self-Report SE (%)	87 ± 7 (frequent nappers) 89 ± 4 (nonnappers) 89 ± 6 (short nappers) 85 ± 6 (long nappers) 87 ± 8 (with insomnia) 91 ± 5 (no insomnia)	86 ± 13 88 ± 6 (frequent nappers) 89 ± 5 (nonnappers) 90 ± 5 (short nappers) 89 ± 8 (long nappers)	83–87 ± 13–19 87 ± 13 (vaginal delivery) 82 ± 13 (cesarean delivery)
SE <85%	No data	No data	67% (actigraphy)
PSG WASO (min)	49 ± 36 33 ± 10[a] 55 ± 36 (primiparous) 45 ± 36 (multiparous)	23 ± 5[a]	62–80 ± 37–44 58 ± 6[a] 77 ± 38 (primiparous) 44 ± 27 (multiparous)
Actigraphy WASO (min)	91 ± 57 86 ± 54 (frequent nappers) 73 ± 33 (nonnappers) 88 ± 59 (short nappers) 97 ± 54 (long nappers) 113 ± 58 (with insomnia) 91 ± 59 (no insomnia)	28–72 ± 10–38 70 ± 40 (frequent nappers) 69 ± 25 (nonnappers) 70 ± 31 (short nappers) 76 ± 45 (long nappers)	54 ± 27 57 ± 21 (good sleepers) 54 ± 23 (poor sleepers) 53 ± 19 (frequent nappers) 56 ± 21 (infrequent nappers) 53 ± 21 (weekdays) 56 ± 28 (weekends)
Self-Report WASO (min)	24 ± 18 24 ± 18 (frequent nappers) 16 ± 12 (nonnappers) 24 ± 19 (short nappers) 25 ± 17 (long nappers) 38 ± 22 (with insomnia) 23 ± 17 (no insomnia)	20 ± 14 20 ± 14 (frequent nappers) 19 ± 12 (nonnappers) 20 ± 14 (short nappers) 20 ± 18 (long nappers)	No data
WASO ≥30 min	98% (actigraphy)	No data	No data

(continued on next page)

Table 4
(continued)

Measure	1st Trimester Mean ± SD	2nd Trimester Mean ± SD	3rd Trimester Mean ± SD
PSG SOL (min)	11 ± 8 (to stage 2) 20 ± 4[a] (to stage 2) 20 ± 17 (3 consecutive stages of sleep)	22 ± 8[a] (to stage 2)	14 ± 12[a] (to stage 1) 13 ± 11 (to stage 2) 25 ± 4[a] (to stage 2) 18 ± 13 (no criteria)
Actigraphy SOL (min)	15 ± 11 15 ± 13 (frequent nappers) 11 ± 6 (nonnappers) 12 ± 9 (short nappers) 19 ± 14 (long nappers) 15 ± 9 (with insomnia) 15 ± 12 (no insomnia)	10–13 ± 6–10	22 ± 16–21 23 ± 20 (weekdays) 21 ± 17 (weekends)
Self-Report SOL (min)	20 ± 15 20 ± 17 (frequent nappers) 17 ± 8 (nonnappers) 17 ± 12 (short nappers) 25 ± 18 (long nappers) 27 ± 21 (with insomnia) 20 ± 14 (no insomnia)	16–27 ± 13–17	23–27 ± 3–23
SOL >20 min	37% (actigraphy)	No data	44% (self-report) (37% difficulty getting to sleep, 63% difficulty falling asleep after waking)
SOL >30 min	No data	No data	23% (actigraphy)

Reported by SE, WASO, and SOL; measured with PSG, actigraphy, and self-report.
[a] SEM rather than SD.
Data from Refs.[2–4,15,23,25–31,38–43,45–47]

Sleep Disturbances

A single study provided information on arousals (Median (Mdn) = 11, range = 8–16) and number of awakenings (mean = 16 ± 5) as measured by PSG in the first trimester.[23] This study also reported that 24% of women had sleep disordered breathing (Apnea–Hypopnea Index (AHI) >5) and 10% a periodic limb movement index (PLMI) >5. The same study reported that 57% self-reported awakening 1 to 2 times per night, 48% had difficulty falling asleep after waking up at night. The main causes of nighttime awakenings were the need to urinate (76%) and care for children or partner (45%). Another study reported the prevalence of snoring to be 29% in the first trimester when measured using the "Do you snore?" item of the Berlin Questionnaire.[24]

For the second trimester, minimal data have been published on sleep disturbances. One study reported an actigraphy sleep fragmentation index of 28 (±10),[28] and another study measured sleep disturbance with the PSQI disturbance subscale (1.6 ± 0.6).[29]

In the third trimester, 2 PSG studies reported on the number of awakenings per hour (19 ± 7 and 37 ± 11).[23,30] Objectively, there are limited data on arousals, with only 1 PSG study presenting data on total arousals per hour (Mdn = 15, range = 11–19), respiratory arousals per hour (Mdn = 2, range = 1–5), and spontaneous arousals per hour (8 ± 5).[23] This study also found that 31% of women had an AHI >5, and 30% of women had a PLMI >5. One study that used actigraphy reported a fragmentation index of 22 (±5).[31] Two subjective studies found that women report between 2 to 3 (±1) awakenings per night.[30,31] Another study indicated self-reported awakenings with the following frequencies: 4% of women with no awakenings, 30% with 1 to 2 awakenings, 44% with 3 to 4 awakenings, and 22% with 5 or more awakenings per night.[23] This same study also provided information on the primary causes of the awakenings, with the need to urinate and feeling uncomfortable as the most prevalent. Women have also reported almost an hour of sleep disruptions per night (59 minutes ± 6 SEM).[15] Only 1 study reported on snoring in the third trimester: 42% reported they never snored, 58% reported they sometimes snored, and 0% reported they always snored.[30] This same study reported on percentages of women reporting restless sleep (17% never, 50% sometimes, 33% always) and bad dreams (25% never, 75% sometimes, 0% always).[30]

Sleep Timing

This review yielded 3 studies on sleep timing in pregnancy, measured with actigraphy and diary self-reports in the first and third trimesters (**Table 5**). In the first trimester, actigraphy and self-report bedtime were after 23:00. There was no information on rise times. On average, in the third trimester, bedtime and sleep onset was after midnight on both weekdays and weekends, and average wake times ranged between 06:50 and nearly 08:00 on weekdays and later on weekends. For all timing values SDs were greater than 60 minutes.

Alertness/Sleepiness

Data on alertness/sleepiness are limited (**Table 6**). In the first and second trimesters, daytime alertness/sleepiness were primarily measured using the ESS, with approximately one-third of women reporting excessive daytime sleepiness. Similar proportions of women reported excessive daytime sleepiness in the third trimester. Measures of fatigue (VAS-F) were also used in studies focused on the third trimester. However, owing to differences in the construction of each scale, it was difficult to compare or summarize findings from these studies.

Sleep Satisfaction/Quality

Perceived sleep satisfaction/quality were all measured using the PSQI, with average scores >5 in the first and third trimesters across all studies, and slightly lower averages in the second trimester. The proportion of women with PSQI scores greater than 5 was approximately 40% in the first and second trimesters. In the third trimester, proportions with scores >5 were higher and ranged from 45% to 76%, depending on how groups of women were defined. **Table 7** details the measures and findings relating to perceived satisfaction/quality of sleep.

DISCUSSION

A scoping review was used to collect and summarize the available research evidence on healthy sleep in each trimester of pregnancy. Consultation with maternal health care providers confirmed the need for empirical information on this issue and, although findings show that some data are available for most dimensions of healthy sleep in each trimester, information is relatively limited.

Table 5
Sleep timing in each trimester

Measure	1st Trimester	2nd Trimester	3rd Trimester
	Mean Time ± SD (min)	Mean Time ± SD (min)	Mean Time ± SD (min)
Actigraphy Bedtime	23:24 ± 72 (with insomnia) 23:15 ± 65 (no insomnia)	No data	No data
Self-Report Bedtime	23:12 ± 60 (with insomnia) 23:19 ± 61 (no insomnia)	No data	00:24 ± 150 22:43 ± 7[a]
Self-Report Wake time	No data	No data	07:46 ± 78 06:50 ± 9[a]
Actigraphy Onset	No data	No data	00:30 ± 60 (week) 00:28 ± 60 (weekdays) 00:39 ± 72 (weekends)
Actigraphy Offset	No data	No data	07:55 ± 72 (week) 07:37 ± 72 (weekdays) 08:30 ± 84 (weekends)

Measured with actigraphy (bedtime, onset, and offset) and self-report (bedtime and wake time).
[a] SEM rather than SD.
Data from Refs.[15,27,40]

Table 6
Sleepiness/alertness in each trimester

Measure	1st Trimester Mean ± SD or %	2nd Trimester Mean ± SD or %	3rd Trimester Mean ± SD or %
ESS (Global)	8.4 ± 3.9	9.0 ± 4.1	8.0 ± 3.8
ESS ≥10 (%)	37%	32% (>10)	37%
FCF (Global)	—	—	51.3 ± 12.0
SSS (Global)	—	—	4.1 ± 1.4
POMS (Fatigue Subscale)	—	—	10.5 ± 7.4 (negative postpartum affect) 11.8 ± 7.0 (positive postpartum affect)
Fatigue (VAS-F 18-item)	—	—	64.2 ± 17.9 (primigravidae) 64.8 ± 19.3 (multigravidae)
Vitality (VAS-F 18-item)	—	—	30.5 ± 13.4 (primigravidae) 26.2 ± 16.9 (multigravidae)
Morning Fatigue (VAS-F 13-item)	—	—	36.2 ± 17.1 (7th mo) 41.6 ± 21.0 (8th mo) 47.9 ± 23.3 (9th mo)
Afternoon Fatigue (VAS-F 13-item)	—	—	74.8 ± 16.3 (7th mo) 74.5 ± 16.2 (8th mo) 77.6 ± 13.2 (9th mo)
Fatigue (VAS-F 7-item)	—	—	4.2 ± 1.3 (overall fatigue) 3.4 ± 1.6 (morning fatigue) 3.6 ± 1.6 (midday fatigue) 4.4 ± 1.2 (afternoon fatigue) 5.8 ± 1.8 (evening fatigue)
Study-Specific Questionnaire	95% (experiencing daytime tiredness)	—	93% (experiencing daytime tiredness)

Measured with ESS, FCF, POMS, SSS, VAS-F and a study-specific questionnaire.
Data from Refs.[23,24,26,29,30,41,42,44–46]

Table 7
Sleep satisfaction/quality in each trimester

Measure	1st Trimester Mean ± SD or %	2nd Trimester Mean ± SD or %	3rd Trimester Mean ± SD or %
PSQI (Global)	5.4–5.6 ± 2.4–2.5	5.2–6.7 ± 2.7–3.1 4.9 ± 2.6 (inactive) 4.2 ± 2.3 (insufficiently active) 4.0 ± 2.4 (sufficiently active)	5.7–8.4 ± 2.8–3.7 5.8 ± 3.2 (vaginal delivery) 6.7 ± 3.3 (Cesarean delivery) 7.9 ± 3.4 (frequent nappers) 5.2 ± 3.3 (infrequent nappers)
PSQI Global >5 (%)	45%	37%	45%–66% 48% (vaginal delivery) 66% (cesarean delivery) 76% (frequent nappers) 36% (infrequent nappers)
ISQ (Met Criteria) (%)	13%	—	—
SHPS (Global)	—	—	63.3 ± 11.7

Measured with PSQI, ISQ, and SHPS.
Data from Refs.[4,24–26,28,29,31,40,42,43,45,47,48]

The growth in the number of studies published on this topic since 2011 points to an increased awareness of the importance of healthy sleep in pregnancy, and to an increased need for information on the topic from pregnant women and their health care providers.

Most of the available data on healthy sleep in pregnancy focuses on sleep duration, the architecture of sleep, and sleep continuity/efficiency. There is limited information on daytime sleepiness/alertness, and on subjective perceptions of sleep satisfaction/quality. Very little information is available on sleep timing. Recent literature points to the importance of stable sleep timing in health[32]; however, little is known about how sleep timing might change across pregnancy, and what the consequences may be for maternal and child health. This is certainly an area deserving of further research attention.

Another aspect of sleep, potentially relevant to sleep health during pregnancy, is the position in which women slept. Position was only reported in 1 of the studies included in this review. Given the possible relationship between sleep position and stillbirth,[33–35] position is an important aspect of sleep that should be described for pregnant women, and about which women and health care providers are seeking information.

This review does not aim to compare dimensions of healthy sleep across trimesters. However, several longitudinal studies were identified. PSG-recorded TST in a laboratory setting was similar across all 3 trimesters,[2] whereas PSG recorded in the home indicated that women obtained more sleep in the first trimester than the third trimester.[3] Two studies showed that sleep continuity/efficiency were reduced in the third trimester.[2,23] Brunner and colleagues[2] found that WASO was higher in the third trimester compared with the second trimester, despite comparable TST. Wilson and colleagues[23] examined changes between the first and third trimesters using PSG and found that SOL was similar; however, arousals, awakenings, AHI >5, and PLMI >5 were all higher in the third trimester, and time spent in the supine position was halved. Self-report data from this study showed that SOL >20 minutes was greater in the third trimester and reports of >5 awakenings per night doubled from the first to third trimester. No other studies reviewed used statistical comparisons to examine changes in sleep across trimesters.

A strength of this study is the use of the framework proposed by Arksey and O'Malley[22] for conducting a scoping review and the incorporation of Buysse's[21] definition of sleep health, which places a positive focus on sleep and considers sleep health as a multifaceted concept. None of the studies in this review were specifically designed with Buysse's[21] recent definition in mind; therefore, no single paper provided data for all dimensions of sleep in each trimester of pregnancy.

Studies provided different amounts of detail on exclusion and inclusion criteria, which, in some instances, produced uncertainty on how women were screened. Given that mood disorders have a strong and consistent relationship with alterations in sleep in pregnancy,[12–14] the authors of this review decided that these aspects of health needed to be clearly described in the screening process for a publication to be included. Many other aspects of maternal health and infant health have also been associated with changes in sleep (eg, gestational diabetes, hypertension, small for gestational age infants, preterm infants)[5–10]; however, most studies did not specifically state all the conditions for which women were excluded (see **Fig. 1**). Instead, they referred to women being healthy, having an uncomplicated pregnancy, or being free of chronic illnesses. The authors' approach may have resulted in studies being included that did not sufficiently screen women for all health conditions currently shown to be related to altered sleep; however, requiring this criterion would have resulted in only 3 studies for this scoping review. This review may have also excluded studies that did screen for sleep and mood disorders but did not state this explicitly in the methods. Future studies should focus on healthy samples of pregnant women and researchers should clearly specify the health issues considered in the screening process.

Related to screening and enrolling pregnant participants for research is the issue of ongoing health for women participating in longitudinal studies. No studies included in this review discussed screening women throughout the course of the study to ensure they remained free of health complications. As a consequence, it is possible that women developed health issues later in pregnancy (ie, hypertension or preeclampsia) that could affect sleep or could be associated with changes in sleep.

Another limitation of this scoping review is that 38% (n = 9) of the publications were conducted in Taiwan and 54% were conducted in the United States, biasing results toward cultural practices in those areas of the world. There may be cultural differences in sleep practices (ie, napping) during pregnancy that would influence the findings presented in this review. Furthermore, half of the studies had small sample sizes (<40), which may limit the generalizability of the results.

The authors have provided information on the range (and variability) of values presented for each dimension of sleep but have not made judgements or recommendations on when maternal health care professionals should refer women to other clinicians for further assessment or treatment. It is argued that recommendations should be made only after using a consensus approach, similar to the process for developing other guidelines.[36,37] A consensus group would also consider if there were sufficient data currently available on which to base such guidelines. Unfortunately, even if guidelines were in place, many countries may not have clearly defined treatment pathways for pregnant women with sleep problems or disorders. In New Zealand, for example, there are clinical sleep services but the public health system often experiences long waiting times. It would important for pregnant women to be given priority in such circumstances.

SUMMARY

Although data on each of the 5 dimensions of sleep detailed in Buysse's[21] definition of sleep health are presented in this scoping review, diverse and extensive evidence of healthy sleep in pregnancy is limited. Most studies are relatively recent, with 92% of studies originating from only 2 countries and from a limited group of investigators and cohorts. Comparable data on sleep duration and measures of continuity/efficiency are available; however, reports of sleep timing, perceived sleep satisfaction/quality, and alertness/sleepiness measures are lacking. The data presented in this scoping review indicate that sleep in each trimester of pregnancy is highly variable between women but does not support the idea of large changes in sleep across pregnancy in healthy pregnant woman. There is some evidence of more disturbed sleep in the third trimester but at this stage there is limited information from which to draw firm conclusions. Further research is needed to clearly differentiate between healthy sleep and insufficient or disturbed sleep in which intervention might be necessary. Knowing when to intervene if women need help with their sleep is vital in ensuring the short-term and long-term health and wellbeing of mothers and their children.

REFERENCES

1. Kennedy HP, Gardiner A, Gay C, et al. Negotiating sleep: a qualitative study of new mothers. J Perinat Neonatal Nurs 2007;21(2):114–22.

2. Brunner DP, Münch M, Biedermann K, et al. Changes in sleep and sleep electroencephalogram during pregnancy. Sleep 1994;17(7):576–82.

3. Lee KA, Zaffke ME, McEnany G. Parity and sleep patterns during and after pregnancy. Obstetrics Gynecol 2000;95(1):14–8.

4. Tsai S-Y, Lee P-L, Lin J-W, et al. Cross-sectional and longitudinal associations between sleep and health-related quality of life in pregnant women: a prospective observational study. Int J Nurs Stud 2016;56:45–53.

5. Micheli K, Komninos I, Bagkeris E, et al. Sleep patterns in late pregnancy and risk of preterm birth and fetal growth restriction. Epidemiology 2011;22(5):738.

6. Okun ML, Schetter CD, Glynn LM. Poor sleep quality is associated with preterm birth. Sleep 2011;34(11):1493–8.

7. Facco F, Grobman W, Kramer J, et al. Self-reported short sleep duration and frequent snoring in pregnancy: impact on glucose metabolism. Am J Obstet Gynecol 2010;203(2):142–5.

8. Qiu C, Enquobahrie D, Frederick IO, et al. Glucose intolerance and gestational diabetes risk in relation to sleep duration and snoring during pregnancy: a pilot study. BMC Womens Health 2010;10:17.

9. Williams MA, Miller RS, Qiu C, et al. Associations of early pregnancy sleep duration with trimester-specific blood pressures and hypertensive disorders in pregnancy. Sleep 2010;33(10):1363–71.

10. O'Brien LM, Bullough AS, Owusu JT, et al. Pregnancy-onset habitual snoring, gestational hypertension, and preeclampsia: prospective cohort study. Am J Obstet Gynecol 2012;207(6):487–9.

11. Lee KA, Gay C. Sleep in late pregnancy predicts length of labor and type of delivery. Am J Obstet Gynecol 2004;191(6):2041–6.

12. Dorheim SK, Bjorvatn B, Eberhard-Gran M. Insomnia and depressive symptoms in late pregnancy: a population-based study. Behav Sleep Med 2012;10(3):152–66.

13. Okun ML, Kiewra K, Luther JF, et al. Sleep disturbances in depressed and nondepressed pregnant women. Depress Anxiety 2011;28(8):676–85.

14. Swanson LM, Pickett SM, Flynn H, et al. Relationships among depression, anxiety, and insomnia symptoms in perinatal women seeking mental health treatment. J Womens Health (Larchmt) 2011;20(4):553–8.

15. Wolfson AR, Crowley SJ, Anwer U, et al. Changes in sleep patterns and depressive symptoms in first-time mothers: last trimester to 1-year postpartum. Behav Sleep Med 2003;1(1):54–67.

16. Farrell P, Richards G. Recognition and treatment of sleep-disordered breathing: an important component of chronic disease management. J Transl Med 2017;15(1):114.

17. Jike M, Itani O, Watanabe N, et al. Long sleep duration and health outcomes: a systematic review, meta-analysis and meta-regression. Sleep Med Rev 2018;39:25–36.

18. Cappuccio F, Miller M. Sleep and cardio-metabolic disease. Curr Cardiol Rep 2017;19(11):110.

19. Canadian Society for Exercise Physiology. Canadian 24-hour movement guidelines for children and youth: an integration of physical activity, sedentary behavior, and sleep. 2016. Available at: www.csep.ca/guidelines. Accessed February 3, 2018.

20. New Zealand Ministry of Health. Sit less, move more, sleep well: physical activity guidelines for children and young people. 2017. Available at: https://www.health.govt.nz/system/files/documents/pages/physical-activity-guidelines-for-children-and-young-people-may17.pdf. Accessed February 3, 2018.

21. Buysse DJ. Sleep health: can we define it? Does it matter? Sleep 2014;37(1):9–17.

22. Arksey H, O'Malley L. Scoping studies: towards a methodological framework. Int J Social Res Methodol 2005;8(1):19–32.

23. Wilson DL, Barnes M, Ellett L, et al. Decreased sleep efficiency, increased wake after sleep onset and increased cortical arousals in late pregnancy. Aust N Z J Obstet Gynaecol 2011;51(1):38–46.

24. Tsai S-Y, Lee P-L, Lin J-W, et al. Persistent and new-onset daytime sleepiness in pregnant women: a prospective observational cohort study. Int J Nurs Stud 2017;66:1–6.

25. Tsai SY, Lin JW, Kuo LT, et al. Nighttime sleep, daytime napping, and labor outcomes in healthy pregnant women in Taiwan. Res Nurs Health 2013;36(6):612–22.

26. Tsai S-Y, Lin J-W, Kuo L-T, et al. Daily sleep and fatigue characteristics in nulliparous women during the third trimester of pregnancy. Sleep 2012;35(2):257–62.

27. Tsai SY, Kuo LT, Lai YH, et al. Factors associated with sleep quality in pregnant women: a prospective observational study. Nurs Res 2011;60(6):405–12.

28. Crowley S, O'Buckley T, Schiller C, et al. Blunted neuroactive steroid and HPA axis responses to stress are associated with reduced sleep quality and negative affect in pregnancy: a pilot study. Psychopharmacology 2016;233(7):1299–310.

29. Strange LB, Parker KP, Moore ML, et al. Disturbed sleep and preterm birth: a potential relationship? Clin Exp Obstet Gynecol 2009;36(3):166–8.

30. Hertz G, Fast A, Feinsilver SH, et al. Sleep in normal late pregnancy. Sleep 1992;15(3):246–51.

31. Tsai S-Y, Kuo L-T, Lee C-N, et al. Reduced sleep duration and daytime naps in pregnant women in Taiwan. Nurs Res 2013;62(2):99–105.

32. Landhuis C, Poulton R, Welch D, et al. Childhood sleep time and long-term risk for obesity: a 32-year prospective birth cohort study. Pediatrics 2008;122:955–60.

33. Gordon A, Raynes-Greenow C, Bond D, et al. Sleep position, fetal growth restriction, and late-pregnancy stillbirth. The Sydney Stillbirth Study. Obstet Gynecol 2015;125:347–55.

34. Stacey T, Thompson JMD, Mitchell EA, et al. Association between maternal sleep practices and risk of late stillbirth: a case-control study. BMJ 2011;342:d3403.

35. Cronin RS, Okesene-Gafa K, Thompson JMD, et al. Survey of maternal sleep practices in late pregnancy in a multi-ethnic sample in South Auckland, New Zealand. BMC Pregnancy Childbirth 2017;17(1):190.

36. Hirshkowitz M, Whiton K, Albert SM, et al. National Sleep Foundation's updated sleep duration recommendations: final report. Sleep Health 2015;1:233–43.

37. Ohayon M, Wickwire EM, Hirshkowitz M, et al. National Sleep Foundation's sleep quality recommendations: first report. Sleep Health 2017;3:6–19.

38. Haney A, Buysse DJ, Okun ML, et al. Sleep disturbance and cardiometabolic risk factors in early pregnancy: a preliminary study. Sleep Med 2014;15:444–50.

39. Ebert RM, Wood A, Okun ML. Minimal effect of daytime napping behavior on nocturnal sleep in pregnant women. J Clin Sleep Med 2015;11(6):635–43.

40. Okun ML, Buysse DJ, Hall MH. Identifying insomnia in early pregnancy: validation of the Insomnia Symptoms Questionnaire (ISQ) in pregnant women. J Clin Sleep Med 2015;11(6):645–54.

41. Lee KA, McEnany G, Zaffke ME. REM sleep and mood state in childbearing women: sleepy or weepy? Sleep 2000;23(7):877–85.

42. Tsai S-Y, Lin J-W, Wu W-W, et al. Sleep disturbances and symptoms of depression and daytime sleepiness in pregnant women. Birth 2016;43(2):176–83.

43. Tsai S-Y, Lee C-N, Wu W-W, et al. Sleep hygiene and sleep quality of third-trimester pregnant women. Res Nurs Health 2016;39(1):57–65.

44. Elek SM, Hudson DB, Fleck MO. Expectant parents' experience with fatigue and sleep during pregnancy. Birth 1997;24(1):49–54.

45. Tzeng Y-L, Chen S-L, Chen C-F, et al. Sleep trajectories of women undergoing elective Cesarean section: effects on body weight and psychological well-being. PLoS One 2015;10(6):1–15.

46. Waters MA, Lee Kathryn A, Lee KA. Differences between primigravidae and multigravidae mothers in sleep disturbances, fatigue, and functional status. J Nurse Midwifery 1996;41(5):364–7.

47. Baker JH, Okun ML, Rothenberger SD, et al. Exercise during early pregnancy is associated with greater sleep continuity. Behav Sleep Med 2016;14:1–14.

48. Hux VJ, Roberts JM, Okun ML. Higher allostatic load in early pregnancy is associated with chronic stressors and poorer sleep quality. Sleep Med 2017;33:85–90.

Management Strategies for Restless Legs Syndrome/Willis-Ekbom Disease During Pregnancy

Corrado Garbazza, MD*, Mauro Manconi, MD, PhD

KEYWORDS

- Restless legs syndrome • Willis-Ekbom disease • Pregnancy • Sleep

KEY POINTS

- Restless legs syndrome/Willis-Ekbom disease (RLS/WED) is a common sensorimotor sleep disorder, with a prevalence and severity peaking during the third trimester of pregnancy and receding around delivery.
- The exact causal mechanisms of restless legs syndrome have not been completely identified. Possible pathogenetic hypotheses include pregnancy-related endocrine and metabolic changes, and genetic factors.
- An accurate diagnosis of RLS is essential and should particularly consider other frequent complications of pregnancy that may mimic its symptoms.
- Management strategies should be personalized and based on an individual assessment of symptoms severity and impact, as well as of risks and benefits for the patient.
- Nonpharmacologic treatments should be considered first. If pharmacologic interventions are needed, medications should be used at the lowest effective dose and for the shortest duration possible.

INTRODUCTION

Restless legs syndrome (RLS), also known as Willis-Ekbom disease (WED), is a common sensorimotor disorder characterized by a strong, nearly irresistible urge to move the limbs during rest, which improves with movement, and worsens during the evening and night.[1] About 70% of patients with RLS complain about sleep onset insomnia and, in 80% to 90% of the affected individuals, periodic leg movements during sleep (PLMS) can be detected, whose impact on sleep quality is still being investigated.[2] When periodic leg movements during sleep occur without RLS symptoms, but are associated with sleepiness and/or insomnia,

the diagnosis of periodic limb movement disorder should be considered.

Prevalence rates of periodic limb movement disorder during pregnancy are still lacking. Around 5% to 10% of the general population suffers from RLS,[3,4] with women being affected twice as often as men.[2] Pregnant women are particularly at risk to develop a new onset and often transient form of RLS, or to experience a worsening of a preexisting RLS. A recent meta-analysis found a mean prevalence of RLS during pregnancy of 21%, with variability by geographic region, ranging from 14% in the Western Pacific Region, to 20% and 22% in

Disclosure Statement: The authors declares no relationship with a commercial company that has a direct financial interest in subject matter or materials discussed in article or with a company making a competing product.
Sleep and Epilepsy Center, Neurocenter of Southern Switzerland, Civic Hospital of Lugano (EOC), Via Tesserete 46, Lugano CH-6903, Switzerland
* Corresponding author.
E-mail address: corrado.garbazza@eoc.ch

Sleep Med Clin 13 (2018) 335–348
https://doi.org/10.1016/j.jsmc.2018.05.001
1556-407X/18/© 2018 Elsevier Inc. All rights reserved.

the American and European regions, respectively, and up to 30% in the Eastern Mediterranean region.[5] Pregnancy-related RLS peaks in the third trimester of gestation, affecting up to one-third of women, and usually remits around delivery.[6–8] Chen and colleagues[5] found prevalence rates of 8%, 16%, and 22% in the first, second, and third trimesters, respectively, and the pooled estimated prevalence of RLS after delivery was 4%.

In women already affected by RLS before pregnancy (preexisting RLS) the symptoms usually worsen in severity during pregnancy and are more likely to persist after delivery, compared with women with new-onset RLS during pregnancy.[9] Most pregnant women affected by RLS are unaware of the diagnosis and do not receive adequate information and reassurance by clinicians, who often tend to underestimate the problem.

PATHOGENETIC MECHANISMS

The question of why pregnancy triggers or worsens RLS remains unanswered. Some pathogenetic hypotheses have been postulated, but further investigation is still needed. These include endocrine changes, iron and folate metabolism, genetics, and other factors.

Endocrine Changes

Endocrine-related changes in pregnancy, such as an increase in estradiol, progesterone, and prolactin, all peaking in the third trimester, may play a role in inducing RLS. Estradiol and progesterone dramatically decrease around delivery, when RLS usually disappears, whereas prolactin, which is inhibited by dopamine, maintains a pulsatile secretion during lactation. Higher levels of estradiol were found in a small population of pregnant women with RLS compared to with women without RLS.[10] Also, the use of estrogen-based therapies in nonpregnant women may be associated with a significantly higher incidence of RLS.[11]

Iron and Folate Metabolism

During pregnancy, iron, ferritin, and serum folate levels decrease, possibly because of their dilution in a greater total blood volume and due to increased fetal requirements.[12] Iron is an important cofactor in the synthesis of dopamine,[13] whose deficiency may be involved in the pathogenesis of RLS.[14] Low serum ferritin before or during early pregnancy has been found to be a predictor of RLS occurring during gestation[15] and iron supplementation may be considered in

the treatment of patients with RLS and low serum ferritin, including during late pregnancy and lactation.[16]

Folate also plays a role in the synthesis of dopamine via the regeneration of tetrahydrobiopterin.[17,18] Lee and colleagues[19] showed that, even before pregnancy, a decreased serum folate level, rather than indicators of iron status, was associated with RLS in pregnant women. However, because RLS symptoms rapidly decrease after delivery, whereas iron and folate levels normalize much more gradually,[20] the contribution of these 2 factors to the pathogenesis of RLS during pregnancy remains unclear. Moreover, oral folate and iron supplementation during pregnancy seems to be ineffective in preventing RLS symptoms.[8]

Genetics

The hypothesis that pregnancy may trigger the onset of symptoms in women already genetically predisposed to develop RLS is supported by 3 findings:

1. Familial RLS is a much more common trait in pregnant women with RLS than in women without the syndrome[8,21,22] and compared with other secondary forms of RLS;
2. Most women with a preexisting form of RLS experience a worsening of symptoms during pregnancy[8]; and
3. A new-onset disease during pregnancy predisposes affected women to develop a chronic, idiopathic form of RLS in the future.[9,23]

Although several allelic variants are known to be associated with idiopathic RLS,[24] further genetic analyses in women with pregnancy-related RLS are needed to better characterize the genetic component of RLS during gestation.

Other Factors

A number of other possible causal factors of RLS during pregnancy has been investigated. These factors include comorbidity with other sleep disturbances, such as respiratory disorders[23]; insomnia and excessive daytime sleepiness; psychological conditions exacerbating RLS symptoms, such as anxiety, stress, and fatigue; positional discomfort; and lower limb hypoxia or edema.[8,15,25,26]

CONSEQUENCES OF RESTLESS LEG SYNDROME IN PREGNANCY

The severity of RLS/WED symptoms during pregnancy ranges from very mild to quite severe.

However, severe to very severe symptoms, as assessed by the International Restless Legs Syndrome Study Group (IRLSSG) rating scale, were reported in 45% and 54% of pregnant women in 2 recent studies,[27–29] whereas in another study 75% of the affected women had at least moderate symptoms.[3] The impact of idiopathic RLS on the quality of life of the affected patients is significant.[30,31] RLS during pregnancy is a risk factor for developing negative consequences for women, including insomnia, birth complications, and mood disorders.

1. Insomnia. The prevalence of insomnia is higher in pregnant women with RLS than in healthy controls.[8] RLS during gestation leads to excessive daytime sleepiness, poor daytime function, and poor sleep quality.[32] These consequences, in turn, represent risk factors for negative pregnancy outcomes, such as preterm birth.[33]
2. Birth complications. Few researchers have investigated the links between RLS and birth complications. Some have found a significant association between pregnancy-related RLS and preeclampsia, gestational diabetes, hypertension, eclampsia, gestational age at birth, and birth weight,[34–36] whereas others have found no correlation.[37]
3. Mood disorders. RLS causes psychological distress[38] and, when occurring in pregnant women, increases the risk of developing perinatal depression.[39]

CLINICAL COURSE AND RECURRENCE OF RESTLESS LEG SYNDROME

About one-third of women with pregnancy-related RLS report a prior diagnosis of the syndrome or already experienced RLS symptoms at some time before pregnancy.[8] In 70% to 80% of these patients, RLS worsens during pregnancy.[8] In fact, the incidence of RLS clearly increases across gestation, reaching the highest rate in the third trimester, and then remitting around delivery. Very few women continue suffering from RLS after giving birth,[8,28] and in most cases the clinical course of RLS during the perinatal period is benign.

However, the long-term course of the disease must be carefully monitored. Cesnik and colleagues[9] showed that women who suffered from pregnancy-related RLS have a 4-fold higher risk to develop an idiopathic form of RLS over a 7-year follow-up period, compared with women who did not experience RLS during pregnancy. Moreover, more than 60% of women with RLS onset during a first pregnancy, also experience the syndrome during a second pregnancy, although this probability is

only about 3% in women who did not suffer from RLS during a previous pregnancy.[9] Sarberg and colleagues[23] obtained similar results with a sample of women followed for 3 years after pregnancy. These findings from 2 long-term prospective studies substantially support the hypothesis of a genetic predisposition behind the pregnancy-related form of RLS.[40]

The role of parity in RLS is still not completely clear. Nulliparous women have the same risk to develop RLS/WED as age-matched men, but there is an increased risk for women after one pregnancy (odds ratio, 1.98), 2 pregnancies (odds ratio, 3.04), and 3 or more pregnancies (odds ratio, 3.57).[15,41] This increased risk with parity partly accounts for the gender differences in the prevalence of idiopathic RLS.

MANAGEMENT OVERVIEW

The first step toward an effective management of RLS during pregnancy is an accurate clinical diagnosis, which is based on an individual assessment of diagnostic criteria, severity, frequency, and impact of symptoms, as well as of the risks and benefits for the patient. There are 3 key factors that may contribute to the underestimation of the importance of an accurate RLS management during pregnancy.

1. Poor knowledge of the syndrome entity, which often leads to missed or wrong diagnoses.
2. The transient character of RLS symptoms, which usually worsen during pregnancy and remit around delivery. This factor results in RLS being considered as a pseudophysiologic pregnancy-related phenomenon, often not distinguished from other common conditions associated with pregnancy. These conditions, such as ankle edema, fatigue, positional discomfort, or insomnia, are common and therefore not considered as deserving particular attention or care.
3. The false opinion that RLS cannot have a significant effect on pregnant women. In contrast, RLS may present with severe symptoms and has potentially negative consequences on pregnancy outcomes. Moreover, even in cases of a mild clinical presentation of the syndrome, which does not require treatment, RLS should be diagnosed and women should receive support and education to better understand their symptoms and to reduce the related worries and anxiety.

PATIENT EVALUATION
Diagnostic Criteria and Differential Diagnosis

The diagnosis of pregnancy-related RLS is essentially clinical and based on the updated consensus criteria of the IRLSSG,[16] which are the same used for the idiopathic form of RLS.[42] In fact, the idiopathic and pregnancy-related forms of RLS share the main features and a comparable anatomic distribution of symptoms. Some lines of evidence support a similar clinical approach for the diagnosis of RLS regardless of pregnancy status[16]:

- High familial tendency for RLS in pregnant women affected by the syndrome[8,22,23];
- Common occurrence of RLS during pregnancy in familial clusters of RLS[43];
- Positive history of transient RLS in previous pregnancies; and
- Increased risk for pregnant women with transient RLS to develop an idiopathic RLS form later on in life.[9]

In addition to the 5 main standard diagnostic criteria, other clinical features can help to confirm the suspicion of RLS. These factors include the presence of periodic limb movements, the treatment response to dopaminergic agents, the familiarity for RLS/WED, and the lack of profound daytime sleepiness.[16] Moreover, clinicians should be aware that, compared with the idiopathic form of RLS, during pregnancy the diagnosis of RLS may be more difficult owing to possible mimics that must be taken into account in the differential diagnosis. The most frequent conditions that may mimic or overlap with RLS are listed in **Table 1**.[16]

After a diagnosis of RLS has been established, possible other symptomatic causes of the syndrome need to be ruled out by a careful assessment. Before judging pregnancy as the main or unique triggering factor of RLS, clinical assessment should include the following 3 considerations:

1. A careful pharmacologic history must be obtained to identify possible RLS inducing or exacerbating drugs like antidepressants, neuroleptics and antiemetics.[31,44,45]
2. Particular attention should be given to comorbidities with other sleep disorders, especially sleep apnea and primary insomnia.[46–48] A careful evaluation of the 5 essential diagnostic criteria, together with the supportive criteria, and eventually with a polysomnographic recording is warranted, as suspected overlap with other sleep disorders can guide clinicians to an accurate diagnosis.
3. A positive medical history of neurologic or systemic conditions such as multiple sclerosis, spinal lesions, radiculopathy or peripheral neuropathy, diabetes, iron deficiency anemia, rheumatoid arthritis, or chronic obstructive pulmonary disease should be considered.

Table 1
Differential diagnosis of RLS/WED during pregnancy

Common Mimics	Less Common Mimics
Leg cramps	Arthritis
Positional discomfort	Other orthopedic disorders
Venous stasis	Peripheral neuropathy
Leg edema	Radiculopathy
Compression and stretch neuropathies	Myelopathy
Sore leg muscles	Myopathy
Ligament sprain/ tendon strain	Fibromyalgia
Positional ischemia (numbness)	Complex regional pain syndrome
Dermatitis	Drug-induced akathisia
Bruises	Sickle cell disease

Abbreviations: RLS, restless legs syndrome; WED, Willis-Ekbom disease.

(*Adapted from* Picchietti DL, Hensley JG, Bainbridge JL, et al; International Restless Legs Syndrome Study Group (IRLSSG). Consensus clinical practice guidelines for the diagnosis and treatment of restless legs syndrome/Willis-Ekbom disease during pregnancy and lactation. Sleep Med Rev 2015;22:67; with permission.)

Assessment of Severity

RLS/WED symptoms may present with a wide range of severity and impact on the quality of life of pregnant women.[31,49] According to the 2014 consensus diagnostic criteria, RLS should be considered clinically relevant when causing "significant distress or impairment in social, occupational, educational, or other important areas of functioning by its impact on sleep, mood, cognition, health, daily activities, behavior, or energy/vitality."[16] Regarding the severity of RLS/WED symptoms, research studies consider "at least twice a week and moderate-to-severe distress" indicative of a moderate to severe form of RLS/WED.[2]

The IRLSSG has validated an international rating instrument, the Restless Legs Syndrome Rating Scale (IRLS),[50] consisting of 10 questions listed in a self-administered questionnaire, with a final score ranging between 0 and 40. A score between 10 and 20 corresponds to moderate, between 20 and 30 to severe, and greater than 30 to very severe symptoms. In a recent study on RLS during pregnancy, 53.5% of women reported severe or very severe RLS symptoms based on the IRLS.[27] Another useful instrument to assesses the impact of RLS on daily life, emotional well-being, social life, and work life in clinical setting is represented by the Restless Legs Syndrome Quality of Life questionnaire,[51] in which 13 of 18 items are scored on a 5-point scale. Scores are then transformed to a 0 to 100 scale, with lower scores indicating a worse quality of life.

NONPHARMACOLOGIC TREATMENT OPTIONS

Before deciding for a potentially unsafe pharmacologic approach, possible nonpharmacologic strategies for RLS during pregnancy and lactation should be considered.[16] In mild cases, a simple reassurance by the clinician on the nature and prognosis of RLS symptoms can be sufficient to avoid excessive concerns.[52]

Self-Management Treatment Strategies

- Sleep hygiene rules need to be reviewed with the patient and reinforced at frequent intervals.
- Alcohol and tobacco, even if not directly linked to RLS, should be avoided or limited because of their negative impact on sleep quality (and on the developing fetus).
- Moderate, safe aerobic physical exercise, preferably not too close to bedtime, should be encouraged, based on its beneficial effects on idiopathic RLS.[53,54]
- Low-impact activity, such as yoga, water aerobics, or walking, is warranted, prior consent of the healthcare provider.[16]
- Legs massage may be beneficial in primary RLS and potentially helpful during pregnancy.

IRON SUPPLEMENTATION

There is solid evidence from several studies supporting a causal relationship between iron deficiency and idiopathic RLS.[55–67] Thus, recent treatment guidelines recommend oral iron supplementation if serum ferritin levels are less than 50 to 75 µg/L.[68–70] During pregnancy, maternal serum ferritin decreases to about 50% at midgestation and remain low also in late pregnancy, when RLS symptoms are more frequent or severe. This decrease is due to the expansion of the maternal red blood cell mass, as well as the growth of the fetus and placental structures.[71]

Oral Iron Supplements

Oral supplements of iron are considered safe during pregnancy and lactation and may have potential benefits for both mother and infant.[71–73] Thus, iron supplementation is generally suggested in all

pregnant women when ferritin is less than 30 µg/L.[25] If RLS occurs during pregnancy, the clinical guidelines recommend administering ferrous sulfate at a dose of 65 mg elemental iron, 1 to 2 times daily when ferritin levels decrease to less than 75 µg/L.[49]

Concurrent intake of vitamin C and taking iron without food can facilitate iron absorption, but the safety of vitamin C use during pregnancy is still debated and should, therefore, be avoided.[74] Although direct evidence of a beneficial effect of iron supplementation for RLS during pregnancy is scarce,[43,75,76] it should be taken into account that an overload of iron is dangerous for women and can even be fatal for the infant. Thus, ferritin levels should be rechecked regularly after starting an iron supplementation therapy.

Intravenous iron administration

Intravenous (IV) iron administration may be considered for the treatment of refractory RLS during the second or third trimester of pregnancy and the postpartum period when oral iron administration failed, and ferritin values are less than 30 µg/L.[49] Since the demands of iron during pregnancy are high, and intestinal absorption of iron can be decreased in some women, IV administration of iron may represent a valid alternative.

Caution must be used because of possible, rare, but severe anaphylactic reactions, especially if women receive IV iron for the first time.[73] However, IV iron supplementation during pregnancy is generally considered safe. For idiopathic RLS, IV iron has shown mostly positive results.[64,67,77,78] In addition, a few open-label studies have been performed to test the efficacy of IV iron in RLS during pregnancy, reporting encouraging results and no serious adverse events.[43,75,76] Some studies also support its use during lactation, because breast milk iron levels seem not to be increased after IV infusion.[79] However, further, large-scale, randomized, controlled studies with IV and oral iron in both idiopathic and pregnancy-related RLS forms are needed.

Supplementation with Magnesium, Folate, and Vitamins C, D, and E

Despite their discrete safety during pregnancy, no adequate evidence for the efficacy of vitamins (folate, C, D, and E) or magnesium are available for RLS. Folate is a common supplement in pregnant women because of its protective property against neuronal tube defects. However, except for a single, small study, no solid evidence supports the effectiveness of folate in RLS.[19,80]

PHARMACOLOGIC TREATMENT OPTIONS

To date, randomized, controlled trials of pharmacologic treatments for RLS during pregnancy are lacking. Current knowledge of this topic generally refers to studies conducted on idiopathic RLS. A task force of the IRLSSG recently published consensus guidelines on the available management strategies for RLS during pregnancy and lactation to be used in clinical practice.[16] These are discussed in the following paragraphs and summarized in **Table 2**.

The following 3 general recommendations regarding pharmacologic approaches to pregnancy-related RLS should be considered:

1. Currently approved drugs for the treatment of idiopathic RLS, with differences depending on

Table 2
Recommended management strategies for RLS/WED during pregnancy and lactation

Class of Treatment	Drug/Intervention	Recommendation	Indication
Nonpharmacologic	Moderate intensity exercise, yoga, massage, pneumatic compression devices, treating obstructive sleep apnea, avoidance of aggravating factors	Yes	Pregnancy, lactation
Nutraceuticals	Valerian or Chinese herbal preparations	Insufficient evidence	Pregnancy, lactation
Vitamin/mineral supplementation	Oral iron	If serum ferritin <75 µg/L	Pregnancy, lactation
	IV iron	If failure of oral iron supplementation and serum ferritin <30 µg/L	Refractory RLS/WED during the second or third trimester of pregnancy and lactation
	Magnesium, folate, vitamins C, D, and E	Insufficient evidence	Pregnancy, lactation
Benzodiazepines/ benzodiazepine receptor agonists	Low-dose clonazepam	Up to 0.5 mg/d at night; avoidance of concurrent use with diphenhydramine or anticonvulsants during pregnancy	Refractory RLS/WED during the second and third trimester of pregnancy and lactation
Alpha-2-delta ligands	Gabapentin	300–900 mg in the evening or at night	Refractory RLS/WED during lactation
Dopaminergics	Carbidopa/levodopa	25/100–50/200 mg extended release in the evening or at night; avoidance of combination of levodopa with benserazide. Caveat: Dopaminergics inhibit lactation.	Refractory RLS/WED during pregnancy
Opioids	Low-dose oxycodone	5–10 mg/d	Very severe, very refractory RLS/WED after the first trimester pregnancy
	Low-dose tramadol	50–100 mg/d	Very severe, very refractory RLS/WED during lactation.
Other medications	Trazodon, clonidine, carbamazepine	Insufficient evidence	Pregnancy, lactation

Abbreviations: IV, intravenous; RLS, restless leg syndrome; WED, Willis-Ekbom disease.

national authorities, include ropinirole, pramipexole, rotigotine, enacarbil, and levodopa;
other compounds are used off-label.

2. Because of the scarce knowledge about side
effects or potential dangers for the fetus,
these medications are not recommended for
use during pregnancy. Therefore, a pharmacologic treatment is indicated only in women
with a clinically significant RLS, for example,
occurring more than twice a week, with an
IRLS score greater than 20 (severe or very severe disease), and in women who already
failed to respond to a previous nonpharmacologic intervention, including iron administration, when needed.[16]

3. Any drug treatment should be prescribed at
the lowest effective dose, for the shortest
possible duration, and possibly not during the
first trimester of pregnancy, when the risk of
embryonal malformations is greatest. In case
of occasional RLS symptoms, an on-demand
treatment can be considered. Once a drug therapy is started, the patients must be followed
regularly at short intervals by their healthcare
provider.

Dopaminergic Medications

Dopamine agonists are considered the first-line
treatment in idiopathic RLS.[68,69,81,82] These medications are generally well-tolerated in patients with
RLS. However, owing to the long-term risk of
augmentation and the scarcity of safety data about
their use during pregnancy, caution is required.

Levodopa
As a monotherapy or in combination with carbi-
dopa, levodopa has been used during pregnancy
in some cases of juvenile Parkinson disease or
Segawa syndrome, as well as in a prospective
case series on different dopamine agonists prescribed for the treatment of RLS.[83–85] Overall, no
major malformations or other adverse pregnancy
outcomes were observed in these patients. However, the combination of levodopa with benserazide should be avoided because of possible
adverse effects of benserazide on fetal skeletal
development.[72]

Pramipexole, ropinirole, and rotigotine
Safety data on the use of these drugs during pregnancy are limited,[72,85,86] and the IRLSSG task
force concluded that there is "insufficient evidence
to reach consensus."

Bromocriptine and cabergoline
Bromocriptine and cabergoline have been used
largely during the first trimester of pregnancy for

treatment of hyperprolactinemia. These 2 ergoline
derivatives, as well as pergolide, can induce severe fibrotic reactions[87] and should be avoided
for RLS during pregnancy.

It should be stressed that all dopaminergic
agents are inhibitors of prolactin secretion via D2
receptors and may interfere with lactation. Thus,
they are not indicated for breastfeeding women.
However, if the use of carbidopa/levodopa is
limited to pregnancy, prolactin levels rebound
quickly after discontinuation and lactation can be
established.[72]

Alpha-2-Delta Ligand Therapy

Given their positive effects and tolerance profile,
gabapentin enacarbil, gabapentin, and pregabalin
are second-line or in some conditions even first-
line treatments for chronic idiopathic
RLS.[68,69,81,82,88] However, insufficient safety data
about these medications during pregnancy did
not permit to reach consensus on their use in pregnant women with RLS.[72]

A previous recommendation on the use of
gabapentin for pregnancy-related RLS, which
was supported by safety data from studies in
patients with epilepsy,[89–93] has been questioned
and finally withdrawn, based on the observation
that a very high dose of gabapentin
(400 mg/kg) intraperitoneally administered in
mice was associated with an impaired synaptogenesis.[94] In humans, one study showed no effect on head circumference in newborns
exposed to gabapentin monotherapy during
pregnancy.[95] Because gabapentin has been
linked to lower mean serum folate levels, folic
acid supplementation of 4 mg/d is recommended during pregnancy, to potentially decrease
the risk of neural tube defects.[96,97] No adverse
effects were observed in neonates of women
treated with gabapentin, probably because infants are estimated to receive only 1% to 4%
of the maternal weight-adjusted dose through
the maternal milk.[98–100] Therefore, the use of
gabapentin is currently limited to refractory
forms of RLS/WED during lactation.

Benzodiazepines and Benzodiazepine Receptor Agonists

Clonazepam
This benzodiazepine is used as a second-line or
third-line treatment for idiopathic RLS after dopamine agonists and alpha-2-delta ligands.[69,70] It is
particularly effective in reducing arousals, facili-
tating and stabilizing sleep, and partially controlling the sensory symptoms of RLS.[101–103] As a
precaution, it is avoided during the first trimester

of pregnancy, like other medications, even if clonazepam, and benzodiazepine in general, seem to have no significant teratogenic risk.[72,104–106] Although an early case study reported sedation and periodic breathing in a newborn,[107] subsequent case series did not describe sedation or withdrawal symptoms in infants of pregnant or breastfeeding women taking clonazepam.[95,105,108,109] In any case, caution when initiating treatment, avoidance of combination with other central nervous system depressants, including alcohol, and careful observation of the infant is warranted, especially if born prematurely or ill.[108] A suggested strategy to reduce the risk of maternal and infant sedation may be to limit the dose to no more than 0.5 mg/d and administer at night.

Temazepam

This benzodiazepine is still in use for idiopathic RLS, but is not indicated during pregnancy. Animal data and a case report also showed an increased fetal mortality when temazepam is combined with diphenhydramine.[110]

Eszopiclone and zolpidem

These 2 benzodiazepine receptor agonists are approved for the treatment of insomnia, but literature on their safety during pregnancy is too limited to support their use in clinical practice. All these medications are likely to cause greater maternal sedation than clonazepam and may be associated with amnesia or confusional behaviors. The efficacy data for the treatment of idiopathic RLS are scarce.[111]

Opioids

Opioids represent a third-line strategy in the treatment of severe cases of idiopathic RLS. Although these drugs seem to be very effective in controlling RLS symptoms,[68–70,112] their use as a first-line therapy is complicated by side effects and risk of addiction/abuse. Opioids during pregnancy have been regularly used in cases of pain or heroin addiction, but no studies about pregnancy-related RLS are available thus far. These medications should not be administered during the first trimester because of the risk of malformations in the infants, including congenital heart disease, as shown in one large study on opioid analgesics during the first trimester,[113] but not in another investigation.[114] Three more reasons for concern are:

1. The sedative effects on the mothers, especially those carrying the ultrafast metabolism genetic variant CYP2D6, that can lead to overdose-like reactions in individuals taking normal doses,[115] and in the breastfed infant.[116–118] However, oxycodone does not seem to cause this reaction.[119,120]

2. Neonatal abstinence syndrome, or neonatal opioid withdrawal syndrome, is a serious condition affecting newborns of mothers, who regularly used opioids during pregnancy,[121] especially heroin or methadone.[122]

3. There is a possible relationship between opioids treatment during pregnancy and lactation and sudden infant death syndrome.[123,124]

Among all opioids, oxycodone and tramadol may be considered for the treatment of very severe, very refractory RLS/WED during pregnancy or lactation, respectively.

Oxycodone

This opioid showed solid efficacy, good tolerability, and no significant risk of addiction in a recent large trial.[112] Therefore, low-dose oxycodone (5–10 mg/d) may be used during pregnancy in extremely rare, very severe, and very refractory cases of RLS during the second or third trimester, as defined by a score of higher than 30 on the IRLS and failure to respond to at least one nonpharmacologic intervention, iron (if ferritin <75 µg/L), and one nonopioid pharmacologic treatment.

Tramadol

This atypical weak mu-receptor agonist may also be effective in idiopathic RLS.[68–70,125] According to a recent review, tramadol use in pregnancy and lactation "appears unlikely to cause harm to healthy term infants."[126] Moreover, because the amount of drug trasferring into the breast milk and reaching the infant is unknown, low doses of tramadol (50–100 mg/d), should be preferred to classical opioids for use during lactation.[16]

SUMMARY

RLS/WED is a common disorder during pregnancy, affecting up to one-third of women, with a typical peak of symptoms in the third trimester and a rapid decrease around delivery. The pathophysiology of pregnancy-related RLS has not been completely elucidated, but some factors, such as endocrine and metabolic changes during gestation, as well as a genetic predisposition, are likely to play a major causal role.

RLS/WED can significantly impact the health and well-being of the affected mother and her infant, with clinical distress, negative pregnancy outcomes, and long-term consequences. A careful clinical evaluation of the patient, including pharmacologic history, genetic factors, and possible comorbid conditions that may simulate or overlap with RLS, is the essential basis for a correct management of the syndrome during pregnancy. A range of pharmacologic and non-pharmacologic or self-management strategies are available in clinical practice and their use should be individualized, to maximize benefits and reduce risks for the affected patients (**Fig. 1**).

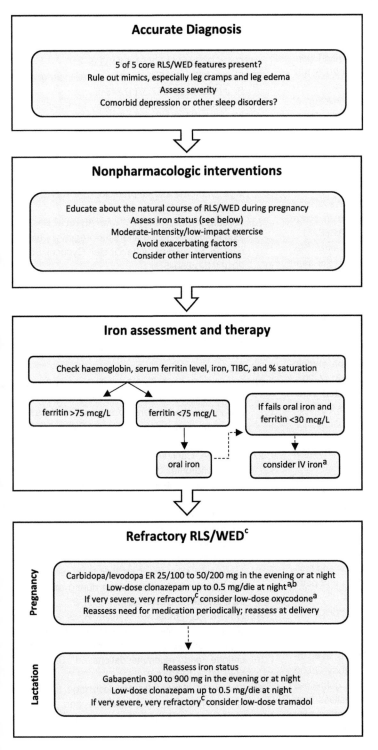

Fig. 1. Algorithm for the diagnosis and management of restless leg syndrome/Willis-Ekbom disease (RLS/WED) during pregnancy and lactation. Dotted arrows: proceed only after assessment of severity, risks, and benefits by provider and patient. [a] After the first trimester. [b] Avoid concurrent use with diphenhydramine or anticonvulsants. [c] Refractory: an inadequate response to at least 2 nonpharmacologic intervention and iron (if ferritin <75 μg/L), tried over an adequate period of time. [d] Very severe, very refractory: a score of greater than 30 on the International RLS Study Group rating scale and failure to respond to at least 1 nonpharmacologic treatment, iron (if ferritin <75 μg/L), and 1 nonopioid pharmacologic treatment. % saturation, percent iron saturation; ER, extended release; IV, intravenous; TIBC, total iron-binding capacity. (*Adapted from* Picchietti DL, Hensley JG, Bainbridge JL, et al; International Restless Legs Syndrome Study Group (IRLSSG). Consensus clinical practice guidelines for the diagnosis and treatment of restless legs syndrome/Willis-Ekbom disease during pregnancy and lactation. Sleep Med Rev 2015;22:72; with permission.)

REFERENCES

1. American Academy of Sleep Medicine. International classification of sleep disorders. 3rd edition. Darien (IL): American Academy of Sleep Medicine; 2014.
2. Garcia-Borreguero D, Cano-Pumarega I. New concepts in the management of restless legs syndrome. BMJ 2017;356:j104.
3. Allen RP, Walters AS, Montplaisir J, et al. Restless legs syndrome prevalence and impact: REST general population study. Arch Intern Med 2005;165: 1286–92.
4. Ohayon MM, O'Hara R, Vitiello MV. Epidemiology of restless legs syndrome: a synthesis of the literature. Sleep Med Rev 2012;16(4):283–95.
5. Chen SJ, Shi L, Bao YP, et al. Prevalence of restless legs syndrome during pregnancy: a systematic review and meta-analysis. Sleep Med Rev 2017 [pii: S1087-0792(17)30108-9].
6. Minár M, Habánová H, Rusňák I, et al. Prevalence and impact of restless legs syndrome in pregnancy. Neuro Endocrinol Lett 2013;34(5):366–71.
7. Berger K, Luedemann J, Trenkwalder C, et al. Sex and the risk of restless legs syndrome in the general population. Arch Intern Med 2004;164(2): 196–202.
8. Manconi M, Govoni V, De Vito A, et al. Restless legs syndrome and pregnancy. Neurology 2004;63(6): 1065–9.
9. Cesnik E, Casetta I, Turri M, et al. Transient RLS during pregnancy is a risk factor for the chronic idiopathic form. Neurology 2010;75(23):2117–20.
10. Dzaja A, Wehrle R, Lancel M, et al. Elevated estradiol plasma levels in women with restless legs during pregnancy. Sleep 2009;32:169–74.
11. Budhiraja P, Budhiraja R, Goodwin JL, et al. Incidence of restless legs syndrome and its correlates. J Clin Sleep Med 2012;8(2):119–24.
12. Srivanitchapoom P, Pandey S, Hallett M. Restless legs syndrome and pregnancy: a review. Parkinsonism Relat Disord 2014;20(7):716–22.
13. Allen R. Dopamine and iron in the pathophysiology of restless legs syndrome (RLS). Sleep Med 2004; 5(4):385–91.
14. Connor JR, Patton SM, Oexle K, et al. Iron and restless legs syndrome: treatment, genetics and pathophysiology. Sleep Med 2017;31:61–70.
15. Tunç T, Karadağ YS, Doğulu F, et al. Predisposing factors of restless legs syndrome in pregnancy. Mov Disord 2007;22(5):627–31.
16. Picchietti DL, Hensley JG, Bainbridge JL, et al, International Restless Legs Syndrome Study Group (IRLSSG). Consensus clinical practice guidelines for the diagnosis and treatment of restless legs syndrome/Willis-Ekbom disease during pregnancy and lactation. Sleep Med Rev 2015;22:64–77.
17. Kaufman S. Some metabolic relationships between biopterin and folate: implications for the "methyl trap hypothesis". Neurochem Res 1991; 16:1031–6.
18. Bottiglieri T, Hyland K, Laundy M, et al. Folate deficiency, biopterin and monoamine metabolism in depression. Psychol Med 1992;22:871–6.
19. Lee KA, Zaffke ME, Baratte-Beebe K. Restless legs syndrome and sleep disturbance during pregnancy: the role of folate and iron. J Womens Health Gend Based Med 2001;10(4):335–41.
20. Fenton V, Cavill I, Fisher J. Iron stores in pregnancy. Br J Haematol 1977;37(1):145–9.
21. Sikandar R, Khealani BA, Wasay M. Predictors of restless legs syndrome in pregnancy: a hospital based cross sectional survey from Pakistan. Sleep Med 2009;10:676–8.
22. Balendran J, Champion D, Jaaniste T, et al. A common sleep disorder in pregnancy: restless legs syndrome and its predictors. Aust N Z J Obstet Gynaecol 2011;51:262–4.
23. Sarberg M, Josefsson A, Wiréhn AB, et al. Restless legs syndrome during and after pregnancy and its relation to snoring. Acta Obstet Gynecol Scand 2012;91(7):850–5.
24. Jiménez-Jiménez FJ, Alonso-Navarro H, García-Martín E, et al. Genetics of restless legs syndrome: an update. Sleep Med Rev 2017 [pii:S1087-0792(17)30154-5].
25. Goodman JD, Brodie C, Ayida GA. Restless leg syndrome in pregnancy. BMJ 1988;297(6656): 1101–2.
26. Suzuki K, Ohida T, Sone T, et al. The prevalence of restless legs syndrome among pregnant women in Japan and the relationship between restless legs syndrome and sleep problems. Sleep 2003;26: 673–7.
27. Alves DA, Carvalho LB, Morais JF, et al. Restless legs syndrome during pregnancy in Brazilian women. Sleep Med 2010;11:1049–54.
28. Hubner A, Krafft A, Gadient S, et al. Characteristics and determinants of restless legs syndrome in pregnancy: a prospective study. Neurology 2013; 80:738–42.
29. Vahdat M, Sariri E, Miri S, et al. Prevalence and associated features of restless legs syndrome in a population of Iranian women during pregnancy. Int J Gynaecol Obstet 2013;123:46–9.
30. Walters AS, Frauscher B, Allen R, et al. Review of quality of life instruments for the restless legs syndrome/Willis-Ekbom disease (RLS/WED): critique and recommendations. J Clin Sleep Med 2014;10:1351–7.
31. Earley CJ, Silber MH. Restless legs syndrome: understanding its consequences and the need for better treatment. Sleep Med 2010;11(9): 807–15.

32. Dunietz GL, Lisabeth LD, Shedden K, et al. Restless legs syndrome and sleep-wake disturbances in pregnancy. J Clin Sleep Med 2017;13(7):863–70.

33. Okun ML, Schetter CD, Glynn LM. Poor sleep quality is associated with preterm birth. Sleep 2011;34: 1493–8.

34. Ramirez JO, Cabrera SA, Hidalgo H, et al. Is preeclampsia associated with restless legs syndrome? Sleep Med 2013;14:894–6.

35. Innes KE, Kandati S, Flack KL, et al. The association of restless legs syndrome to history of gestational diabetes in an Appalachian primary care population. J Clin Sleep Med 2015;11(10): 1121–30.

36. Ma S, Shang X, Guo Y, et al. Restless legs syndrome and hypertension in Chinese pregnant women. Neurol Sci 2015;36:877–81.

37. Sharma SK, Nehra A, Sinha S, et al. Sleep disorders in pregnancy and their association with pregnancy outcomes: a prospective observational study. Sleep Breath 2016;20(1):87–93.

38. Castillo PR, Mera RM, Fredrickson PA, et al. Psychological distress in patients with restless legs syndrome (Willis-Ekbom disease): a population-based door-to-door survey in rural Ecuador. BMC Res Notes 2014;7:911.

39. Wesstrom J, Skalkidou A, Manconi M, et al. Pre-pregnancy restless legs syndrome (Willis-Ekbom disease) is associated with perinatal depression. J Clin Sleep Med 2014;10:527–33.

40. Hensley JG. On "heredity of restless legs syndrome in a pregnant population". J Obstet Gynecol Neonatal Nurs 2014;43:270–1.

41. Uglane MT, Westad S, Backe B. Restless legs syndrome in pregnancy is a frequent disorder with a good prognosis. Acta Obstet Gynecol Scand 2011;90:1046–8.

42. Allen RP, Picchietti DL, Garcia-Borreguero D, et al, International Restless Legs Syndrome Study Group. Restless legs syndrome/Willis-Ekbom disease diagnostic criteria: updated International Restless Legs Syndrome Study Group (IRLSSG) consensus criteria–history, rationale, description, and significance. Sleep Med 2014;15(8):860–73.

43. Xiong L, Montplaisir J, Desautels A, et al. Family study of restless legs syndrome in Quebec, Canada: clinical characterization of 671 familial cases. Arch Neurol 2010;67:617–22.

44. Moller C, Wetter TC, Koster J, et al. Differential diagnosis of unpleasant sensations in the legs: prevalence of restless legs syndrome in a primary care population. Sleep Med 2010;11:161–6.

45. Hensley JG. Leg cramps and restless legs syndrome during pregnancy. J Midwifery Womens Health 2009;54:211–8.

46. Terzi H, Terzi R, Zeybek B, et al. Restless legs syndrome is related to obstructive sleep apnea symptoms during pregnancy. Sleep Breath 2015; 19:73–8.

47. Oyiengo D, Louis M, Hott B, et al. Sleep disorders in pregnancy. Clin Chest Med 2014;35:571–87.

48. Facco FL, Kramer J, Ho KH, et al. Sleep disturbances in pregnancy. Obstet Gynecol 2010;115: 77–83.

49. Dodel R, Happe S, Peglau I, et al. Health economic burden of patients with restless legs syndrome in a German ambulatory setting. Pharmacoeconomics 2010;28:381–93.

50. Walters AS, LeBrocq C, Dhar A, et al, International Restless Legs Syndrome Study Group. Validation of the international restless legs syndrome study Group rating scale for restless legs syndrome. Sleep Med 2003;4(2):121–32.

51. Abetz L, Vallow SM, Kirsch J, et al. Validation of the restless legs syndrome quality of life questionnaire. Value Health 2005;8(2):157–67.

52. Manconi M, García-Borreguero D, editors. Restless legs syndrome/Willis Ekbom disease. New York: Springer Science+Business Media LLC; 2017. https://doi.org/10.1007/978-1-4939-6777-3_18.

53. Lakasing E. Exercise beneficial for restless legs syndrome. Practitioner 2008;252:43–5.

54. Aukerman MM, Aukerman D, Bayard M, et al. Exercise and restless legs syndrome: a randomized controlled trial. J Am Board Fam Med 2006;19: 487–93.

55. Earley CJ, Barker PB, Horska A, et al. MRI-determined regional brain iron concentrations in early- and late-onset restless legs syndrome. Sleep Med 2006;7:458–61.

56. Godau J, Klose U, Di Santo A, et al. Multiregional brain iron deficiency in restless legs syndrome. Mov Disord 2008;23:1184–7.

57. Earley CJ, Connor JR, Beard JL, et al. Ferritin levels in the cerebrospinal fluid and restless legs syndrome: effects of different clinical phenotypes. Sleep 2005;28:1069–75.

58. Connor JR, Boyer PJ, Menzies SL, et al. Neuropathological examination suggests impaired brain iron acquisition in restless legs syndrome. Neurology 2003;61:304–9.

59. Connor JR, Ponnuru P, Wang XS, et al. Profile of altered brain iron acquisition in restless legs syndrome. Brain 2011;134:959–68.

60. O'Keeffe ST, Gavin K, Lavan JN. Iron status and restless legs syndrome in the elderly. Age Ageing 1994;23:200–3.

61. Sun ER, Chen CA, Ho G, et al. Iron and the restless legs syndrome. Sleep 1998;21:371–7.

62. Frauscher B, Gschliesser V, Brandauer E, et al. The severity range of restless legs syndrome (RLS) and augmentation in a prospective patient cohort: association with ferritin levels. Sleep Med 2009;10: 611–5.

63. Allen RP, Auerbach S, Bahrain H, et al. The prevalence and impact of restless legs syndrome on patients with iron deficiency anemia. Am J Hematol 2013;88:261–4.

64. Grote L, Leissner L, Hedner J, et al. A randomized, double-blind, placebo controlled, multi-center study of intravenous iron sucrose and placebo in the treatment of restless legs syndrome. Mov Disord 2009;24:1445–52.

65. Wang J, O'Reilly B, Venkataraman R, et al. Efficacy of oral iron in patients with restless legs syndrome and a low-normal ferritin: a randomized, double-blind, placebo-controlled study. Sleep Med 2009; 10:973–5.

66. Ondo WG. Intravenous iron dextran for severe refractory restless legs syndrome. Sleep Med 2010; 11:494–6.

67. Allen RP, Adler CH, Du W, et al. Clinical efficacy and safety of IV ferric carboxymaltose (FCM) treatment of RLS: a multi-centred, placebo-controlled preliminary clinical trial. Sleep Med 2011;12: 906–13.

68. Silber MH, Becker PM, Earley C, et al. Willis-Ekbom disease foundation revised consensus statement on the management of restless legs syndrome. Mayo Clin Proc 2013;88:977–86.

69. Aurora RN, Kristo DA, Bista SR, et al. The treatment of restless legs syndrome and periodic limb movement disorder in Adults–An update for 2012: practice parameters with an evidence-based systematic review and meta-analyses. Sleep 2012; 35:1039–62.

70. Garcia-Borreguero D, Ferini-Strambi L, Kohnen R, et al. European guidelines on management of restless legs syndrome: report of a joint task force by the European Federation of Neurological Societies, the European Neurological Society and the European Sleep Research Society. Eur J Neurol 2012; 19:1385–96.

71. Bothwell TH. Iron requirements in pregnancy and strategies to meet them. Am J Clin Nutr 2000;72: 257S–64S.

72. Briggs GG, Freeman RK, Yaffe SJ. Drugs in pregnancy and lactation. 9th edition. Philadelphia: Lippincott Williams & Wilkins; 2011.

73. Pavord S, Myers B, Robinson S, et al. UK guidelines on the management of iron deficiency in pregnancy. Br J Haematol 2012;156: 588–600.

74. Swaney P, Thorp J, Allen I. Vitamin C supplementation in pregnancy–does it decrease rates of preterm birth? A systematic review. Am J Perinatol 2014;31:91–8.

75. Vadasz D, Ries V, Oertel WH. Intravenous iron sucrose for restless legs syndrome in pregnant women with low serum ferritin. Sleep Med 2013; 14:1214–6.

76. Schneider J, Krafft A, Bloch A, et al. Iron infusion in restless legs syndrome in pregnancy. J Neurol 2011;258:55.

77. Cho YW, Allen RP, Earley CJ. Lower molecular weight intravenous iron dextran for restless legs syndrome. Sleep Med 2013;14:274–7.

78. Birgegård G, Schneider K, Ulfberg J. High incidence of iron depletion and restless leg syndrome (RLS) in regular blood donors: intravenous iron sucrose substitution more effective than oral iron. Vox Sang 2010;99:354–61.

79. Hale T. Medications and mothers' milk online. Amarillo (TX): Hale Publishing; 2013. Available at: http://www.medsmilk.com.

80. Botez MI, Lambert B. Folate deficiency and restless-legs syndrome in pregnancy. N Engl J Med 1977;297:670.

81. Garcia-Borreguero D, Kohnen R, Silber MH, et al. The long-term treatment of restless legs syndrome/Willis-Ekbom disease: evidence-based guidelines and clinical consensus best practice guidance: a report from the International Restless Legs Syndrome Study Group. Sleep Med 2013; 14:675–84.

82. Aurora RN, Kristo DA, Bista SR, et al. Update to the AASM clinical practice guideline: "the treatment of restless legs syndrome and periodic limb movement disorder in adults–an update for 2012: practice parameters with an evidence-based systematic review and meta-analyses". Sleep 2012;35:1037.

83. Serikawa T, Shimohata T, Akashi M, et al. Successful twin pregnancy in a patient with Parkinson-associated autosomal recessive juvenile parkinsonism. BMC Neurol 2011;11:72.

84. Watanabe T, Matsubara S, Baba Y, et al. Successful management of pregnancy in a patient with Segawa disease: case report and literature review. J Obstet Gynaecol Res 2009;35:562–4.

85. Dostal M, Weber-Schoendorfer C, Sobesky J, et al. Pregnancy outcome following use of levodopa, pramipexole, ropinirole, and rotigotine for restless legs syndrome during pregnancy: a case series. Eur J Neurol 2013;20:1241–6.

86. Mucchiut M, Belgrado E, Cutuli D, et al. Pramipexole-treated Parkinson's disease during pregnancy. Mov Disord 2004;19:1114–5.

87. Andersohn F, Garbe E. Cardiac and noncardiac fibrotic reactions caused by ergot-and nonergot-derived dopamine agonists. Mov Disord 2009;24: 129–33.

88. Allen RP, Chen C, Garcia-Borreguero D, et al. Comparison of pregabalin with pramipexole for restless legs syndrome. N Engl J Med 2014; 370:621–31.

89. Montouris G. Gabapentin exposure in human pregnancy: results from the Gabapentin Pregnancy Registry. Epilepsy Behav 2003;4:310–7.

90. Djokanovic N, Garcia-Bournissen F, Koren G. Medications for restless legs syndrome in pregnancy. J Obstet Gynaecol Can 2008;30:505–7.

91. Hernandez-Diaz S, Smith CR, Shen A, et al. Comparative safety of antiepileptic drugs during pregnancy. Neurology 2012;78:1692–9.

92. Holmes LB, Hernandez-Diaz S. Newer anticonvulsants: lamotrigine, topiramate and gabapentin. Birth Defects Res A Clin Mol Teratol 2012;94: 599–606.

93. Molgaard-Nielsen D, Hviid A. Newer-generation antiepileptic drugs and the risk of major birth defects. JAMA 2011;305:1996–2002.

94. Eroglu Ç, Allen NJ, Susman MW, et al. Gabapentin receptor a2d-1 is a neuronal thrombospondin receptor responsible for excitatory CNS synaptogenesis. Cell 2009;139:380–92.

95. Almgren M, K€allen B, Lavebratt C. Population-based study of antiepileptic drug exposure in utero: influence on head circumference in newborns. Seizure 2009;18:672–5.

96. Linnebank M, Moskau S, Semmler A, et al. Antiepileptic drugs interact with folate and vitamin B12 serum levels. Ann Neurol 2011;69: 352–9.

97. Cheschier N. ACOG practice bulletin. Neural tube defects. Number 44, July 2003. (Replaces committee opinion number 252, March 2001). Int J Gynaecol Obstet 2003;83:123–33.

98. Ohman I, Vitols S, Tomson T. Pharmacokinetics of gabapentin during delivery, in the neonatal period, and lactation: does a fetal accumulation occur during pregnancy? Epilepsia 2005;46: 1621–4.

99. Ohman I, Tomson T. Gabapentin kinetics during delivery, in the neonatal period, and during lactation. Epilepsia 2009;50(Suppl. 10):108.

100. Kristensen JH, Ilett KF, Hackett LP, et al. Gabapentin and breastfeeding: a case report. J Hum Lact 2006;22:426–8.

101. Manconi M, Ferri R, Zucconi M, et al. Dissociation of periodic leg movements from arousals in restless legs syndrome. Ann Neurol 2012;71:834–44.

102. Saletu M, Anderer P, Saletu-Zyhlarz G, et al. Restless legs syndrome (RLS) and periodic limb movement disorder (PLMD): acute placebo-controlled sleep laboratory studies with clonazepam. Eur Neuropsychopharmacol 2001; 11:153–61.

103. Montagna P, Sassoli de Bianchi L, Zucconi M, et al. Clonazepam and vibration in restless legs syndrome. Acta Neurol Scand 1984;69: 428–30.

104. Lin AE, Peller AJ, Westgate MN, et al. Clonazepam use in pregnancy and the risk of malformations. Birth Defects Res A Clin Mol Teratol 2004;70: 534–6.

105. Weinstock L, Cohen LS, Bailey JW, et al. Obstetrical and neonatal outcome following clonazepam use during pregnancy: a case series. Psychother Psychosom 2001;70:158–62.

106. Wikner BN, Stiller C-O, Bergman U, et al. Use of benzodiazepines and benzodiazepine receptor agonists during pregnancy: neonatal outcome and congenital malformations. Pharmacoepidemiol Drug Saf 2007;16:1203–10.

107. Fisher JB, Edgren BE, Mammel MC, et al. Neonatal apnea associated with maternal clonazepam therapy: a case report. Obstet Gynecol 1985;66: 34S–5S.

108. Kelly LE, Poon S, Madadi P, et al. Neonatal benzodiazepines exposure during breastfeeding. J Pediatr 2012;161:448–51.

109. Birnbaum CS, Cohen LS, Bailey JW, et al. Serum concentrations of antidepressants and benzodiazepines in nursing infants: a case series. Pediatrics 1999;104:e11.

110. Kargas GA, Kargas SA, Bruyere HJ Jr, et al. Perinatal mortality due to interaction of diphenhydramine and temazepam. N Engl J Med 1985;313: 1417–8.

111. Hwang T-J, Ni H-C, Chen H-C, et al. Risk predictors for hypnosedative-related complex sleep behaviors. J Clin Psychiatry 2010;71:1331–5.

112. Trenkwalder C, Benes H, Grote L, et al. Prolonged release oxycodone-naloxone for treatment of severe restless legs syndrome after failure of previous treatment: a double-blind, randomised, placebo-controlled trial with an open-label extension. Lancet Neurol 2013;12: 1141–50.

113. Broussard CS, Rasmussen SA, Reefhuis J, et al. Maternal treatment with opioid analgesics and risk for birth defects. Am J Obstet Gynecol 2011; 204:314.e1-11.

114. Nezvalova-Henriksen K, Spigset O, Nordeng H. Effects of codeine on pregnancy outcome: results from a large population-based cohort study. Eur J Clin Pharmacol 2011;67:1253–61.

115. Smith HS. Opioid metabolism. Mayo Clin Proc 2009;84:613–24.

116. Timm NL. Maternal use of oxycodone resulting in opioid intoxication in her breastfed neonate. J Pediatr 2013;162:421–2.

117. Lam J, Kelly L, Ciszkowski C, et al. Central nervous system depression of neonates breastfed by mothers receiving oxycodone for postpartum analgesia. J Pediatr 2012;160:33–7.e2.

118. Sauberan JB, Anderson PO, Lane JR, et al. Breast milk hydrocodone and hydromorphone levels in mothers using hydrocodone for postpartum pain. Obstet Gynecol 2011;117:611–7.

119. Andreassen TN, Eftedal I, Klepstad P, et al. Do CYP2D6 genotypes reflect oxycodone

requirements for cancer patients treated for cancer pain? A cross-sectional multicentre study. Eur J Clin Pharmacol 2011;68:55–64.

120. Klimas R, Witticke D, El Fallah S, et al. Contribution of oxycodone and its metabolites to the overall analgesic effect after oxycodone administration. Expert Opin Drug Metab Toxicol 2013;9:517–28.

121. Hudak ML, Tan RC. Neonatal drug withdrawal. Pediatrics 2012;129:e540–60.

122. Patrick SW, Schumacher RE, Benneyworth BD, et al. Neonatal abstinence syndrome and associated health care expenditures: United States, 2000-2009. JAMA 2012;307:1934–40.

123. Burns L, Conroy E, Mattick RP. Infant mortality among women on a methadone program during pregnancy. Drug Alcohol Rev 2010;29:551–6.

124. Klonoff-Cohen H, Lam-Kruglick P. Maternal and paternal recreational drug use and sudden infant death syndrome. Arch Pediatr Adolesc Med 2001;155:765–70.

125. Lauerma H, Markkula J. Treatment of restless legs syndrome with tramadol: an open study. J Clin Psychiatry 1999;60:241–4.

126. Bloor M, Paech MJ, Kaye R. Tramadol in pregnancy and lactation. Int J Obstet Anesth 2012;21:163–7.

Sleep-Disordered Breathing in Pregnancy

Lakshmy Ayyar, MD, Fidaa Shaib, MD, Kalpalatha Guntupalli, MD*

KEYWORDS

- Obstructive sleep apnea • Pregnancy • Sleep-disordered breathing • Snoring • Preeclampsia
- Gestational diabetes

KEY POINTS

- Sleep-disordered breathing manifests predominantly with snoring and/or obstructive sleep apnea during pregnancy.
- The gold standard for diagnosis in pregnancy is overnight, attended, in-laboratory polysomnography.
- Continuous positive airway pressure therapy is the preferred first-line therapy for obstructive sleep apnea.
- Untreated sleep-disordered breathing has been associated with preeclampsia, gestational hypertension, gestational diabetes, and severe maternal morbidity.
- Early identification and treatment are key factors in improving maternal and fetal outcomes.

INTRODUCTION

Sleep and pregnancy are 2 unique states with dynamic and characteristic physiologic changes. Sleep physiology renders the body vulnerable to the occurrence of breathing impairment in rapid eye movement sleep but is protected during slow-wave sleep. The physiologic changes that evolve during pregnancy pose an increased risk to the development of respiratory impairment with consequences that will ultimately affect pregnancy and its outcome.

Sleep-disordered breathing (SDB) is a group of respiratory abnormalities that occur as a result of impaired airflow and gas exchange due to upper airway narrowing or inefficiency of the ventilatory systems. Obstructive SDB is a spectrum of respiratory impairment due to partial narrowing or complete collapse of the upper airway. Sleep-related breathing disorders are categorized in the latest version of International Classification of Sleep Disorders-3 into snoring, obstructive sleep apnea (OSA), central sleep apnea, and sleep-related hypoventilation.[1] SDB is a common disorder in both men and women but remains underdiagnosed, especially in women.[2]

Although the respiratory physiologic changes and sleep state instability associated with pregnancy might suggest an increased risk for central sleep apnea, the prevalence of central sleep apnea in the pregnant population is low.[3] Preexisting sleep-related hypoventilation can impose an additional stress on the pregnant patient and the fetus. This article focuses on snoring and OSA in pregnancy and their impact on maternal and fetal health.

Clinically, OSA is manifested by the occurrence of daytime sleepiness, loud snoring, witnessed breathing interruptions, or awakenings due to gasping or choking. The diagnosis is confirmed by the presence of at least 5 obstructive respiratory events (apneas, hypopneas, or respiratory effort–related arousals) per hour of sleep in the presence of sleep-related symptoms or comorbidities or 15 or more obstructive respiratory events per hour of sleep.[4]

Section of Pulmonary, Critical Care, and Sleep Medicine, Baylor College of Medicine, One Baylor Plaza, Houston, TX 77030, USA
* Corresponding author.
E-mail address: kkg@bcm.edu

Sleep Med Clin 13 (2018) 349–357
https://doi.org/10.1016/j.jsmc.2018.04.005
1556-407X/18/© 2018 Elsevier Inc. All rights reserved.

SDB can worsen during pregnancy or can be induced by pregnancy-related changes of the upper airway, lung mechanics, and control of breathing.[5] In addition, there is increasing prevalence of obesity in women of reproductive age, which in turn increases the risk of developing OSA. SDB has been consistently associated with adverse pregnancy outcomes, including gestational hypertensive disorders and gestational diabetes.[6] Therefore, a timely diagnosis and management is crucial in improving maternal and fetal outcomes.

EPIDEMIOLOGY

The exact prevalence of SDB in pregnancy, diagnosed by polysomnography (PSG), is not well defined. Large prospective studies with precise definitions and estimates are lacking.

Several studies report that snoring steadily increases during pregnancy.[7,8] The prevalence of snoring has been estimated to be between 10% and 46%.[9,10] This wide range is mainly because of variability in study designs and objective or self-report measures of snoring, because women are less likely to report snoring than men.[11] Longitudinal studies have shown that habitual snoring (3 or more nights per week) increases from 7% to 11% in the first trimester to 16% to 25% in the third trimester.[12] The limited self-reporting of habitual versus occasional snoring and body position may limit the reliability of snoring as a presenting symptom of SDB in pregnant women.

Prevalence of OSA with daytime sleepiness is estimated to be approximately 3% to 7% for adult men and 2% to 5% for adult women. These estimates are similar when compared between different continents.[13] In pregnant women, the prevalence of OSA with apnea–hypopnea index (AHI) greater than 5 has been reported to be 3.6% in early pregnancy and 8.3% in midpregnancy.[14]

PATHOPHYSIOLOGY

Several physiologic changes in pregnancy are likely to predispose to development of SDB (**Box 1**). On the other hand, concurrent protective factors are also present (**Box 2**) that probably account for the overall low incidence of OSA in pregnancy.[5,15] It remains unclear as to what ultimately tips the balance toward development of clinically significant SDB in a pregnant woman.

Increasing age and obesity remain independent risk factors for development of SDB. Hypertensive pregnant women who snore are at increased risk for unrecognized SDB.[16] Moreover, high-risk women with chronic hypertension, gestational diabetes, a history of preeclampsia, and/or a twin

---

> **Box 1**
> **Potential risk factors for sleep-disordered breathing in pregnancy**
>
> Reduction in upper airway size[60,61] likely due to
> - Increased fluid retention
> - Weight gain
>
> Nasal obstruction[62,63]
> - Increased edema from high estrogen
> - Nasal congestion/rhinitis
>
> Lung mechanics[21]
> - Reduced functional residual capacity and residual volume
> - Increased minute ventilation
>
> Fragmented sleep
> - Frequent awakenings due to pregnancy-related discomfort lowering arousal threshold

gestation are at increased risk for developing SDB that continues to increase during the course of their pregnancy.[17] Active and passive smoking have also been associated with snoring, breathing problems, and sleep disturbances.[18]

The effect of body position on sleep during pregnancy is worth noting. Left lateral sleep is the preferred sleep position for pregnant women mainly because of relief of pressure of the gravid uterus on the inferior vena cava and resulting favorable hemodynamic effects. In general, SDB is worse in the supine position, and severity

---

> **Box 2**
> **Protective factors for sleep-disordered breathing in pregnancy**
>
> High progesterone level leading to
> - Increased upper airway dilator muscle activity
> - Enhanced chemo-responsiveness
>
> Improved delivery of oxygen leading to
> - Right-shifted oxyhemoglobin dissociation curve
> - Increase in maternal heart rate and stroke volume
>
> Less time in supine position
>
> *Adapted from* Facco FL, Parker CB, Reddy UM, et al. Association between sleep-disordered breathing and hypertensive disorders of pregnancy and gestational diabetes mellitus. Obstet Gynecol 2017;129(1):31–41; and Bourjeily G. Sleep disorders in pregnancy. Obstet Med 2009;2(3):100–6; with permission.

improves with lateral position due to effect on lung dynamics and upper airway dimensions.[19] Several studies have shown an association between maternal sleep position and late stillbirth, with 3.7 increased risk of stillbirth in a multicenter case control study.[20] This is an area that needs further investigation to better understand the contribution of positional SDB.

PATIENT EVALUATION
Clinical Manifestations

Available literature does not clearly differentiate between clinical presentation for OSA in pregnant and nonpregnant population. The classic symptoms of OSA are described in **Box 3**.

Pregnant women with a higher body mass index (BMI) are more likely to snore than women with lower BMI.[21] Symptoms of daytime hypersomnolence increase in pregnancy, with reported Epworth Sleepiness Scale (ESS) scores greater than 10 in 30% to 40% of healthy pregnant women.[22]

In general, women are likely to be delayed in receiving a diagnosis of OSA due to their low self-reports of classic symptoms. Women also tend to have a different spectrum of symptoms from men that are often overlooked. These symptoms include daytime fatigue, morning headaches, and symptoms of depression.[2]

Sleepiness in pregnancy is not specific to SDB. Daytime sleepiness and nonrestorative sleep are often caused by alternative factors such as increased frequency of urination, fetal movement, or general discomfort.[23] Sleep disruption is probably considered a normal part of pregnancy that contributes to underreporting of symptoms.

Diagnosis

Screening questionnaires
There are a variety of questionnaires available to screen for OSA, such as Berlin Questionnaire (BQ), ESS, and STOP-BANG. Although these tools

---

Box 3
Classic symptoms of obstructive sleep apnea
Snoring
Awakening with a sensation of choking or gasping
Pauses in breathing reported by partner
Excessive daytime sleepiness
Morning headaches
Awakening with a dry mouth
Restless sleep
Frequent nocturnal awakenings

---

could reliably predict the presence of severe OSA in the specific patient groups that were studied, they have limited utility for screening in the general population.[24]

A recent systematic review assessed the performance of screening questionnaires during pregnancy and reported sufficient data on 2 questionnaires, the ESS and the BQ. The sensitivity and specificity of the ESS were only 0.44 and 0.62, respectively.[25] The BQ had pooled sensitivity of 0.66 (95% CI 0.45–0.83) and specificity of 0.62 (95% CI 0.48–0.75). Sensitivity of the BQ increased if diagnosis was based on PSG (0.90) and respiratory disturbance index (0.90) and sensitivity decreased if screening was performed in early pregnancy (0.47 at $\leq$20 weeks gestation). In a recent questionnaire-based study by Louis and colleagues[26] among nulliparous women, frequent snoring, chronic hypertension, increased maternal age, BMI, neck circumference, and systolic blood pressure were associated with increased risk for SDB at any point during the course of pregnancy. This work provides a 3-variable logistic regression model that includes age, body mass index and frequent snoring that could serve as a predictive tool for SDB among nulliparous women diagnosed by home sleep testing.[26]

In summary, screening tools have poor predictive value and are not recommended for use in pregnant women.

Objective testing
There are no studies addressing the best method of objective testing for suspected SDB in pregnancy. The Home Sleep Apnea Test (HSAT), with unattended portable monitoring, has been shown to be reliable in diagnosing OSA in patients with moderate to high pretest probability and no significant comorbid medical or sleep disorders.[27] There is insufficient data for their validity and reliability in pregnant women,[28] and the role for HSAT using traditional airflow monitoring devices in this population is yet to be determined.

There is emerging evidence over recent years for use of WatchPAT in pregnant women. WatchPAT is a portable diagnostic device approved by Food and Drug Administration that monitors peripheral arterial tonometry by measuring arterial volume changes at the fingertip. A single-center study validated the WatchPAT against full overnight 22-channel home PSG in pregnant women in third trimester and demonstrated high sensitivity and specificity.[29] This is an area of ongoing research and will likely evolve to more wide spread use in the future.

Of note, despite the fact that attended and unattended sleep studies record sleep position, there is a tendency for sleep in the supine position on attended sleep studies that might exaggerate the degree of SDB. Conversely, unattended sleep studies tend to underestimate severity of SDB due to overestimation of sleep time.

In summary, at the current time the gold standard for diagnosis of SDB in pregnancy remains a full night of PSG in the laboratory setting.

Who to test?

As mentioned earlier, SDB is probably underdiagnosed in pregnant women. Studies suggest that habitual snoring, older age, chronic hypertension, and high prepregnancy BMI could be reliable indicators for preexisting SDB in early pregnancy.[30,31] These risk factors should alert health care providers to have a high level of suspicion of SDB and to evaluate women's sleep history with a plan for early referral to a sleep specialist. Women with preexisting SDB also need frequent reassessment throughout the pregnancy, particularly after the first 6 months.[12]

COMPLICATIONS

In the general population, SDB has been strongly associated with a broad range of cardiovascular morbidities, including systemic hypertension, coronary artery disease, cardiac arrhythmias, heart failure, and stroke.[32,33] In addition, patients with OSA are also at increased risk for Type 2 diabetes, insulin resistance, and nonalcoholic fatty liver disease, independent of obesity and other risk factors.[34,35]

These effects are likely compounded during pregnancy given the vast physiologic changes that occur during a short period of time. SDB has been associated with development of preeclampsia and gestational hypertension.[6,14] There is also strong evidence linking SDB and gestational diabetes.[6,14,36] In addition, preterm birth and low birth weight have been associated with maternal SDB.[36,37] In a recent systematic review and meta-analysis, Brown and colleagues[38] showed that pregnant women with SDB are older with greater BMI compared with those without SDB. The presence of SDB in this population was associated with preterm birth, low birth weight, increased assisted vaginal delivery, and elective or emergent cesarean section. Moreover, there was an increased risk of delivery of infants with low Apgar scores, stillbirth, or neonatal nursery admission.[38]

The mechanisms linking SDB to adverse pregnancy outcomes have not yet been fully elucidated. Possible pathways for impact of SDB on poor maternal and fetal outcomes include recurrent episodes of placental hypoxemia, changes in vascular tone, oxidative stress, endothelial dysfunction, and increased sympathetic activity.[39]

Maternal Effects

Preeclampsia and gestational hypertension

Preeclampsia refers to the new onset of hypertension and proteinuria, or hypertension and end-organ dysfunction with or without proteinuria, after 20 weeks gestation in a previously normotensive woman.[40] Gestational hypertension refers to hypertension without proteinuria or other signs of preeclampsia that develops after 20 weeks gestation.[40] They are associated with significant maternal and neonatal morbidity and mortality.

Snoring has been shown to be associated with higher rates of pregnancy-induced hypertension and preeclampsia. In a cohort of 502 women, Franklin and colleagues[9] found that snoring was an independent risk factor for both hypertension and preeclampsia, even when adjusted for age and weight.

Several studies have shown the association between OSA and development of preeclampsia and gestational hypertension. A systematic review including retrospective and small cohort studies reported a two-fold increase in preeclampsia among women with SDB (**Table 1**).[6] A more recent large prospective cohort study including 3306 nulliparous women who underwent HSAT in early pregnancy and midpregnancy demonstrated increased risk for preeclampsia in women diagnosed with OSA (see **Table 1**).[14] The largest cohort study of 791 women with PSG-diagnosed OSA reported that women with preexisting OSA diagnosed before pregnancy had an increased risk of preeclampsia (adjusted odds ratio 1.6), compared with women without an SDB diagnosis.[36] The ongoing Sleep-Disordered Breathing substudy of the Nulliparous Pregnancy Outcomes Study: Monitoring Mothers-to-be (nuMoM2b) study is further investigating the role of SDB during pregnancy as a risk factor for adverse pregnancy outcomes.[41]

Gestational diabetes mellitus

The prevalence of gestational diabetes mellitus (GDM) rises with increasing rates of maternal obesity. GDM is associated with numerous adverse maternal, fetal, and neonatal outcomes. There is insufficient evidence linking snoring alone with development of GDM. In contrast, SDB is associated with GDM. Two systematic reviews and meta-analyses of observational studies reported that SDB was associated with a 2- to 3-fold increased odds of GDM.[6,42] This was also

Table 1
Sleep-disordered breathing and adverse pregnancy outcomes

Author, Year	Sample	Adjusted OR (95% CI)	
Chen et al,[36] 2012	n = 791 Taiwan		
Preeclampsia		1.60 (2.16–11.26)	
Luque-Fernandez et al,[42] 2013	9 studies Meta-analysis		
GMD		3.06 (1.89–4.96)	
Pamidi et al,[6] 2014	31 studies Meta-analysis		
Pre-eclampsia		2.34 (1.60–3.09)	
GDM		1.86 (1.29–2.37)	
Low birth weight		1.39 (1.14–1.65)[a]	
Bourjeily et al,[44] 2017	US discharge data 1.5 million pregnancies		
Preeclampsia		2.22 (1.94–2.54)	
GDM		1.51 (1.34–1.72)	
Facco et al,[14] 2017	n = 3306 US nulliparous	Early pregnancy	Mid-pregnancy
Preeclampsia		1.94 (1.07–3.51)	1.95 (1.18–3.23)
GDM		3.47 (1.95–6.19)	2.79 (1.63–4.77)

Abbreviations: OR, odds ratio; CI, confidence interval; GMD, gestational diabetes mellitus.
[a] Unadjusted OR.

supported by more recent evidence from a prospective cohort study of nulliparous women who underwent in-home SDB assessments in early (6–15 weeks of gestation) and midpregnancy (22–31 weeks of gestation). This study found a strong and independent association between SDB and preeclampsia, hypertensive disorders of pregnancy, and GDM as shown in **Table 1**.[14]

Severe maternal morbidity
A large database study done in the United States from 1998 to 2009 used hospital discharge codes to demonstrate that the rate of OSA among pregnancy-related discharges increased significantly over the 10-year period and coincided with the increase in obesity rates. OSA was associated with increased likelihood of preeclampsia, eclampsia, cardiomyopathy, pulmonary embolism, and early-onset of labor delivery in addition to maternal mortality. These associations persisted even after statistical adjustment for potential confounders including obesity.[43]

This association between OSA and pregnancy complications is further supported by recent data from the National Perinatal Information Center in the United States. Bourjeily and colleagues[44] showed that when compared with pregnant women without OSA, pregnant women with OSA have a significantly higher risk of pregnancy-specific complications, including gestational hypertensive conditions and gestational diabetes in addition to cardiomyopathy, pulmonary edema, congestive heart failure, and hysterectomy. OSA diagnosis was also associated with a prolonged hospital stay and significantly increased risk for admission to an intensive care unit.[44]

Fetal effects
The studies linking SDB to adverse fetal outcomes have shown equivocal results, likely due to small sample sizes, lack of objective measures, and effects of confounders such as maternal obesity, diabetes, and hypertension. The effect of intermittent hypoxia and cyclic placental ischemia is thought to be the possible mechanism for adverse effects on the fetus.[45]

Habitual snoring has been linked to intrauterine growth retardation and low infant Apgar scores.[9] Several studies reported no differences in birth weight between women with and without SDB. Pamidi and colleagues[6] found a link between SDB and low-birth weight (see **Table 1**); however, the validity of their outcome is limited by potential confounding variables. Case reports and small studies have identified recordable fetal heart decelerations, but this was not supported by findings in a larger prospective study of 20 women with PSG-diagnosed OSA.[46]

The increased risk of preterm birth in pregnant women with SDB is supported by several population-based studies.[36,37,47] However, these preterm births may often be medically indicated due to confounding maternal comorbidities than spontaneous.

Pregnancy in Patients with Preexisting Sleep-Disordered Breathing

There are no studies demonstrating the effect of pregnancy on women with previously diagnosed SDB. On the other hand, evidence from a small longitudinal study indicates that OSA diagnosed during late pregnancy markedly improves following delivery, with changes in both AHI and oxygen saturation.[48] This further confirms that the severity of sleep apnea varies before, during the course of pregnancy, and the postpartum period, and one-time assessment will not be sufficient to understand the relationship. With increasing rates of obesity and early identification of SDB, this is an area with vast potential for future research that would enable both researchers and clinicians to further understand the long-term implications and interventions for SDB in this population.

MANAGEMENT GOALS

There are no specific guidelines for treatment of SDB in pregnancy. The treatment options and recommendations are similar to guidelines for the general population[4] where the goals of therapy for SDB are

- Resolution of signs and symptoms, especially those related to daytime function
- Improvement in sleep quality
- Normalization of AHI and oxygen saturation levels

Pregnancy-specific goals also include minimizing maternal and fetal complications and improving overall birth outcomes. Fetal well-being is paramount during pregnancy, and this should be taken into consideration, although there is a lack of studies that directly relate intermittent hypoxia to fetal outcomes.

TREATMENT OPTIONS
Self-management Strategies

All women should be counseled on behavioral modifications, as listed in **Box 4**. Weight loss is recommended in the general population, but this is not always an appropriate option during pregnancy. However, women with predisposing risk

---

> **Box 4**
> **Behavioral strategies for improving sleep-disordered breathing in pregnancy**
>
> Control weight gain
>
> Sleeping position: left lateral or elevated head of bed
>
> Avoidance of smoking, alcohol, and caffeine
>
> Treat nasal congestion
>
> Regular exercise
>
> Follow good sleep hygiene measures

---

factors should be counseled on achieving normal weight before pregnancy, and this can also be reinforced in the postpartum period.

Women with position-dependent SDB without significant desaturation or comorbidities might benefit from positional therapy with positioning belts or pillows, to promote sleep in the left lateral position or upper body elevated position at 45°.[49]

Pharmacologic Strategies

There are no medications to prevent or treat SDB. However, emerging literature suggests a role for hormones in the pharmacologic treatment of SDB. Progesterone, a respiratory stimulant, has been shown to be lower in pregnant women with SDB compared with those without even when accounting for BMI and gestational age.[50]

Nonpharmacologic Strategies

Continuous positive airway pressure
Continuous positive airway pressure (CPAP) is generally safe and well tolerated during pregnancy. CPAP may be initiated after an in-laboratory titration, or an auto-titrating device may be used with close follow-up. Auto-titrating CPAP may be better suited to pregnant patients, because it allows the clinician to increase the range of therapeutic pressures during the course of pregnancy. However, there are no trials comparing benefits of fixed pressure versus auto-titrating CPAP in pregnant women.

The goal of CPAP therapy is to eliminate abnormal respiratory events or reduce to AHI less than 5 and prevent recurrent oxygen desaturation. Regular follow-up with review of objective adherence data is also necessary in all pregnant women who initiate CPAP.[51] It is estimated that adherence rates to CPAP in pregnancy are between 50% and 60%, which is similar to the general population.[52]

Does CPAP help? Both the acute and chronic effects of CPAP have been studied in subgroups of pregnant patients. CPAP reportedly improves maternal and fetal outcomes for women with OSA, preeclampsia or risk factors such as chronic hypertension. Small studies of pregnant women with OSA have shown improvement in inspiratory flow limitation, nocturnal oxygen saturation, blood pressure, cardiac output, fetal movements, and total peripheral arterial resistance during sleep.[53–56] No significant adverse events have been reported with use of CPAP in pregnant women.

In severe cases of OSA with preexisting obesity or multiple gestation, bilevel positive airway pressure therapy may need to be considered.[5] Oxygen supplementation is not recommended as a primary treatment for OSA, and its effectiveness has not been studied in pregnancy.[4]

In summary, although the CPAP intervention studies are limited by small numbers of patients, the results are promising and support a potential hemodynamic benefit for CPAP therapy in patients with preeclampsia. Close monitoring of treatment efficacy throughout the course of pregnancy is very important in the management of OSA in pregnancy.

Oral appliances

Oral appliances are devices intended to protrude and stabilize the mandible to maintain a patent airway during sleep. They have been proved effective for patients with snoring and mild to moderate OSA.[57] However, oral appliances are impractical during pregnancy, because multiple fitting sessions would be necessary in a short period of time.[58] At this time, there is no evidence to recommend use of oral appliances in pregnant women.

Surgery

In the general population, surgical options such as uvulopalatopharyngoplasty are effective in about half of patients with OSA.[58] The risks associated with surgery are likely to be exaggerated during pregnancy, and surgical options for OSA are not routinely recommended. Tracheostomy has been described in a pregnant woman with OSA,[59] but it is likely unnecessary except under unusual circumstances.

RECURRENCE

The severity of SDB may improve following delivery due to weight loss and attenuation of upper airway edema.[39,48] The severity of SDB and the management plan need to be reassessed by a sleep specialist for women with preexisting SDB, women diagnosed with new-onset SDB, or women suspected of SDB during pregnancy.[12] Patients with OSA who were receiving therapy should resume treatment as soon as possible after delivery.

Repeat PSG may be indicated once the new mother has reached her stable weight.[28] The prescription for CPAP may also need to be adjusted depending on her symptoms and PSG results.

SUMMARY

The prevalence of SDB is increasing due to the increase in maternal obesity. Pregnant women often present with fatigue or daytime sleepiness than the classic symptoms of OSA. Habitual snoring, older age, chronic hypertension, and high prepregnancy BMI serve as indicators of increased risk for SDB, and clinical assessment should occur on a frequent basis during antenatal care. The gold standard for diagnosis of OSA is an overnight laboratory PSG that documents an AHI greater than 5 per hour of sleep. Early and timely treatment with close monitoring is crucial, because untreated SDB is associated with preeclampsia and gestational diabetes. CPAP is the preferred, first-line therapy for pregnant women with SDB.

REFERENCES

1. International classification of sleep disorders. 3rd edition. Darien (IL): American Academy of Sleep Medicine; 2014.
2. Kapsimalis F, Kryger MH. Gender and obstructive sleep apnea syndrome, part 1: clinical features. Sleep 2002;25(4):412–9. Available at: https://www.ncbi.nlm.nih.gov/pubmed/12071542.
3. Bourjeily G, Sharkey KM, Mazer J, et al. Central sleep apnea in pregnant women with sleep disordered breathing. Sleep Breath 2015;19(3):835–40.
4. Epstein LJ, Kristo D, Strollo PJ Jr, et al. Clinical guideline for the evaluation, management and long-term care of obstructive sleep apnea in adults. J Clin Sleep Med 2009;5(3):263–76. Available at: https://www.ncbi.nlm.nih.gov/pubmed/19960649.
5. Izci Balserak B, Lee K. Sleep disturbances during pregnancy. In: Kryger HM, Roth T, Dement WC, editors. Principles and practice of sleep medicine. 5th edition. Philadelphia: WB Saunders; 2010. p. 1573–8.
6. Pamidi S, Pinto LM, Marc I, et al. Maternal sleep-disordered breathing and adverse pregnancy outcomes: a systematic review and metaanalysis. Am J Obstet Gynecol 2014;210(1):52.e1-e4.
7. Izci B, Riha RL, Martin SE, et al. The upper airway in pregnancy and pre-eclampsia. Am J Respir Crit Care Med 2003;167(2):137–40.
8. Guilleminault C, Querra-Salva M, Chowdhuri S, et al. Normal pregnancy, daytime sleeping, snoring and blood pressure. Sleep Med 2000;1(4):289–97. Available at: https://www.ncbi.nlm.nih.gov/pubmed/11040461.

9. Franklin KA, Holmgren PA, Jonsson F, et al. Snoring, pregnancy-induced hypertension, and growth retardation of the fetus. Chest 2000;117(1):137–41. Available at: https://www.ncbi.nlm.nih.gov/pubmed/10631211.

10. Loube DI, Poceta JS, Morales MC, et al. Self-reported snoring in pregnancy. Association with fetal outcome. Chest 1996;109(4):885–9. Available at: https://www.ncbi.nlm.nih.gov/pubmed/8635365.

11. Lin CM, Davidson TM, Ancoli-Israel S. Gender differences in obstructive sleep apnea and treatment implications. Sleep Med Rev 2008;12(6):481–96.

12. Izci Balserak B. Sleep disordered breathing in pregnancy. Breathe (Sheff) 2015;11(4):268–77.

13. Punjabi NM. The epidemiology of adult obstructive sleep apnea. Proc Am Thorac Soc 2008; 5(2):136–43.

14. Facco FL, Parker CB, Reddy UM, et al. Association between sleep-disordered breathing and hypertensive disorders of pregnancy and gestational diabetes mellitus. Obstet Gynecol 2017;129(1): 31–41.

15. Bourjeily G. Sleep disorders in pregnancy. Obstet Med 2009;2(3):100–6.

16. O'Brien LM, Bullough AS, Chames MC, et al. Hypertension, snoring, and obstructive sleep apnoea during pregnancy: a cohort study. BJOG 2014;121(13): 1685–93.

17. Facco FL, Ouyang DW, Zee PC, et al. Sleep disordered breathing in a high-risk cohort prevalence and severity across pregnancy. Am J Perinatol 2014;31(10):899–904.

18. Ohida T, Kaneita Y, Osaki Y, et al. Is passive smoking associated with sleep disturbance among pregnant women? Sleep 2007;30(9):1155–61. Available at: https://www.ncbi.nlm.nih.gov/pubmed/17910387.

19. Joosten SA, Edwards BA, Wellman A, et al. The effect of body position on physiological factors that contribute to obstructive sleep apnea. Sleep 2015; 38(9):1469–78.

20. McCowan LME, Thompson JMD, Cronin RS, et al. Going to sleep in the supine position is a modifiable risk factor for late pregnancy stillbirth; findings from the New Zealand multicentre stillbirth case-control study. PLoS One 2017;12(6):e0179396.

21. Maasilta P, Bachour A, Teramo K, et al. Sleep-related disordered breathing during pregnancy in obese women. Chest 2001;120(5):1448–54. Available at: https://www.ncbi.nlm.nih.gov/pubmed/11713118.

22. Pien GW, Fife D, Pack AI, et al. Changes in symptoms of sleep-disordered breathing during pregnancy. Sleep 2005;28(10):1299–305. Available at: https://www.ncbi.nlm.nih.gov/pubmed/16295215.

23. Izci B, Martin SE, Dundas KC, et al. Sleep complaints: snoring and daytime sleepiness in pregnant and pre-eclamptic women. Sleep Med 2005;6(2): 163–9.

24. Jonas DE, Amick HR, Feltner C, et al. Screening for obstructive sleep apnea in adults: evidence report and systematic review for the US preventive services task force. JAMA 2017;317(4):415–33.

25. Tantrakul V, Numthavaj P, Guilleminault C, et al. Performance of screening questionnaires for obstructive sleep apnea during pregnancy: a systematic review and meta-analysis. Sleep Med Rev 2017;36: 96–106.

26. Louis JM, Koch MA, Reddy UM, et al. Predictors of sleep-disordered breathing in pregnancy. Am J Obstet Gynecol 2018;218(5):521.e1-12.

27. Collop NA, Anderson WM, Boehlecke B, et al. Clinical guidelines for the use of unattended portable monitors in the diagnosis of obstructive sleep apnea in adult patients. Portable monitoring task force of the American Academy of Sleep Medicine. J Clin Sleep Med 2007;3(7):737–47. Available at: https://www.ncbi.nlm.nih.gov/pubmed/18198809.

28. Louis J, Pien GW. Obstructive sleep apnea in pregnancy. Waltham (MA): Uptodate; 2017. Available at: www.uptodate.com/contents/obstructive-sleep-apnea-in-pregnancy.

29. O'Brien LM, Bullough AS, Shelgikar AV, et al. Validation of Watch-PAT-200 against polysomnography during pregnancy. J Clin Sleep Med 2012;8(3):287–94.

30. Pien GW, Pack AI, Jackson N, et al. Risk factors for sleep-disordered breathing in pregnancy. Thorax 2014;69(4):371–7.

31. O'Brien LM, Bullough AS, Owusu JT, et al. Pregnancy-onset habitual snoring, gestational hypertension, and preeclampsia: prospective cohort study. Am J Obstet Gynecol 2012;207(6):487.e1-9.

32. Bradley TD, Floras JS. Obstructive sleep apnoea and its cardiovascular consequences. Lancet 2009;373(9657):82–93.

33. Gottlieb DJ, Yenokyan G, Newman AB, et al. Prospective study of obstructive sleep apnea and incident coronary heart disease and heart failure: the sleep heart health study. Circulation 2010;122(4): 352–60.

34. Kent BD, Grote L, Ryan S, et al. Diabetes mellitus prevalence and control in sleep-disordered breathing: the European Sleep Apnea Cohort (ESADA) study. Chest 2014;146(4):982–90.

35. Musso G, Cassader M, Olivetti C, et al. Association of obstructive sleep apnoea with the presence and severity of non-alcoholic fatty liver disease. A systematic review and meta-analysis. Obes Rev 2013; 14(5):417–31.

36. Chen YH, Kang JH, Lin CC, et al. Obstructive sleep apnea and the risk of adverse pregnancy outcomes. Am J Obstet Gynecol 2012;206(2):136.e1-5.

37. Louis JM, Auckley D, Sokol RJ, et al. Maternal and neonatal morbidities associated with obstructive sleep apnea complicating pregnancy. Am J Obstet Gynecol 2010;202(3):261.e1-5.

38. Brown NT, Turner JM, Kumar S. The intrapartum and perinatal risks of Sleep-Disordered Breathing in pregnancy: a systematic review and meta-analysis. Am J Obstet Gynecol 2018. https://doi.org/10.1016/j.ajog.2018.02.004.

39. Izci-Balserak B, Pien GW. Sleep-disordered breathing and pregnancy: potential mechanisms and evidence for maternal and fetal morbidity. Curr Opin Pulm Med 2010;16(6):574–82.

40. American College of Obstetricians and Gynecologists, Task Force on Hypertension in Pregnancy. Hypertension in pregnancy. Report of the American College of Obstetricians and Gynecologists' task force on hypertension in pregnancy. Obstet Gynecol 2013;122(5):1122–31.

41. Haas DM, Parker CB, Wing DA, et al. A description of the methods of the Nulliparous Pregnancy Outcomes Study: monitoring mothers-to-be (nuMoM2b). Am J Obstet Gynecol 2015;212(4):539.e1-e24.

42. Luque-Fernandez MA, Bain PA, Gelaye B, et al. Sleep-disordered breathing and gestational diabetes mellitus: a meta-analysis of 9,795 participants enrolled in epidemiological observational studies. Diabetes Care 2013;36(10):3353–60.

43. Louis JM, Mogos MF, Salemi JL, et al. Obstructive sleep apnea and severe maternal-infant morbidity/mortality in the United States, 1998-2009. Sleep 2014;37(5):843–9.

44. Bourjeily G, Danilack VA, Bublitz MH, et al. Obstructive sleep apnea in pregnancy is associated with adverse maternal outcomes: a national cohort. Sleep Med 2017;38:50–7.

45. Kapsimalis F, Kryger M. Obstructive sleep apnea in pregnancy. Sleep Med Clin 2(4):603–13.

46. Olivarez SA, Maheshwari B, McCarthy M, et al. Prospective trial on obstructive sleep apnea in pregnancy and fetal heart rate monitoring. Am J Obstet Gynecol 2010;202(6):552.e1-7.

47. Bin YS, Cistulli PA, Ford JB. Population-based study of sleep apnea in pregnancy and maternal and infant outcomes. J Clin Sleep Med 2016;12(6):871–7.

48. Edwards N, Blyton DM, Hennessy A, et al. Severity of sleep-disordered breathing improves following parturition. Sleep 2005;28(6):737–41. Available at: https://www.ncbi.nlm.nih.gov/pubmed/16477961.

49. Zaremba S, Mueller N, Heisig AM, et al. Elevated upper body position improves pregnancy-related OSA without impairing sleep quality or sleep architecture early after delivery. Chest 2015;148(4):936–44.

50. Lee J, Eklund EE, Lambert-Messerlian G, et al. Serum progesterone levels in pregnant women with obstructive sleep apnea: a case control study. J Womens Health (Larchmt) 2017;26(3):259–65.

51. Guilleminault C, Kreutzer M, Chang JL. Pregnancy, sleep disordered breathing and treatment with nasal continuous positive airway pressure. Sleep Med 2004;5(1):43–51. Available at: https://www.ncbi.nlm.nih.gov/pubmed/14725826.

52. Sawyer AM, Gooneratne NS, Marcus CL, et al. A systematic review of CPAP adherence across age groups: clinical and empiric insights for developing CPAP adherence interventions. Sleep Med Rev 2011;15(6):343–56.

53. Edwards N, Blyton DM, Kirjavainen T, et al. Nasal continuous positive airway pressure reduces sleep-induced blood pressure increments in preeclampsia. Am J Respir Crit Care Med 2000;162(1):252–7.

54. Poyares D, Guilleminault C, Hachul H, et al. Pre-eclampsia and nasal CPAP: part 2. Hypertension during pregnancy, chronic snoring, and early nasal CPAP intervention. Sleep Med 2007;9(1):15–21.

55. Guilleminault C, Palombini L, Poyares D, et al. Pre-eclampsia and nasal CPAP: part 1. Early intervention with nasal CPAP in pregnant women with risk-factors for pre-eclampsia: preliminary findings. Sleep Med 2007;9(1):9–14.

56. Pamidi S, Kimoff RJ. Maternal sleep-disordered breathing. Chest 2018;153(4):1052–66.

57. Ramar K, Dort LC, Katz SG, et al. Clinical practice guideline for the treatment of obstructive sleep apnea and snoring with oral appliance therapy: an update for 2015. J Clin Sleep Med 2015;11(7):773–827.

58. Pien GW, Schwab RJ. Sleep disorders during pregnancy. Sleep 2004;27(7):1405–17. Available at: https://www.ncbi.nlm.nih.gov/pubmed/15586794.

59. Hastie SJ, Prowse K, Perks WH, et al. Obstructive sleep apnoea during pregnancy requiring tracheostomy. Aust N Z J Obstet Gynaecol 1989;29(3 Pt 2): 365–7. Available at: https://www.ncbi.nlm.nih.gov/pubmed/2619690.

60. Pilkington S, Carli F, Dakin MJ, et al. Increase in Mallampati score during pregnancy. Br J Anaesth 1995;74(6):638–42. Available at: https://www.ncbi.nlm.nih.gov/pubmed/7640115.

61. Izci B, Vennelle M, Liston WA, et al. Sleep-disordered breathing and upper airway size in pregnancy and post-partum. Eur Respir J 2006;27(2):321–7.

62. Ellegard E, Karlsson G. Nasal congestion during pregnancy. Clin Otolaryngol Allied Sci 1999;24(4): 307–11. Available at: https://www.ncbi.nlm.nih.gov/pubmed/10472465.

63. Young T, Finn L, Palta M. Chronic nasal congestion at night is a risk factor for snoring in a population-based cohort study. Arch Intern Med 2001;161(12): 1514–9. Available at: https://www.ncbi.nlm.nih.gov/pubmed/11427099.

The Role of Circadian Rhythms in Postpartum Sleep and Mood

Kari Grethe Hjorthaug Gallaher, MD[a],*,
Anastasiya Slyepchenko, HBSc[b,c],
Benicio N. Frey, MD, MSc, PhD[c,d], Kristin Urstad, PhD[e],
Signe K. Dørheim, MD, PhD[a]

KEYWORDS

- Postpartum • Perinatal • Circadian rhythms • Sleep • Depression • Maternal mental distress

KEY POINTS

- Altered circadian rhythms during pregnancy and postpartum can affect postpartum mood.
- Circadian rhythm disturbances are strongly correlated with depression, social factors, and mother's exposure to light.
- Randomized controlled trial designs are needed to test effects of circadian rhythm interventions on postpartum mental health outcomes.

INTRODUCTION

Pregnancy and the postpartum period are characterized by sleep disturbances and poor sleep quality. In most cases, sleep quality worsens during the last trimester, and mothers experience shorter and more interrupted sleep in the first few months after delivery.[1] The arrival of the newborn places new demands on the mother and may change the rhythms of nighttime and daytime activities. Over the last decade or so, there has been an increasing number of studies describing maternal sleep both during pregnancy and during postpartum (also called the perinatal period) and how sleep disturbances may be linked to higher risk of mood disorders.[1–4]

Circadian rhythms are closely linked to sleep, wakefulness, and health and are therefore essential to examine when investigating different aspects of sleep disturbance among perinatal women.[5] Circadian rhythms are generated by a central pacemaker, the suprachiasmatic nucleus, a self-sustained timing system that is highly regulated and synchronized to elements of the external environment (zeitgebers), such as light and social activities.[6] Altered circadian rhythms have been hypothesized to be associated with mood disorders in the general population[5,7] and may be an important factor to consider in the context of mental illness that develops in the perinatal period. In order to develop effective strategies for preventing and treating sleep disturbances linked to altered circadian rhythms, an important first step is to provide a structured overview of existing literature in the area of circadian rhythms in the perinatal period. Hence, the aim of this systematic review was to provide a summary of studies looking at how circadian rhythms are affected and contribute to sleep problems during pregnancy and postpartum, with special focus on the postpartum period.

[a] Department of Psychiatry, Stavanger University Hospital, Gerd Ragna Bloch Thorsens Gate 8, 4011 Stavanger, Norway; [b] Neuroscience Graduate Program, McMaster University, 1280 Main Street West, Hamilton, ON L8S 4L8, Canada; [c] Women's Health Concerns Clinic, St Joseph's Healthcare Hamilton, 100 West 5th Street, Hamilton, ON L8N 3K7, Canada; [d] Department of Psychiatry and Behavioural Neurosciences, McMaster University, 100 West 5th Street, Hamilton, ON L8N 3K7, Canada; [e] Faculty of Health Sciences, University of Stavanger, Kitty Kjellandshus, 4021 Stavanger, Norway
* Corresponding author.
E-mail address: karigrethe@gmail.com

Sleep Med Clin 13 (2018) 359–374
https://doi.org/10.1016/j.jsmc.2018.04.006
1556-407X/18/© 2018 Elsevier Inc. All rights reserved.

Overview of Sleep in the Postpartum Period

According to a large longitudinal study, more than 50% of women with insomnia during the third trimester of pregnancy continue to have insomnia at 8 weeks postpartum, whereas an additional 23% of women without insomnia during pregnancy develop insomnia during the postpartum period.[8] Longitudinal studies of the perinatal period show a variety of sleep changes during this time. From late pregnancy to the early postpartum period, there is typically a decrease in sleep duration and sleep efficiency, accompanied by an increase in wake after sleep onset (WASO), according to both actigraphy and self-report studies.[1,9] From the early postpartum period to approximately 3 months postpartum, sleep duration and sleep efficiency tend to increase, whereas WASO decreases, although these continue to differ from women who are not pregnant.[9] It has been estimated that it is only after 6 months postpartum that mothers fully recover their own pre-pregnancy sleep pattern.[10]

Postpartum Sleep and Mood Disorders

Approximately 6% to 13% of women in high-income countries experience postpartum depression, and the prevalence in low- and middle-income countries may be even higher.[11,12] Around 8.5% experience distressing postpartum anxiety.[13]

Insomnia and depressive symptoms are associated both before[14] and after delivery in a bidirectional and additive relationship. Several investigators have recently reviewed this topic.[2–4,14] A common finding in these reviews is that self-reported poor sleep during both pregnancy and the postpartum period has been linked to increased risk for or worsening of postpartum depression,[3,4] whereas the relationship between objectively poor sleep, measured by actigraphy or polysomnography, and postpartum depression is more difficult to determine.[3,14] Lawson and colleagues[3] concluded that there was not enough evidence to conclude whether there is a link between sleep problems postpartum, anxiety or psychosis. Bhati and colleagues[2] found that effect sizes relating sleep disturbance with postpartum depression ranged between 0.4 and 1.7 across studies, indicating strong relationships between sleep disturbances and postpartum depression but the definitions and measurements of postpartum sleep "disturbance" varied greatly among the included articles.

Insomnia in pregnancy may seem to be a predictor for postpartum depressive symptoms, but several studies have found that insomnia did not remain a risk factor when controlling for lifetime depression.[1,15] Sleep problems, especially insomnia, may alternatively be an early marker of recurrence of depression or precipitate depression in women susceptible to this disorder. Furthermore, despite this strong relationship between poor sleep and depression, nonpharmacologic interventions for maternal sleep have proved effective for improving maternal sleep and infant sleep, but not for improving maternal depression.[16] This emphasizes the need to address and treat both conditions separately and not assume that depression is merely a symptom of poor sleep.

Although sleep disturbances are a key early warning sign of depression, there is growing evidence that circadian rhythm disturbances may have a role in the cause of depression in the general population.[17,18] For instance, depressed individuals display more variability in salivary melatonin levels over a 30-day period and have higher mean melatonin levels than their nondepressed counterparts.[19] Expression of melatonin receptor 1 in the suprachiasmatic nucleus of the hypothalamus seems to be increased in depressed patients.[20]

Purpose

Currently, knowledge of how circadian rhythms change and may be associated with mood in the postpartum period is limited. In light of increasing evidence of associations between sleep, circadian rhythms, and mood disorders in the general population, the authors conducted a systematic review of studies of circadian rhythm disturbances, sleep, and mood among women in the postpartum period.

METHODS
Selection Criteria

All types of studies of circadian rhythms in women of all ages in the first year postpartum were considered relevant for inclusion. The authors' main focus was on studies of circadian rhythms in postpartum mothers, but longitudinal studies looking at circadian rhythms from pregnancy to the postpartum period were also reviewed, whereas studies restricted to pregnancy only were not included. They also included studies looking at the mutual influence of circadian rhythms in mothers and infants in the first year postpartum. The authors limited their scope to studies performed in humans.

Search Strategy

The authors performed a literature search in the PubMed/Medline database and included longitudinal, cross-sectional, etiologic, biological, and intervention studies to examine circadian rhythms in postpartum women. Searches were performed using the following search terms: (pregnan* OR prenatal OR antenatal OR perinatal OR gestation* OR parity OR gravidity OR peripartum OR postpartum OR puerperium OR postnatal) AND (circadian OR nyctohemeral OR nyctemeral OR diurnal OR 24 hour rhythm OR day night rhythms OR actigraphy OR actiwatch OR polysomnography) AND sleep. This was combined with search terms (prenatal sleep OR postnatal sleep OR antenatal sleep OR peripartum sleep OR postpartum sleep OR maternal sleep OR perinatal sleep).

The time period for this search was from 1980 to November 2017 and limited to Danish, English, Norwegian, or Swedish languages. In addition, the authors manually searched the references of the selected full-text articles to identify additional relevant articles. Based on the search, 2 of the authors (KGHG and AS) independently made a list of titles and abstracts for articles to be read in full-text. The 2 lists were then compared, and agreed on full-text articles were then read by both researchers. Any discrepancies were resolved through discussion. Articles were included if they met the selection criteria.

RESULTS
Search Results

The search resulted in 850 hits (**Fig. 1**), which were evaluated for content regarding perinatal sleep and circadian rhythms. Of these, 43 articles were read in full-text to determine whether they fulfilled the inclusion criteria, yielding 15 articles. Three additional articles were found from manual searches of the reference lists of these selected articles, resulting in 18 articles for inclusion in the current review.

Study Characteristics

The 18 studies included in this review were conducted between 2002 and 2016. Six studies were from Asia, 2 from Canada, and 10 from United States. Number of participants ranged from 10 to 101. Two studies were randomized controlled trials (RCTs), of which one was a pilot study. Eleven were longitudinal and 7 were cross-sectional studies in different populations. The articles are presented in **Table 1**.

After reading through the full texts of the selected articles, 4 main themes emerged: (1) studies describing circadian rhythms among healthy mothers; (2) studies of associations between circadian rhythms and mother/infant interaction; (3) studies of the relationship between circadian rhythms and maternal mood; and (4) interventions to improve circadian rhythms and associated mental distress. Some articles described more than one topic and hence were discussed under more than one theme.

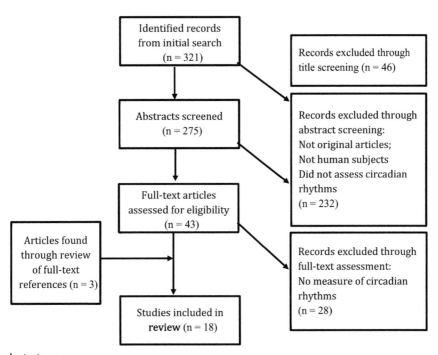

Fig. 1. Search strategy.

Table 1
Studies investigating circadian rhythms over the postpartum period

Study	Study Design	n	Measures and Interventions	Time Point	Results
Bennett et al,[22] 2009	Longitudinal RCT	Women with postpartum depression (n = 18)	Use of blue light-blocking glasses and bulbs for 2 mo	1 and 2 mo post-treatment. Time postpartum not specified	Women who used glasses and bulbs that blocked blue light recovered more quickly than women who used placebo glasses and bulbs
Krawzcak et al,[26] 2016	Longitudinal observational	83: women with (n = 38) and without (n = 45) history of mood disorder	PSQI BRIAN	3rd trimester; 6–12 wk postpartum	Change in biological rhythms, but not sleep, during perinatal period predicted postpartum mood changes in healthy pregnant and pregnant women with a history of mood disorders
Krawzcak et al, 2016[25]	Longitudinal observational	33: women with (n = 15) and without (n = 18) history of mood disorder	21-d actigraphy, PSQI BRIAN	3rd trimester; 6–12 wk postpartum	Changes in both subjective biological rhythms and objective sleep efficiency predicted changes in depressive symptoms across the perinatal period
Lee & Kimble,[24] 2009	Cross-sectional observational	Healthy primiparas with infants in NICU (n = 20)	GSDS; 48-h actigraphy; sleep diary	2 wk postpartum	Postpartum sleep was related to circadian variables and light exposure. Higher light exposure was linked to better sleep, physical and mental health outcomes. Higher amplitude and circadian quotient correlated with longer total sleep time

Lee et al,[23] 2010	Cross-sectional observational	Healthy women with infant in NICU (n = 72)	48–72 h actigraphy; sleep diary	2 wk postpartum	Postpartum circadian variables correlated with sleep variables, fatigue, daytime dysfunction. Mothers with lower circadian quotient had shorter sleep, worse sleep quality
Lee, et al,[27] 2012	Cross-sectional observational	Healthy primiparas with infant in NICU (n = 51)	48–72 h actigraphy; sleep diary	2 wk postpartum	Low daytime light exposure in postpartum mothers—average 66.2 lux. Circadian quotient correlated with total sleep time
Lee et al,[29] 2013	Longitudinal interventional	Mothers with low birth-weight infant in NICU: Treatment group (n = 16); Controls (n = 14)	Bright light therapy: 3 d actigraphy; sleep diary; GSDS	2 wk postpartum, 3 wk post-treatment	No statistically significant differences in pre- and posttreatment between groups. Clinically significant: increased nocturnal total sleep time, increased circadian quotient; morning fatigue and depressive symptoms present in treatment group
Matsumoto et al,[9] 2003	Longitudinal observational	20: healthy pregnant women (n = 10); nonpregnant women (n = 10)	Actigraphy from 34 wk gestation to 16 wk postpartum or 2 wk for nonpregnant women; sleep logs	34 wk gestation to 2 wk postpartum	Mean amplitude of circadian rhythms decreased from pregnancy to postpartum and increased until day 71–93 postpartum. 12-h rhythm higher in pregnancy than at 71–93 d postpartum. 12-h and 8-h rhythms decreased throughout pregnancy

(continued on next page)

Table 1
(continued)

Study	Study Design	n	Measures and Interventions	Time Point	Results
McBean & Montgomery-Downs,[27] 2015	Longitudinal observational	Healthy primiparas (n = 71)	12-wk actigraphy from 1 wk postpartum; real-time PDA-based sleep diary; chronotype questionnaire adapted from MEQ	2 and 12 wk postpartum	Women with rhythmic daily patterns of fatigue had better mental health outcome in regard to reduced stress, had earlier chronotype.
Nishihara, et al,[31] 2002	Longitudinal, observational	Healthy, primiparas (n = 11) and their infants (n = 11)	3–5 d actigraphy	3, 6, 9, 12 wk postpartum	In mothers and infants, amplitude of 24-h peak increases from 6th to 12th wk. Both mothers and infants had a 4-h peak from 6 wk on for infants. Mothers had 4-h and 24-h peaks at 3 wk postpartum
Nishihara, et al,[32] 2012	Longitudinal observational	Healthy, primiparas (n = 10) and their infants (n = 10)	3–5 d actigraphy	33, 36 wk gestation (mothers); 2, 6, 12 wk postpartum	Mothers and infants had smallest 24-h peak at 2 wk, increased 6-12 wks postpartum. Does not reach pregnancy values Mothers had 24-h peak at 33 and 36 wk gestation

Parry et al,[34] 2008	Cross-sectional observational	Pregnant (n = 25); postpartum (n = 25) with and without depression	Plasma melatonin in dim light; every 30 min from 6:00 PM to 11:00 AM	Pregnancy ≤34 wk; postpartum ≤1 y	Pregnant and postpartum women with depression might have disturbed regulation of the melatonin generating system. Women with personal or family history of depression have earlier onset and offset of melatonin synthesis during pregnancy but not postpartum. Morning melatonin levels were higher in postpartum women with depression
Sharkey et al,[35] 2013	Longitudinal observational	Women with history of major depressive disorder (n = 12)	7-d actigraphy; sleep diary; MEQ; salivary melatonin to measure DLMO every 30 min in the evening	33 wk gestation; 6 wk postpartum	Most women had dim light melatonin onset phase shifts from pregnancy to postpartum. During postpartum women were going to bed closer to melatonin secretion onset. Mood correlated with circadian phase and chronotype

(continued on next page)

Table 1
(continued)

Study	Study Design	n	Measures and Interventions	Time Point	Results
Thomas et al,[30] 2014	Longitudinal observational	Healthy women (n = 43) and their infants (n = 43)	3 d actigraphy, sleep diary	4, 8, 12 wk postpartum	Mothers had constant mesor, acrophase throughout study; increased amplitude at wk 4-8, increased IS, decreased IV. Circadian variables correlated between mothers and infants at wk 4. Correlation between mothers and infants increased for circadian variables by wk 12.
Thomas & Burr,[33] 2006	Cross-sectional observational	58: postpartum (n = 38) Nonpregnant nulliparous (n = 20) with no postpartum depression	Urinary 6-sulfatoxy-melatonin across 24 h, measure at each voiding; sleep diary	4–10 wk postpartum	Postpartum women had lower mean and maximum levels of 6-sulfatoxymelatonin and lower percent rise (i.e. maximum = baseline/baseline ×100)

Study	Design	Sample	Measures	Timing	Findings
Tsai et al,[38] 2009	Cross-sectional observational	Healthy primiparas (n = 22) and their infants (n = 22)	7-d actigraphy; sleep diary	<10 wk postpartum	Correlation between maternal and infant light exposure. Greater exposure to light in mothers than infants. Light exposure had modest circadian pattern. Mothers and infants spend >70% of daytime and 99% of nighttime exposed to <50 lux
Tsai, et al,[39] 2011	Cross-sectional observational	Healthy primiparas (n = 22) and their infants (n = 22)	7-d actigraphy; sleep diary	<10 wk postpartum	Mothers and their infants were more active during day than night. Mothers and infants had correlated circadian activity patterns.
Yamazaki et al,[40] 2005	Longitudinal observational	101 first-time parent couples	7-d Monk's Social Rhythm Metric; 7-d sleep logs	32, 36 wk gestation; 4–5 wk postpartum	Mothers' sleep-wake rhythm autocorrelation decreased from pregnancy to postpartum. Mothers who slept alone with baby, rather than with baby and father had decreased social rhythm during perinatal period

Abbreviation: Neonatal intensive care unit.

Measures of Circadian Rhythm in Postpartum Women in the Included Studies

Box 1 contains descriptions of sleep and circadian rhythm measures discussed in this article. Wrist actigraphy was the most common measure of daily rhythm, specifically circadian activity rhythm (CAR) or rest-activity rhythms (12 studies).[9,23–25,27–32,35,38,39]

Circadian Rhythms in Healthy Mothers

We found 7 articles describing circadian rhythm variables during the postpartum period in healthy women. One study compared postpartum melatonin secretion patterns with controls, 1 study reported longitudinal changes in BRIAN scores, and 6 studies performed cosinor analyses of actigraphy data collected during the postpartum period.[23–25,27,30,39]

Thomas and Burr[33] compared urinary 6-sulfatoxymelatonin secretion patterns between women at 4 to 10 weeks postpartum and nonpregnant women. Over 24 hours, postpartum women had lower mean and lower maximum levels of 6-sulfatoxymelatonin levels, along with a lower percent rise, indicating a different secretion pattern of melatonin in postpartum women than controls.

In 6 actigraphy studies, acrophase for CAR varied from 15:12 to 17:01 during the postpartum period.[23–25,27,30,39] There was no effect of postpartum week on acrophase.[30] But Thomas and colleagues[30] found that amplitude and rhythm fit or strength increased from 4 to 12 weeks postpartum, whereas acrophase and mesor remained relatively constant. IS increased in this sample between 4 to 12 weeks postpartum, and IV decreased, indicating progressive stabilization of CAR during the postpartum period.

Krawczak and colleagues[25,26] evaluated self-reported rhythm disruptions in 45 healthy women from the third trimester of pregnancy to 6 to 12 weeks postpartum. They found an increase (worsening) in BRIAN scores from pregnancy to postpartum. In a smaller subsample from this study, 18 healthy women wore an actigraph from pregnancy to postpartum.[26] Mesor and acrophase decreased; amplitude, circadian quotient, and IV increased; and IS did not change. However, no statistical analyses were performed to compare pregnancy and postpartum values.[25]

In a longitudinal actigraphy study from 34 weeks gestation to 16 weeks postpartum, Matsumoto and colleagues[9] found that CAR amplitude decreased from pregnancy to postpartum and increased until 10 to 13 weeks postpartum. A 12-h rhythm was higher in pregnancy than at 10 to 13 weeks postpartum, and 8-h rhythms decreased throughout the postpartum period, indicating greater variability in CAR after delivery in the postpartum period compared with that during pregnancy, and CAR had not normalized to the level of nonpregnant controls at this time point. During the early postpartum period, mothers slept at more irregular intervals while adjusting to a new routine with their infants. The sleep variables measured during this study indicated that mothers were taking longer naps during the day in the early postpartum, and length of daytime naps decreased throughout the postpartum period, likely accounting for the increase in 12-h rhythms.[9]

In an investigation of self-reported CAR and social rhythm patterns from pregnancy to postpartum in 101 mother-infant dyads in Japan, researchers found that mothers' sleep-wake rhythm decreased from pregnancy to postpartum, indicating a less regular CAR for postpartum mothers. The Japanese mothers who slept with their baby had lower social rhythm scores on the Monk Social Rhythm Metric than mothers who slept with both the baby and the father.[40]

Sleep Disturbances Associated with Altered Daily Activity Rhythms

In a series of studies using actigraphy in women with infants in a neonatal intensive care unit, Lee and colleagues[23,24,27] investigated CARs in mothers during 48 to 72 hours at 2 weeks postpartum. In one of these cross-sectional studies, higher amplitude and lower mesor were correlated with better sleep and less morning fatigue,[23] whereas in another study, higher circadian quotient was related to more sleep.[27] Later acrophase was related to worse sleep disturbance and worse daytime dysfunction. A stronger 24-h rhythm, derived through autocorrelation analysis, which indicates a more stable CAR was associated with better sleep and less daytime dysfunction. Finally, when participants with strong and weak rhythms were compared, the mothers with lower (worse) circadian quotients had the most objective and self-reported sleep disturbance.[23]

Mother and Infant Circadian Rhythms

Infant circadian sleep-wake rhythms are typically established during the first 3 months of life, depending largely on light exposure and maternal factors. Animal studies have found maternal activity to exert a large influence on the process of circadian rhythm establishment, commencing intra utero.[21] Five studies measured CAR using actigraphy in mother-infant dyads during the postpartum period.[30–32,38,39]

Box 1
Measures of circadian rhythm and sleep

Objective measures

Actigraphy: activity data obtained from a device typically worn on the wrist; used in a nonintrusive and nondisruptive manner for several days/weeks to assess an individual's activity and sleep in a home environment. The device provides a naturalistic estimate of CAR based on continuous 24-hr wrist movement.

- Sleep variables: total sleep time, number and duration of night awakenings, sleep efficiency, wake after sleep onset, and sleep onset latency.
- CAR variables include cosinor wave analysis, nonparametric analysis of actigraphy rhythms, and auto-correlation analysis.
  - Cosinor wave analysis: uses a cosine curve to fit linear regression for a period of 24 hours. Analysis is used to determine a variety of circadian parameters including the following:
    1. Mesor—the midline estimate of the rhythm (Y intercept), indicating 24-h adjusted mean activity.
    2. Amplitude—the difference between the peak value and the mesor; it may also be calculated as the difference between the peak and the nadir.
    3. Acrophase—the clock time of the peak value; important in assessing chronotype (morningness or eveningness) and circadian rhythms that are phase delayed or phase advanced.
    4. Circadian quotient—the ratio of amplitude to mesor; this ratio is useful when comparing individuals who have different amplitudes
  - Nonparametric analysis: yields data about stability and variability:
    1. Interdaily stability (IS)—measure of coupling of the circadian rhythm to external environmental signals, such as light. Obtained from evaluating regularity of activity data throughout each day of recording. Ranges from 0 to 1, higher values indicate greater stability.
    2. Intradaily variability (IV)—measure of the fragmentation of the rhythm within the day, determined from extent and frequency of transitions between activity and rest. Ranges from 0 to 2; higher values indicate greater variability.
    3. L5—average start of period of 5 hours of least activity within 24 hours.
    4. M10—measure of average start of the 10 most active hours within 24 hours.
    5. Amplitude—calculated from L5 and M10, represents quantity of activity. Ranges from 0 to 1; higher values indicate greater difference between highest and lowest activity phases.
  - Autocorrelation analysis: used to find best-fitting period length of a rhythm.

    This method analyzes data across a range of period lengths, but typically 24-h periods. The correlation coefficients calculated in this analysis represent the extent to which data from each period correlate with data for the subsequent period. A diagram (periodogram) is then produced with correlation coefficients plotted against different period lengths. The highest peak, with the highest correlation strength, corresponds to the best-fitting period length. In addition to circadian (24-h) period lengths, ultradian (less than 24-h) and infradian (more than 24-h) period lengths such as weekly or months rhythms may also be described using this analysis.

Melatonin: precise measure of an individual's endogenous circadian rhythm obtained from melatonin in plasma, saliva, or urine.[33,34] Melatonin is synthesized by the pineal gland from serotonin, as directed by the suprachiasmatic nucleus of the hypothalamus. This hormone regulates circadian rhythms, beginning its secretion 2 to 4 hours before sleep onset and sharply declining by morning. Environmental light–dark cycles control melatonin secretion to entrain daily rhythms with the day–night cycle.

- Dim light melatonin onset (DLMO)—Melatonin measures are better performed under low-light conditions because light as low as 200 lux can suppress melatonin secretion.

Self-report measures

- Horne-Ostberg Morningness-Eveningness Questionnaire (MEQ)—assesses natural tendency of an individual to sleep and be active during a particular time of day (chronotype). Scores distinguish morning ("lark") from evening ("owl") chronotype.[41]
- Biological Rhythms Interview of Assessment in Neuropsychiatry (BRIAN)—assesses key domains of biological rhythm disturbance, including sleep, social, activity, and eating patterns.[39]
- Monk's Social Rhythm Metric (SRM)—a daily, diarylike instrument used to estimate social rhythms over a 1-week duration. Assesses regularity of social rhythms.[36]
- Pittsburgh Sleep Quality Index (PSQI)—measure of sleep quality over the past month; assesses habitual bedtimes.[37]
- General Sleep Disturbance Scale (GSDS)—measure of sleep disturbance over the past week.[24,29]

Nishihara and colleagues reported that infants at 2 and 3 weeks of age had begun to establish a 24-h peak in their CAR. The rhythm was lowest at 2 weeks, and by 3 weeks various ultradian rhythms were present in the infants, but mothers had their lowest 24-h amplitude. From 6 to 12 weeks of age, they observed acrophase peaks at 4-h intervals thought to be a feeding rhythm. The 24-h peak continued to strengthen from 6 to 12 weeks in both mothers and infants,[31,32] although this 24-h peak did not reach the mothers' pregnancy amplitudes.[32]

In mothers and infants between 4 and 12 weeks postpartum, researchers found that CAR stability (IS) increased while variability (IV) decreased, indicating stabilization of daily rhythms.[30] The mothers had a stable postpartum mesor and acrophase; however amplitude increased from week 4 to week 8. There was a moderate correlation between mother-infant CARs at week 4, which increased by week 12 for some variables, indicating increasing synchronization between mothers and infants throughout the postpartum period.[30]

Tsai and colleagues[38] characterized light exposure patterns in a sample of 22 postpartum mothers and their infants. During 2 to 10 weeks postpartum, mothers and infants spent 71% to 80% of their day exposed to less than 50 lux of light, similar to a dimly lit room. They spent 2% to 5% of their daytime exposed to at least 1000 lux, which is approximately the illuminance of overcast daylight. Mothers and infants were exposed to less than 50 lux for more than 98% of the night. There was a modest circadian nature to light exposure in mothers and infants, and light exposure in mothers and infants was highly correlated throughout the day. In a further analysis of these data looking at CAR patterns, investigators found a daily activity rhythm for mothers and infants, and these mothers-infant rhythms were correlated. These findings indicate an early onset of recognizable CAR patterns in infants and suggest that the mother's activity plays an important role in entraining these early rhythms in her infant.[39]

Circadian Rhythms and Postpartum Mood Disorders

Five studies focused on circadian rhythms related to mood disorders in postpartum women.[25,26,28,34,35] In the first prospective study, sleep and rhythms were described in relation to depressive symptoms, as measured by the Edinburgh Postnatal Depression Scale, from pregnancy to the postpartum period in women with and without mood disorders. Changes in BRIAN scores from pregnancy to 6 to 12 weeks postpartum predicted worsening of depressive symptoms in both groups. Disrupted rhythms during the perinatal period increased the risk for deteriorating postpartum mood in women with and without a history of mood disorders.[26] In a subset of these women who underwent actigraphy monitoring, the mothers with a history of mood disorder had high self-reported rhythm disruption (BRIAN) scores, a greater increase in CAR amplitude from pregnancy to postpartum, and more sleep disturbance across the perinatal period. Higher self-reported rhythm disruption scores and lower sleep efficiency predicted worsening of depressive symptoms from pregnancy to postpartum.[25]

Another study explored the association between daily fatigue patterns, CAR measured by wrist actigraphy, and mental health among postpartum women with no history of mood disorders. Women with strong daily patterns of fatigue reported less stress. There was a decreased level of activity during the rest period in both groups, most notable in the high-risk group, and the women in the high-risk group initiated their activity 1 hour later than the low-risk group. Poor day-to-day CAR stability may correlate to higher risk of fatigue.[28]

Only 2 studies used melatonin measures to estimate the endogenous circadian rhythm and both had small samples.[34,35] Parry and colleagues[34] explored differences in plasma melatonin levels for pregnant and postpartum women with and without a personal or family history of depression. Morning melatonin levels were significantly lower in the 10 pregnant women with major depression compared with 15 healthy pregnant women. Melatonin levels were significantly higher in postpartum women with major depression compared with healthy postpartum women.

Sharkey and colleagues[35] examined circadian phase shifts from salivary DLMO to sleep onset over the perinatal period and associations with depressed mood in 12 women with a history of major depressive disorders. Women wore a wrist actigraph and light sensor and completed sleep diaries. They were also assessed with the Hamilton Depression Rating Scale during 3 separate weeks of the perinatal period. To estimate melatonin secretion, they collected saliva samples at 33 weeks of gestation and 6 weeks postpartum. Nine of the twelve women had circadian phase shifts of more than or equal to 30 minutes from third trimester of pregnancy to 6 weeks postpartum. At this time point, mothers were falling asleep closer to the onset of melatonin secretion than in pregnancy. There was an association between DLMO measures and depressed mood, suggesting that changes in prenatal circadian rhythm may influence the development of postpartum mood disorders.[35]

Potential Interventions Involving Light Exposure

Light exposure has been linked to better sleep in 2 studies that showed more circadian rhythm disturbances in women who had reduced exposure to light.[24,27] The authors found 2 intervention studies that tested the effects of light on postpartum depression.[22,29] In the study by Bennet and colleagues,[22] women with postpartum depression were equipped with glasses and light bulbs that block blue light. The mothers in the control group were equipped with glasses and blue light bulbs that looked dark in color but did not block the rays causing melatonin suppression. After 2 months, more women in the intervention group (87.5%) had recovered compared with controls (75%).[22] However, there was no description of how these women were diagnosed with postpartum depression, no measures of sleep were included, and there was no description of how recovery was defined or operationalized.

In the other intervention study, Lee and colleagues[29] examined the effects of bright light therapy on sleep and depressive symptoms in mothers of low birth-weight infants from a neonatal intensive care unit (NICU).[29] Having an infant in intensive care can lead to poor maternal sleep due to both stress and dim light in the hospital setting, and both of these factors affect circadian rhythms. They performed a double-blind randomized control trial (RCT) in which 15 mothers received 30 minutes of daily bright light therapy + sleep hygiene booklet and 15 mothers received red light + nutrition booklet (control group). Mothers in the treatment group had improved CAR, depressive symptoms, and stress compared with controls, although none of the results reached statistical significance over the 3-week time period. This suggests that the improvement was either statistically underpowered or not clinically significant. The investigators recommended replicating the study in postpartum women with circadian rhythm disturbances using larger numbers of participants and longer time periods.[29]

DISCUSSION

The aim of this systematic review was to provide an overview of studies looking at how circadian rhythms are altered during the perinatal period and how they may contribute to poor sleep or mood disorders in the first year postpartum. The review showed that circadian rhythms tend to worsen immediately after delivery and then stabilize over time by the 12th week postpartum. Circadian rhythms are influenced by social factors among postpartum women, and the infant's circadian rhythm and the mother's circadian rhythm synchronize during the first few weeks postpartum. Women's activities, in particular exposure to light, also influence their circadian rhythms. Circadian rhythm disturbances are strongly correlated with mood disorders in postpartum women, particularly depressive symptoms.

Few studies investigated light exposure in postpartum women,[24,27,35,38] and results suggest that light exposure is associated with less circadian rhythm disturbance. Because of the potential for intervention, further research on this topic is warranted. The authors identified only 2 small pilot intervention studies showing that blue light-blocking glasses and bright light therapy are promising therapeutics for regulating circadian rhythms, although no conclusions can be drawn from these studies due to major methodological weaknesses. Both studies had small samples sizes and short-term outcome measures. Further, only one of the intervention studies included baseline data and gave clear description of randomization procedures and intervention.

Most of the studies investigating objective measures of circadian rhythms used actigraphy for time periods ranging from 48 hours to over 16 weeks. Use of sleep logs and actigraphy for a minimum of 1 week is recommended by the Academy of Sleep Medicine to evaluate a range of sleep and circadian disorders.[42] However, most of the included actigraphy studies were performed for only 3 to 5 days or even less.[23,24,27,29–32]

Cosinor analysis of actigraphy data has previously faced criticism as not being representative of the nonsinusoidal nature of rest-activity rhythms, including inability to detect variability in CAR amplitude. Nonparametric CAR analyses have been suggested to be superior to these and autocorrelation methods.[43] DLMO, the gold standard measure of nocturnal melatonin secretion, was investigated in only one of the studies of healthy women.

Sleep parameters are systematically overreported in self-report questionnaires, when compared with objective sleep measures,[44] and among pregnant women self-reported sleep correlates poorly with objective actigraphy sleep measures.[45] However, self-reported sleep through sleep diaries and questionnaires are more readily available for clinicians assessing and treating postpartum women. Thus, studies that use both self-report and objective measures of circadian rhythms simultaneously should be encouraged. Women with worse CAR have been shown to have more nighttime awakenings than women with better CAR, and they had reduced daytime functioning.[24] Descriptions of patterns regarding late bed time, sleep onset latency, nighttime awakenings, or early rise times would be more visible in sleep diaries, and the clinician may therefore focus on this and on sleep during daytime, to determine CAR disturbances. When circadian rhythm disturbance is suspected, women could be advised to increase their daytime activity and also spend more time outside to increase daylight exposure.[29]

The number of studies investigating circadian rhythms in the postpartum period was low. Although the authors' search covered a time period from 1980 to November 2017, they only identified 18 relevant articles, the earliest from 2002. Although they may have missed some articles, the search strategy was done with help of experienced librarians from 2 academic institutions; therefore, they assume that the relevant studies were included. In addition, the sample sizes in most of the studies were low, because the largest study had 101 participants, and some of the studies included in their

review had overlapping samples. In particular, one intervention study completely lacked the methodological details and the pilot RCT was underpowered. This demonstrates a need for more research with better quality.

Furthermore, the authors did not find any qualitative studies as part of their search. Qualitative studies may provide relevant information on the experiences of women living with disturbed circadian rhythms in the perinatal period and may reveal new mechanisms underlying the relationship between circadian rhythm disturbances and perinatal mood. Future studies should include larger sample sizes and use both objective and subjective measures of sleep and circadian rhythms along with validated measures of depression and anxiety. Future investigations should also include the long-term impact of the mutual regulation of mother-infant circadian rhythms.

SUMMARY

Currently, there are few available studies investigating circadian rhythms and sleep parameters among postpartum women, and many existing studies have substantial methodological limitations. Nevertheless, the authors found that circadian rhythm disturbances were strongly correlated with depressive symptoms in postpartum women. It is therefore important to assess and monitor potential circadian rhythm disturbances among postpartum mothers in order to develop and test effective interventions to better prevent and treat perinatal mood disorders.

REFERENCES

1. Dørheim SK, Bjorvatn B, Eberhard-Gran M. Can insomnia in pregnancy predict postpartum depression? A longitudinal, population-based study. PLoS One 2014;9(4):e94674.
2. Bhati S, Richards K. A systematic review of the relationship between postpartum sleep disturbance and postpartum depression. J Obstet Gynecol Neonatal Nurs 2015;44(3):350–7.
3. Lawson A, Murphy KE, Sloan E, et al. The relationship between sleep and postpartum mental disorders: a systematic review. J Affect Disord 2015; 176:65–77.
4. Okun ML. Sleep and postpartum depression. Curr Opin Psychiatry 2015;28(6):490–6.
5. Germain A, Kupfer DJ. Circadian rhythm disturbances in depression. Hum Psychopharmacol 2008;23(7):571–85.
6. Lee ML, Swanson BE, Horacio O. Circadian timing of REM sleep is coupled to an oscillator within the

dorsomedial suprachiasmatic nucleus. Curr Biol 2009;19(10):848–52.

7. Monteleone P, Martiadis V, Maj M. Circadian rhythms and treatment implications in depression. Prog Neuropsychopharmacol Biol Psychiatry 2011;35(7): 1569–74.

8. Sivertsen B, Hysing M, Dørheim SK, et al. Trajectories of maternal sleep problems before and after childbirth: a longitudinal population-based study. BMC Pregnancy Childbirth 2015;15(1):129.

9. Matsumoto K, Shinkoda H, Kang M, et al. Longitudinal study of mothers' sleep-wake behaviors and circadian time patterns from late pregnancy to postpartum–monitoring of wrist actigraphy and sleep logs. Biol Rhythm Res 2003;34(3):265–78.

10. Nowakowski S, Meers J, Heimbach E. Sleep and women's health. Sleep Med Res 2013;4(1):1.

11. Fisher J, Cabral de Mello M, Patel V, et al. Prevalence and determinants of common perinatal mental disorders in women in low-and lower-middle-income countries: a systematic review. Bull World Health Organ 2012;90(2):139–49.

12. Howard LM, Molyneaux E, Dennis C-L, et al. Non-psychotic mental disorders in the perinatal period. Lancet 2014;384(9956):1775–88.

13. Goodman JH, Watson GR, Stubbs B. Anxiety disorders in postpartum women: a systematic review and meta-analysis. J affective Disord 2016;203:292–331.

14. Bei B, Coo S, Trinder J. Sleep and mood during pregnancy and the postpartum period. Sleep Med Clin 2015;10(1):25–33.

15. Marques M, Bos S, Soares MJ, et al. Is insomnia in late pregnancy a risk factor for postpartum depression/depressive symptomatology? Psychiatry Res 2011;186(2):272–80.

16. Owais S, Chow CH, Furtado M, et al. Non-pharmacological interventions for improving postpartum maternal sleep: a systematic review and meta-analysis. Sleep Med Rev 2018. [Epub ahead of print].

17. Melo MC, Abreu RL, Neto VBL, et al. Chronotype and circadian rhythm in bipolar disorder: a systematic review. Sleep Med Rev 2017;34:46–58.

18. Wulff K, Gatti S, Wettstein JG, et al. Sleep and circadian rhythm disruption in psychiatric and neurodegenerative disease. Nat Rev Neurosci 2010;11(8): 589–99.

19. Bouwmans ME, Bos EH, Booij SH, et al. Intra-and inter-individual variability of longitudinal daytime melatonin secretion patterns in depressed and non-depressed individuals. Chronobiol Int 2015; 32(3):441–6.

20. Wu YH, Zhou JN, Balesar R, et al. Distribution of MT1 melatonin receptor immunoreactivity in the human hypothalamus and pituitary gland: colocalization of MT1 with vasopressin, oxytocin, and corticotropin-releasing hormone. J Comp Neurol 2006;499(6): 897–910.

21. Reppert SM, Schwartz WJ. Maternal coordination of the fetal biological clock in utero. Science 1983; 220(4600):969–71.

22. Bennett S, Alpert M, Kubulins V, et al. Use of modified spectacles and light bulbs to block blue light at night may prevent postpartum depression. Med Hypotheses 2009;73(2):251–3.

23. Lee S-Y, Lee KA, Aycock D, et al. Circadian activity rhythms for mothers with an infant in ICU. Front Neurol 2010;1:155.

24. Lee SY, Kimble LP. Impaired sleep and well-being in mothers with low-birth-weight infants. J Obstet Gynecol Neonatal Nurs 2009;38(6):676–85.

25. Krawczak EM, Minuzzi L, Simpson W, et al. Sleep, daily activity rhythms and postpartum mood: a longitudinal study across the perinatal period. Chronobiol Int 2016;33(7):791–801.

26. Krawczak EM, Minuzzi L, Hidalgo MP, et al. Do changes in subjective sleep and biological rhythms predict worsening in postpartum depressive symptoms? A prospective study across the perinatal period. Arch Womens Ment Health 2016;19(4):591–8.

27. Lee S-Y, Grantham CH, Shelton S, et al. Does activity matter: an exploratory study among mothers with preterm infants? Arch Womens Ment Health 2012; 15(3):185–92.

28. McBean AL, Montgomery-Downs HE. Diurnal fatigue patterns, sleep timing, and mental health outcomes among healthy postpartum women. Biol Res Nurs 2015;17(1):29–39.

29. Lee S-Y, Aycock DM, Moloney MF. Bright light therapy to promote sleep in mothers of low-birth-weight infants: a pilot study. Biol Res Nurs 2013; 15(4):398–406.

30. Thomas KA, Burr RL, Spieker S, et al. Mother–infant circadian rhythm: development of individual patterns and dyadic synchrony. Early Hum Dev 2014; 90(12):885–90.

31. Nishihara K, Horiuchi S, Eto H, et al. The development of infants' circadian rest–activity rhythm and mothers' rhythm. Physiol Behav 2002;77(1):91–8.

32. Nishihara K, Horiuchi S, Eto H, et al. Relationship between infant and mother circadian rest-activity rhythm pre-and postpartum, in comparison to an infant with free-running rhythm. Chronobiol Int 2012; 29(3):363–70.

33. Thomas KA, Burr RL. Melatonin level and pattern in postpartum versus nonpregnant nulliparous women. J Obstet Gynecol Neonatal Nurs 2006;35(5):608–15.

34. Parry BL, Meliska CJ, Sorenson DL, et al. Plasma melatonin circadian rhythm disturbances during pregnancy and postpartum in depressed women and women with personal or family histories of depression. Am J Psychiatry 2008;165(12):1551–8.

35. Sharkey KM, Pearlstein TB, Carskadon MA. Circadian phase shifts and mood across the perinatal period in women with a history of major depressive

disorder: a preliminary communication. J affective Disord 2013;150(3):1103–8.

36. Monk TK, Flaherty JF, Frank E, et al. The Social Rhythm Metric: an instrument to quantify the daily rhythms of life. J Nerv Ment Dis 1990;178(2):120–6.

37. Buysse DJ, Reynolds CF, Monk TH, et al. The Pittsburgh Sleep Quality Index: a new instrument for psychiatric practice and research. Psychiatry Res 1989; 28(2):193–213.

38. Tsai S-Y, Barnard KE, Lentz MJ, et al. Twenty-four hours light exposure experiences in postpartum women and their 2–10-week-old infants: an intensive within-subject design pilot study. Int J Nurs Stud 2009;46(2):181–8.

39. Tsai S-Y, Barnard KE, Lentz MJ, et al. Mother-infant activity synchrony as a correlate of the emergence of circadian rhythm. Biol Res Nurs 2011;13(1):80–8.

40. Yamazaki A, Lee KA, Kennedy HP, et al. Sleep-wake cycles, social rhythms, and sleeping arrangement during Japanese childbearing family transition. J Obstet Gynecol Neonatal Nurs 2005;34(3):342–8.

41. Horne JA, Ostberg O. A self-assessment questionnaire to determine morningness-eveningness in human circadian rhythms. Int J Chronobiol 1976;4(2): 97–110.

42. Medicine AAoS. International classification of sleep disorders—third edition (ICSD-3). American Academy of Sleep Medicine 2014.

43. Van Someren EJ, Swaab DF, Colenda CC, et al. Bright light therapy: improved sensitivity to its effects on rest-activity rhythms in Alzheimer patients by application of nonparametric methods. Chronobiol Int 1999;16(4):505–18.

44. Lauderdale DS, Knutson KL, Yan LL, et al. Self-reported and measured sleep duration: how similar are they? Epidemiology 2008;19(6):838–45.

45. Herring SJ, Foster GD, Pien GW, et al. Do pregnant women accurately report sleep time? A comparison between self-reported and objective measures of sleep duration in pregnancy among a sample of urban mothers. Sleep Breath 2013; 17(4):1323–7.

Sleep in Women with Chronic Pain and Autoimmune Conditions
A Narrative Review

Joan L. Shaver, PhD, RN[a],*, Stella Iacovides, PhD[b]

KEYWORDS

- Chronic pain • Autoimmune • Stress-immune • Pain sensitivity • Sleep quality • PSG sleep
- Women

KEY POINTS

- Across clinical conditions that manifest with chronic pain and predominantly in women, lighter and more fragmented sleep and vulnerability to sleep-related disorders are evident.
- Persistent pain is one of the most common reasons patients seek medical care, patients with chronic pain often report sleep difficulties, and patients with persistent insomnia commonly report suffering with pain.
- Chronic pain and poor sleep each involve persistent stress-immune activation with physiologic and behavior changes that signify life-quality threatening morbidity.
- The combined synergistic impact of chronic pain and sleep warrants comprehensive clinical assessment and treatment.
- More research is needed to determine the mechanisms that underlie concurrent poor sleep and chronic pain in women, including the context of menstrual cycles or stages of reproduction.

INTRODUCTION

In this narrative review, we comment on chronic pain and sleep with exemplar papers, published mostly within the last 10 years, for chronically painful conditions manifested predominantly in women. The selected conditions are functional somatic syndromes of chronic pelvic pain (CPP), endometriosis, dysmenorrhea, and fibromyalgia (FM); and the autoimmune (AI) conditions of systemic lupus erythematosus (SLE), rheumatoid arthritis (RA), and multiple sclerosis (MS). We did a PubMed, Medline (Ovid) search from 2007 to 2017, using headings of sleep with pain and immune and pain sensitivity and each of the selected

conditions. We did not select papers by systematic determination of design or measurement quality but rather if the abstract indicated sleep data and predominantly women in the sample. **Box 1** contains the definition of terms used in the text.

Generally, compared with men, women show an excess vulnerability to conditions that are chronically painful and fatiguing. Many conditions exhibit a plethora of symptoms, such as skeletal, gut, or bladder muscle pain; profound fatigue; mental clouding; depressed mood; and almost ubiquitously, sleep disturbance.[1] Generally believed to be at the root of many conditions is stress-immune activation, commonly seen in elevated

Disclosure Statement: The authors have nothing to disclose.
a Biobehavioral Health Science Division, University of Arizona College of Nursing, 1305 North Martin Avenue, Tucson, AZ 85721, USA; b Faculty of Health Sciences, Brain Function Research Group, School of Physiology, University of the Witwatersrand, 7 York Road, Parktown 2193, Johannesburg, South Africa
* Corresponding author.
E-mail address: jshaver@email.arizona.edu

Sleep Med Clin 13 (2018) 375–394
https://doi.org/10.1016/j.jsmc.2018.04.008
1556-407X/18/© 2018 Elsevier Inc. All rights reserved.

Determining the contributors to stress-immune activation is complex as illustrated by a meta-analysis of 72 studies to evaluate sleep quality or sleep patterns as related C-reactive protein (CRP), IL-6, or tumor necrosis factor-α changes.[4] Across sleep deprivation or restriction studies done in healthy individuals, evidence of inflammatory accentuation was sparse. With habitual poor sleep, short sleep duration (<7 hours/night), or extreme long sleep compared with reference groups with normal sleep duration of 7 to 8 hours/night, elevated CRP levels and IL-6 levels (except in short sleep) pertained. None of the sleep variables were related to tumor necrosis factor-α, age was not an influential factor, and results were comparable between men and women. However, a few high-quality studies showed that women were more vulnerable than men to inflammatory activation with sleep difficulties as seen, among other factors, in accentuated CRP, IL-6, and stimulated monocyte production of PICs.[4]

CHRONIC PAIN AND SLEEP DISTURBANCE

People with chronic pain report poor sleep (50%–90%),[5,6] people with insomnia express significant pain, and experimental sleep disruption is associated with augmented pain perceptions.[7] Although a bidirectional relationship between pain and sleep is espoused, data suggest a stronger valence for sleep disturbances driving the development of chronic pain.[5,8] Sleep disturbance can (1) increase vulnerability for new-onset pain when initially pain-free, (2) worsen chance of long-term chronic pain remittance, and (3) impact next day pain expression.[6] Nevertheless, stronger evidence is needed, provoking a call for more longitudinal studies.[9]

In general, patients with significant pain report less total sleep time, long sleep latency, more awakenings, nonrestorative sleep, and daytime sleepiness and fatigue.[10,11] In addition, patients may have sleep-related disorders, such as sleep apnea or restless leg syndrome (RLS).[12] Sleep loss, especially loss of deep sleep, has a significant negative effect on perception of recuperation following a sleep period. Sleep fragmentation, common in chronic pain, may also impact ratings of restoration after sleep, although whether it has a comparable impact to sleep loss is still debated.[13,14] In a review of 29 controlled polysomnography (PSG) studies across various chronic pain populations, the most common disturbance of sleep architecture was sleep continuity disruption.[15] Because perceived arousals or awakenings often fail to coincide in number or duration with

proinflammatory cytokines (PICs), such as interleukins (IL)-1 or -6, and pain dysregulation and hypersensitization. Still to be clarified is whether poor sleep predisposes, precipitates, is a consequence of chronic pain conditions, or some combination thereof, and precisely how sleep regulation and disturbance is intertwined with contributors to prolonged stress-immune activation and pain hypersensitivity.

STRESS-IMMUNE ACTIVATION AND SLEEP

Sleep is altered in the face of stress-immune activation and reciprocally, sleep disturbances can activate the stress-immune system. For example, elevated PIC levels of IL-1 and tumor necrosis factor-α have been associated with more non–rapid eye movement (NREM) sleep. Depleted serotonin (a key sleep regulator and mood factor) or inhibitors of serotonin receptors block IL-1-induced augmented NREM sleep. Manipulations to elevate IL-6 inhibits rapid eye movement (REM) sleep and induces fatigue.[2] When sleep is manipulated, sufficient sleep disturbance coincides with immune cell activation (eg, changes to monocyte, lymphocyte, and neutrophil function and accentuated PIC levels).[3]

recorded events, physical recordings of sleep are necessary to clarify.

SLEEP IN WOMEN WITH SELECTED CHRONICALLY PAINFUL CONDITIONS
Chronic Pelvic Pain

CPP is defined as "intermittent or constant pain in the lower abdomen or pelvis of at least 6 months duration, not occurring exclusively with menstruation or sexual intercourse and not associated with pregnancy."[16] The true prevalence of CPP is difficult to ascertain partly because of its complex nature and the limited knowledge surrounding the condition, and partly because many women consider the pain to be a normal experience for women and thus do not seek health care.[16,17] With a wide array of possible contributors to CPP, including gynecologic, gastrointestinal, urologic, musculoskeletal, and neurologic sources, it is particularly difficult to diagnose and treat.[16]

Most studies of CPP fail to include assessment of sleep, yet, as summarized in **Table 1**, a large proportion of women with CPP report poor sleep quality,[17–19] and short sleep duration.[19] One of these studies used women with dysmenorrhea as their control group.[17] However, 81% of women with CPP also reported dysmenorrhea, making it difficult to determine the relative contributions of the two painful conditions to the sleep difficulties, and flags the need to consider menstrual cycle timing and symptoms when assessing CPP. The only PSG study we uncovered was an older small pilot study showing that women with CPP had more N1 light sleep, more N3 deep sleep, longer REM latency, and less REM-sleep, compared with age-matched healthy women.[20]

Endometriosis

Three studies of women with endometriosis found vulnerability for poor sleep,[21,22] excessive daytime sleepiness,[21] and poor sleep negatively affecting reported pain (see **Table 1**).[22,23] In one study, poorer sleep quality was associated with lower pain thresholds in women with and without endometriosis.[22] Furthermore, following an 8-week randomized control trial of melatonin treatment in women with endometriosis, improved sleep quality was concurrent with reduced pain.[23] Menstrual cycle phase was not mentioned in these studies. Thus, one cannot infer whether poor subjective sleep quality in women with endometriosis, compared with endometriosis-free women, is pain-related, or whether their chronic inflammatory condition or various other manifestations (eg, anxiety and depression[24]) can account for changes in sleep that seem to persist throughout the menstrual cycle. One study mentioned excluding "severe underlying comorbidities" including neurologic and psychiatric comorbidities from their sample; however, details of these criteria were not disclosed.[21]

Primary Dysmenorrhea

Primary dysmenorrhea, or painful menstruation in the absence of pelvic pathology, is experienced by 45% to 95% of menstruating women.[25] Although not typically defined as CPP, manifestations of the two conditions overlap considerably.[17] The experience of recurrent dysmenorrheic pain may predispose women to a chronic pain state, and primary dysmenorrhea seems not to be merely a disorder associated with menstruation.[26] Why some women with dysmenorrhea undergo a transition to a chronic pain state, whereas others do not, is unclear. However, central pain modulation changes in the context of persistent pain with augmented pain sensitivity is likely at play.[26]

Survey data support a link between dysmenorrhea and sleep disturbance[27] and women with dysmenorrhea frequently report daytime fatigue and sleepiness in association with painful uterine cramps.[26] Few investigators have reported on the extent to which dysmenorrhea disturbs reported sleep quality or recorded sleep patterns[28–30] (see **Table 1**). Two PSG-based studies found that women with severe primary dysmenorrhea had a lower sleep efficiency and reduced REM sleep when experiencing menstrual pain compared with control subjects and/or their pain-free phases of the menstrual cycle.[28,30] In contrast, during menstruation, a third study indicated no differences in PSG sleep patterns between women experiencing untreated menstrual pain, women taking pain medication, and control subjects.[29] However, compared with previously mentioned studies (mean age, 21–23 years),[28,30] participants reported less severe menstrual pain and were older (mean age, 35–37 years).[29] Because only 5% of women older than 35 years of age report severe menstrual pain,[31] it is not surprising that no woman in this study reported being awakened during the night because of the pain.

Severity of dysmenorrhea pain seems to influence the extent of sleep disturbance. One survey showed that women with mild dysmenorrhea reported better sleep quality than women reporting moderate or severe dysmenorrhea.[32] Furthermore, insomnia severity was directly associated with dysmenorrhea severity and the association occurred throughout the menstrual cycle, not only during menstruation.[32] Sleep data were self-reported, and not mentioned was timing of pain

Table 1
Reviewed sleep studies related to CPP, endometriosis, dysmenorrhea, and FM

Authors/Sample	Study Type/Specific Aims	Measures	Sleep Findings
Chronic Pelvic Pain			
Cosar et al,[18] 2014 CPP (n = 72) Control subjects (n = 85)	Compare sleep quality in women with CPP with control subjects in women attending a gynecology clinic	PSQI	Significantly higher percentage of women with CPP (80%) had poor sleep quality compared with 55% of control women with poor sleep quality
Singh et al,[19] 2014 Premenopausal women with pelvic problems (n = 838)	Cross-sectional analysis to estimate the prevalence of and determine factors associated with poor sleep quality and short sleep duration (≤6 h) among women with noncancerous gynecologic conditions	Pelvic Problem Impact Questionnaire Patient Health Questionnaire (depression)	34% of women reported poor sleep quality, and 47% of the women reported short sleep duration Poor sleep quality was associated with depression and with pelvic problem impact Short sleep duration was associated with higher pelvic problem impact scores
Zondervan et al,[17] 2001 Randomly selected UK community sample, women of reproductive age (n = 2016)	Cross-sectional survey to determine the community prevalence of CPP and its impact on the lives of women with CPP, compared with women with dysmenorrhea (control subjects)	Nonstandardized questionnaire assessing "sleep problems in the past 4 wk"; specifically: difficulty Falling asleep, frequent awakenings (more than once a night), and nonregenerative sleep (waking up tired/not rested) SF-36 (general health status)	All sleep problems were worse and more frequent in women with CPP compared with women with dysmenorrhea but no other pelvic pain in the previous 3 mo General health (physical and mental components) was significantly worse in CPP vs dysmenorrhea
Dunlap et al,[20] 1998 CPP (n = 11) Age-matched normative data	Pilot study using overnight PSG to determine whether women with CPP have a unique sleep disorder	PSG	Women with CPP had more N1 sleep, less REM-sleep, and increased SWS and longer REM sleep-onset latency

Endometriosis

Study	Aim/Design	Measures	Findings
Maggiore et al,[21] 2017 Endometriosis of the posterior cul-de-sac (n = 145) Age-matched control subjects (n = 145)	Investigate sleep quality, daytime sleepiness, and insomnia in women with endometriosis compared with control subjects	PSQI ESS ISI	Women with endometriosis had a significantly higher prevalence of poor sleep quality and excessive daytime sleepiness, and experienced subthreshold insomnia and moderate clinical insomnia significantly more frequently compared with control women. A multivariate analysis showed that age, body mass index, diagnosis of endometriosis, and pain ratings of dyspareunia, dyschezia, and chronic pelvic pain, were all independent predictors of poor sleep quality
Nunes et al,[22] 2015 Women with laparoscopic and histopathologic diagnosis of endometriosis (n = 257) Endometriosis-free controls (n = 253)	Cross-sectional study assessing sleep quality in women with endometriosis compared with control subjects, and to investigate the correlation between pain and sleep quality	Post-Sleep Inventory VAS (pain)	Women with endometriosis had a poorer sleep quality compared with the control subjects. Poorer sleep scores were associated with lower pain thresholds in both groups of women
Schwertner et al,[23] 2013 Endometriosis (n = 40)	Randomized-controlled trial investigating the efficacy of melatonin (n = 20) vs placebo (n = 20) for 8 wk on endometriosis-related pelvic pain, brain-derived neurotrophic factor, and sleep quality	VAS (sleep and pain)	Melatonin improved sleep quality, and reduced pain scores and brain-derived neurotrophic factor levels

Dysmenorrhea

Study	Aim/Design	Measures	Findings
Sahin et al,[27] 2014 Students (n = 520)	Survey to investigate the frequency of dysmenorrhea in university students and to investigate the relationship between dysmenorrhea and sleep quality	PSQI VAS (dysmenorrhea severity)	Sleep quality was poorer in female students with a history of dysmenorrhea

(continued on next page)

Table 1
(continued)

Authors/Sample	Study Type/Specific Aims	Measures	Sleep Findings
Gagua et al,[33] 2012 Women with dysmenorrhea (n = 276) Control subjects (no dysmenorrhea and with regular ovulatory cycles) (n = 148)	A cross-sectional study that aimed to investigate the prevalence and risk factors of dysmenorrhea in adolescents	Unstandardized sleep questionnaire	Poor sleep hygiene, particularly self-reported short sleep, is negatively associated with dysmenorrhea, and is a risk factor for the development of dysmenorrhea
Woosley & Lichstein,[32] 2014 Women with dysmenorrhea of varying severity (n = 89)	Survey to examine the relationship between dysmenorrhea, insomnia, and sleep across the menstrual cycle in students	Consensus Sleep Diary ISI Brief Pain inventory	Throughout the menstrual cycle, women with mild dysmenorrhea reported better sleep quality than those who experience moderate or severe dysmenorrhea Compared with mild dysmenorrhea, women with severe dysmenorrhea had: ↓SE and ↑SL Severity of insomnia was directly associated with severity of dysmenorrhea, that is, compared with women without insomnia, women with insomnia experienced more severe dysmenorrhea
Baker et al,[28] 1999 Women with severe untreated primary dysmenorrhea (n = 10) HCs (n = 8)	Randomized, controlled study to investigate sleep, nocturnal temperatures, and pain across the menstrual cycle in women with primary dysmenorrhea, compared with control women (free from menstrual-associated disorders)	PSG recordings the first night of menstruation and during the midfollicular and midluteal phases VAS (sleep quality and dysmenorrhea)	During menstruation, compared with both the pain-free phases of their menstrual cycle, and with control subjects, women with dysmenorrhea had: significantly ↓SE, and ↑ combined time spent awake, moving and in N1 (light sleep) When experiencing pain, women with dysmenorrhea had significantly ↓REM sleep, compared with their pain-free menstrual cycle phase Women with dysmenorrhea rated their sleep quality as significantly worse than control subjects during menstruation (ie, in association with their pain), and compared with their own pain-free follicular and luteal phases

			Recorded Sleep Findings	
			Recorded Time/Wake	Recorded Stages
Iacovides et al,[30] 2009 Women with severe primary dysmenorrhea (n = 10)	Randomized, blinded, crossover study, to determine the efficacy of diclofenac potassium, compared with placebo, in alleviating nighttime pain and restoring sleep patterns in women with primary dysmenorrhea	3 overnight PSG recordings, once during the midfollicular phase (no-pain) and twice during menstruation (with pain) VAS (sleep quality and pain)	When experiencing menstrual pain, women dysmenorrhea had: ↓SE, ↓REM sleep, and ↑N1 sleep Compared with the pain-free phase, when women were experiencing pain and receiving placebo, they tended to rate their sleep quality as poorer (56 ± 19 mm vs 70 ± 20 mm), not statistically significant	
Araujo et al,[29] 2011 Women experiencing untreated menstrual pain (n = 8) Women taking medication to relieve menstrual pain (n = 8) HCs (n = 8)	To investigate the impact of menstrual pain on sleep patterns in adult women	PSG recording during menstruation	Overnight PSG recordings were similar regardless of the presence of menstrual pain (present in 66% of women) or use of medication to alleviate menstrual pain	
Fibromyalgia				
Roth et al,[35] 2016 FM (n = 132; 86% women; mA, 48.5); PI (n = 109; 68% women; mA, 47); HCs (n = 52; 73% women; mA, 31)	Descriptive, compare FM with sleep difficulties to PI and pain-free control subjects (no sleep difficulties), from 3 studies	PSG for 2 consecutive nights	FM and PI vs HCs ↓TST ↑SL to persistent sleep ↑WASO ↓sleep bouts FM vs PI ↓SL = WASO	FM and PI vs HCs ↓N3 (deep) sleep FM vs PI ↑N3
Besteiro-Gonzalez et al,[36] 2011 FM (n = 32 women; mA, 50); HCs (n = 20 women; mA, 44)	Cross-sectional, characterize sleep in FM	PSG	FM vs HCs ↓TST, ↑WASO, ↑ number of awakenings ↑ number of PLM	FM vs HCs ↑N2 ↓N3

(continued on next page)

Table 1
(continued)

Authors/Sample	Study Type/Specific Aims	Measures	Sleep Findings		
			Reported Sleep	Recorded Time/Wake	Recorded Stages
Diaz-Piedra et al,[37] 2015 FM (n = 53 women; mA, 46) HCs (n = 36 women; mA, 45)	Cross-sectional, compare PSG and self-report To define predictors of subjective sleep quality	In-home PSG Self-report sleep rating daytime sleepiness, pain, depression and anxiety	FM vs HCs ↓ sleep quality Depression levels, and antidepressant consumption predictive of self-reported sleep quality	FM vs HCs ↓ SE ↑ % time awake More frequent wake bouts	FM vs HCs ↑ N1
			Reported Sleep Quality		
Miro et al,[38] 2011 FM (n = 104 women; mA, 46) HCs (n = 86 women; mA, 45)	Cross-sectional, describe role of sleep as mediator of pain impact on anxiety, dep, daily functioning	PSQI McGill Pain Q, HADS, Chronic Pain Self-Efficacy Scale, Impairment and Functioning	FM vs HCs ↓ Sleep quality ↓ Sleep duration ↑ SL ↓ SE 98% had PSQI score >6; sleep quality and self-efficacy mediated pain and emotional distress		
Munguia-Izquierdo & Legaz-Arrese,[39] 2012 FM (n = 66 women; mA, 49) HCs (n = 48 women; mA, 47)	Cross-sectional, compare sleep quality at home in FM vs HCs; examine factors associated with sleep quality	PSQI BDI STAI FIQ	FM vs HCs 96% = poor sleepers vs 46% FM worse scores on FIQ, total; state and trait anxiety, depression		

Abbreviations: BDI, Beck Depression Inventory; ESS, Epworth Sleepiness Scale; FIQ, fibromyalgia impact questionnaire; HADS, hospital anxiety depression scale; HCs, healthy control subjects; ISI, insomnia severity index; mA, mean age in years (rounded); PLM, periodic leg movement; PSQI, Pittsburgh Sleep Quality Index; SE, sleep efficiency; SF-36, short form-36 health survey; SL, sleep latency; STAI, state-trait anxiety inventory; SWS, slow wave sleep; TST, total sleep time; VAS, visual analogue scale; WASO, wakefulness after sleep onset.

assessments or analgesic medications or whether women had primary or secondary dysmenorrhea. Another cross-sectional study in adolescents reported that poor sleep hygiene and self-reported short sleep in particular, were negatively associated with dysmenorrhea, and both were risk factors for development of dysmenorrhea.[33] More studies are required to determine whether women with primary dysmenorrhea experience sleep disturbances that persist throughout the menstrual cycle.

Fibromyalgia with and Without Chronic Fatigue Syndrome

Widespread pain and other symptoms of FM manifest on a severity spectrum and in the most severe cases, with profound inability to perform activities of daily living and work.[1] More than half of women with FM meet criteria for chronic fatigue syndrome.[34]

Upwards of 70% of people with FM report sleep disturbances (difficulty falling and staying asleep, premature awakening, and fewer hours of sleep).[1] The five FM studies we reviewed (see **Table 1**)[35–39] mostly corroborate prior findings, as did a meta-analysis of 25 FM case-control studies using PSG (published between 1991 and 2015).[40] FM seems to convey a more severe perceived impact on sleep than other conditions. Across studies published since 1990, sleep features in women with FM were compared with those of healthy control subjects (n = 31 studies), rheumatoid arthritis (RA) (n = 7), osteoarthritis (n = 1), or myofascial pain (n = 2).[41] Women with FM consistently showed poor sleep compared with healthy control subjects and, with the exception of one study, had poorer sleep quality than women with other clinical conditions.[41]

Shown also with FM is an excessive prevalence of sleep-related disorders (RLS, periodic leg movement disorder, and sleep-related breathing disorders) and perhaps narcolepsy. In a retrospective study of 74 women with FM or chronic fatigue syndrome who had a multiple sleep latency test, 77% (n = 57) showed abnormal results with 39% (n = 22) having one or more periods of REM sleep onset.[42] For the HLA DQB1*0602 narcolepsy marker, 44% (26/59) of women and 40% (6/15) of men tested positive, warranting close screening for narcolepsy in people with FM or chronic fatigue syndrome.

Poor sleep may convey a risk for developing FM. In a large prospective study in Norway, 12,350 women who reported no FM, musculoskeletal pain, or physical impairments at baseline (1984–86) rated a sleep difficulty item. By the 1995 to 1997 assessment, 327 women had been diagnosed with FM. Compared with those reporting little sleep difficulty at baseline, those reporting more baseline sleep impact showed an adjusted relative risk of 3.43 for FM.[43]

SLEEP IN WOMEN WITH SELECT AUTOIMMUNE CONDITIONS

Given the linkages among stress-immune activation, pain and disturbed sleep are likely to be part of conventional AI conditions. Interestingly, separating chronic pain from an AI condition might not be straightforward and poor sleep may herald the development of AI conditions. In a chart review of women with FM compared with women with chronic pain not caused by FM (n = 116), the prevalence of AI conditions was augmented.[44]

Revealing possible vulnerability for developing AI conditions and poor sleep as a precursor, Taiwanese inpatient and outpatient claims data from January 2000 to December 2003 were analyzed.[45] Compared with 84,996 people with nonapnea sleep disorders, the same number of matched control subjects was followed until an AI diagnosis or death occurred, or the study ended (2010). Patients with a nonapnea sleep disorder were at higher risk (adjusted hazard ratio, 1.47; 95% confidence interval, 1.41–1.53) for developing an AI condition.[45] **Table 2** summarizes exemplar sleep investigations for SLE, RA, and MS. These studies are mainly descriptive, used self-reported sleep measures, had a wide variety of aims, and measured multiple manifestations. Few investigators have included physiologic sleep measures.

Systemic Lupus Erythematosus

SLE is a chronic, multisystem, inflammatory AI disorder that can involve many tissues in the body. We reviewed five sleep studies related to SLE, all using self-report data.[14,46–49] Similar to the 55% to 85% proportion of people with SLE reporting sleep difficulties across studies in a prior review,[50] the proportion across the five studies we reviewed ranged from 55% to 80.5%, mostly defined by a global score greater than 5 on the Pittsburgh Sleep Quality Index.

In a prior review of nine studies (1995–2013), only two measured sleep with PSG.[50] Both revealed lower sleep efficiency and more fragmentation (arousals)[51,52] and one also showed more N1 light sleep and less N3 deep sleep.[51] We found no other PSG studies. However, one published abstract showed that when nine women with SLE were compared with 11 matched control subjects, detectable sleep differences were not evident with actigraphy.[41] To date, indications are that women

Table 2
Sleep studies in systemic lupus erythematosus, rheumatoid arthritis, and multiple sclerosis

Author/Sample	Specific Aims	Measures, Variables	Reported Sleep
Systemic Lupus Erythematosus			
Palagini et al,[46] 2016 SLE (n = 90 women)	Evaluate perceived stress and coping strategies in individuals with SLE and insomnia sx	PSQI Insomnia Severity Index Perceived Stress Scale, Brief COPE, BDI Self-rating Anxiety Scale	66%: insomnia and poor sleep on PSQI Insomnia: ↑ BDI scores, less-effective coping strategies, that is, more behavioral disengagement, self-blame, and emotion-focused
Mirbagher et al,[14] 2016 SLE (n = 77 women; mA, 36.5)	Effects of sleep quality disturbance on HRQoL	PSQI HADS Lupus QoL Disease activity Cumulative damage	57.2% had poor sleep ↓Lupus QoL in older, ↑body mass index, ↑depression and anxiety
Kasitanon et al,[47] 2013 Time series (x3); baseline, 1 mo, and 3 mo SLE (n = 56 women; mA, 35)	Prevalence of poor sleep, factors associated and relationship between sleep and clinical parameters	PSQI Activity index, QoL, damage index, depression, anxiety, fatigue	31; 56%–55%; poor sleep No associations among variables, moderate to severe depression independently related to sleep
Vina et al,[48] 2013 SLE (n = 118; 92% women)	Identify correlates of the MOS Sleep Scale domains	MOS Sleep Scale (6 subscales) BDI STAI SLE Disease Activity Index Damage index	MOS scores lower than general population Depression correlated with 5, anxiety with 4 subscales; sleep adequacy and sleep disturbance independently associated with depression; snoring independently correlated with anxiety; pain
Greenwood et al,[49] 2008 (Australia) SLE (n = 172; 91% women; mA, =52) Seeking rx for sleep problems (n = 223; ~50% women; mA, 49) 456 working people (n = 456; ~7% women; mA, 43)	Assess poor sleep and compare with a working and treatment-seeking sample with insomnia	PSQI	PSQI score >5: 80.5% of SLE, 91.5% of treatment-seeking, and 28.5% of working group SLE: worse sleep on all scores than working group and better sleep than group seeking treatment for insomnia, except for SL
Rheumatoid Arthritis			
Guo et al,[54] 2016 RA (n = 131; 85.5% Chinese women; mA, 55) HCs (n = 104 Chinese; 84.6% women; mA, 55)	Effects of sleep quality on HRQoL in RA patients	PSQI HADS, Pain VAS Health Assessment DAS-28 SF 36	PSQI ≥5: RA = 78.6%; HCs = 18.7% RA differed from HCs in PSQI sleep quality, SL, habitual SE, sleep disorders and use of hypnotics Poor sleepers: ↑disease activity, more severe total/nocturnal pain, ↑ depression and anxiety

(continued on next page)

Table 2
(continued)

Author/Sample	Specific Aims	Measures, Variables	Reported Sleep
Løppenthin et al,[55] 2015 RA (n = 384; 80% women; mA, 59)	Assess sleep quality and correlates of poor sleep in patients with RA	PSQI, ESS MFIS, Health Assessment Q, DAS28-CRP	PSQI ≥5: 61% had poor sleep, mean global PSQI score = 7.54 (SD, 4.17) Poor sleep positively related to mental fatigue, mental fatigue and general fatigue independently associated with sleep quality, SL, TST, SE, and daytime dysfunction
Westhovens et al,[56] 2014 RA (n = 305; mA, 57)	Describe sleep problems and relationship between sleep/disease activity	AIS, PSQI ESS VAS pain, fatigue SF-36 DAS-CRP	Mean (SD) AIS, PSQI, and ESS scores were 6.8 (±4.79), 7.8 (±4.30), and 7.3 (±4.67), positive relationships between disease activity score and perceived sleep quality (AIS/PSQI), negative relationship between disease activity score and daytime sleepiness
			Recorded Sleep
Gjevre et al,[57] 2012 RA ESS >10 (n = 10; 60% women; mA, 58) RA ESS ≤10 (n = 15; 80% women; mA, 62)	Determine whether excess sleepiness is associated with PSG abnormalities	PSG PSQI AHI, ESS Berlin Q – sleep apnea risk, VAS - fatigue, CES-D mHAQ	No PSG factors different by ESS groups No difference in PSG with poor sleep (PSQI ≥5) AHI ≥5 in 80% with ↑ ESS, 60% in normal ESS AHI ≥5: 85% of men, 61% of women
Multiple Sclerosis			
Nociti et al,[58] 2017 MS (n = 102; 61% women; mA, 43)	Assess relationship between sleep and fatigue	PSQI ESS Berlin Q (OSA) IRLSSG Questions MFIS BDI SAS EDSS	Poor sleep: mean PSQI = 7.4 ± 4.0 (n = 57% ≥5) ESS: mean 4.5 ± 4.0 (all n = 15% ≥9) IRLSSG criteria: all n = 14% with score = 4 Poor sleep: more frequently fatigued; have ↑ MFIS global scores, ↑ RLS prevalence, ↑ depression and anxiety scores

(continued on next page)

Table 2
(continued)

Author/Sample	Specific Aims	Measures, Variables	Reported Sleep
Vitkova et al,[59] 2016 MS (n = 153; 76% women; mA, 39)	Identify gender differences in factors of poor sleep quality	PSQI HADS SF-36 (pain item)	No differences in variables by gender Women: mean PSQI = 6.0 ± 3.5 Women: depressed mood/anxiety predicted sleep quality Men: pain main predictor
Braley et al,[60] 2014 MS (n = 195; 66% women; mA, 47)	Determine OSA, OSA risk; relationship of sleep quality to fatigue	ISI ESS FSS STOP-Bang (OSA) EDSS	21% had formal OSA dx 56% of all and 93% with OSA diagnosis had STOP-Bang ≥3, predictor of FSS were ↑ STOP-Bang, nocturnal symptoms, disability scores
Brass et al,[61] 2014 MS (n = 2375; 81% women; mA, 55) 11,400 mailed surveys, 2810 returned	Prevalence of RLS, insomnia, OSA risk; and sleep Associations with fatigue and daytime sleepiness	ISI Sleep hx STOP-BANG Berlin Q. (OSA) IRLSSG Questions ESS FSS	746 (32%) had moderate to severe insomnia 898 (38%) were positive for OSA 866 (37%) for RLS 712 (30%) ESS scores >10; 1555 (66%) FSS ≥36, abnormal fatigue 866 (37%) in met all 4 RLS criteria Abnormal fatigue and sleepiness scores positively related to OSA, insomnia, and RLS
Leonavicius & Adomaitiene,[62] 2014 Relapsing remitting MS (n = 137; 72% women; mA, 45)	Prevalence of sleep disturbances; relationship to depression, anxiety, and QoL	MOS Sleep Scale, HADS, EDSS SF-36 (HRQoL)	45.3% sleep disturbance 22% depressed mood, 20% anxiety Sleep disturbances associated with gender, age, EDSS, depression, anxiety, mental and physical HRQoL scores
Vitkova et al,[63] 2014 MS ≤5 y (n = 66; 78% women; mA, 37) MS >5 y (n = 86; 73% women; mA, 42)	Differences in prevalence, determinants of poor sleep quality	PSQI HADS MFIS Incapacity Status Scale: bladder problems item SF-36: pain item	↑poor sleep (PSQI >5) with MS >5 y (51.2%), MS ≤5 y (34.8%) Associations with poor sleep: MS ≤5 y: anxiety, reduced motivation, mental fatigue associated with poor sleep quality MS >5 y: pain, depression, mental fatigue

(continued on next page)

Table 2
(continued)

Author/Sample	Specific Aims	Measures, Variables	Reported Sleep
Li et al,[65] 2012 Nurses Health Study II cohort (n = 65,544 women; mA, 50) 4-y follow-up	Assess association of MS with RLS, daytime sleepiness	IRLSSG Questions Items: sleep quality Daily activities affected	MS (n = 264; 0.4%): sx ≥5 times/mo; RLS with MS (n = 15.5%), without MS (n = 6.4%) Severe RLS (15 + x/mo) + MS (n = 9.6%) Severe RLS + no MS (n = 2.6%) OR of MS + RLS = 2.72 OR of MS + severe RLS = 4.12 OR of day sleepy = 2.11 47% day sleepy (at least 1x/wk; 10% nearly every day) 172 women with MS and no RLS in 2005; 9 developed RLS (5.2%) during a 4-y, all severe RLS; adjusted relative risk = 3.58
Merlino et al,[68] 2009 MS (n = 120; 72.5% women; mA, 44)	Assess sleep disturbances relationship to comorbidities and QoL	PSQI CCI SF-36 (QoL) EDSS HADS	Poor sleep (n = ~50%): had ↑EDSS, ↑CCI scores, ↑pain, ↓SF-36 scores for physical and mental domains Independent predictors Mental status: sexual and/or bladder dysfunction, global PSQI score For physical status: age, EDSS and global PSQI scores
			Recorded sleep-related disorders
Veauthier et al,[67] 2011 MS fatigued (MFIS ≥45; n = 26; 73% women; mA, 45) MS nonfatigued (MFIS <45; n = 40; 65% women; mA, 42)	Assess relationship between fatigue and sleep disorders	PSG ESS Fatigue VAS, MFIS, FSS BDI Nottingham Health Profile	High fatigue: 96% had sleep-related disorder, 27% SBD; low fatigue: 60% had sleep disorder, 2.5% SBD Sleep disorder risk of fatigue (OR = 18.5) No difference in ESS scores

Abbreviations: AIS, athens insomnia scale; AHI, apnea/hypopnea index; BDI, Beck Depression Inventory; CES-D, Center for Epidemiologic Studies Depression Scale; CCI, Charlson Comorbidity Index; DAS-28, 28 joint disease activity score with erythrocyte sedimentation rate value; DAS-CRP, DAS with C-reactive protein value; EDSS, Expanded Disability Status Scale; ESS, Epworth Sleepiness Scale; FSS, Fatigue Severity Scale; HADS, Hospital Anxiety Depression Scale; HCs, healthy control subjects; HRQoL, health-related quality of life; IRLSSG, International Restless Leg Syndrome Study Group; ISI, Insomnia Severity Index; mA, mean age in years (rounded); MFIS, Multidimensional Fatigue Impact Scale; mHAQ, modified health assessment questionnaire; MOS, Medical Outcomes Study (Rand); OR, odds ratio; OSA, obstructive sleep apnea; PI, primary insomnia; PSQI, Pittsburgh Sleep Quality Index; SBD, sleep-related breathing disorders; SD, standard deviation; SE, sleep efficiency; SF-36, Short Form Health Survey (Rand); SL, sleep latency; STAI, state-trait anxiety inventory; TST, total sleep time; VAS, Visual Analogue Scale.

with SLE perceive their sleep as poor, and in concert with many chronic pain conditions, sleep tends to be lighter and more fragmented.[53]

Rheumatoid Arthritis

We reviewed four studies related to RA published from 2012 to 2016 (see **Table 2**).[1,54–57] One used PSG data but only to compare more or less fatigued RA patients.[57] Prevalence of poor sleep (Pittsburgh Sleep Quality Index score >5) was 61%[55] and 78.6%.[54] In RA patients, reported sleep was poor in quality, with longer onset latency and less efficiency.[54] Poor sleepers had higher disease activity, depression, and anxiety scores and more severe total and nocturnal pain.[54,56] Daytime sleepiness in the face of poor sleep seems to modulate downward with more severe RA disease activity leading to speculations about pain-related cognitive-emotional arousal obviating sleepiness. Intuitively, fatigue and poor sleep correspond but perhaps do separate. For example, following 3 months of therapy with genetically engineered proteins derived from human genes (meant to inhibit specific immune components that spur inflammation), disease-related fatigue improved in 58.6% of 99 patients with RA (72.7% women), whereas no significant improvement in sleep quality was observed.[55]

Multiple Sclerosis

MS is an AI disease of the central nervous system with neurologic manifestations generated by chronic inflammatory demyelination. We reviewed nine sleep studies (see **Table 2**).[58–68] Sleep quality was self-reported in all except one study[67] and poor sleep was prevalent regardless of whether MS duration was greater than 5 years (57%,[58] 45%,[62] 50%[68]) or less than or equal to 5 years (51% and 35%[63]). Studies were aimed at clarifying the association of poor sleep with fatigue,[58,60,67] RLS,[58,61] or sleep-related breathing disorders.[58,60,61] In a review of sleep disorders related to fatigue with MS, the prevalence of RLS, particularly in people with MS and severe disability, was four times higher than in people without MS and authors concluded that treatment of sleep disorders improved fatigue.[69]

IMPLICATIONS FOR CLINICAL PRACTICE

Sleep and pain coexist in the context of many clinical conditions (**Table 3**). Although poor sleep is often thought of as being comorbid with chronic health conditions, such as cardiovascular or neurologic diseases, the conditions in this review generally fail to show organ-specific pathology. Whether chronic pain and sleep disturbances

Table 3
Clinical assessment and treatment implications

Complications in Chronic Pain and Autoimmune Conditions	Clinical Assessment Considerations
Sleep disturbance is common in most clinical populations	Assess for sleep quality; recommend monitoring at home with sleep diary Understand sources of sleep disturbance and whether the disturbance existed before onset of the pain condition Consider referral to sleep specialist
Sleep-related disorders are commonly associated with chronic pain	Screen for sleep-related disorders: RLS, periodic leg movement disorder, obstructive sleep apnea, and narcolepsy Consider referral to sleep specialists
Mood dysfunction, particularly depression, and profound fatigue often coexist, impacting on life functionality	Screen for multiple symptoms with possible treatment of depression/anxiety and/or fatigue Assess and monitor each symptom, including pain, sleep, and mood; detailed self-report pain, mood, and sleep diaries, for 1–2 mo, are useful tools Consider referral to specialists
Most analgesics have direct effects on sleep, independent of their action on pain	Treatment decisions need to balance symptomatic treatment of pain and side effects of sleep disturbances (see **Table 4**)
Given all the complications listed previously	Treatment regimens should be carefully monitored, and frequently re-evaluated

accompany common organ system disease, idiopathic chronic pain, or conventionally defined AI conditions, manifestations, such as depressed mood, impaired cognition, fatigue, and daytime dysfunction, are shared.[12,70] This supports targeting multiple symptoms as an optimal approach,[71] and comprehensive assessment will likely reveal clusters of symptoms,[72] raising the need for greater understanding of integrated systemic drivers and common mechanisms to generate a single comprehensive morbidity definition in conjunction with warranted pathophysiologic insights. Also obvious is the need for assessment and treatment of multiple symptoms, including, pain, poor sleep, depressed mood, and fatigue.

Importantly, treatment regimens, whether pharmacologic and/or cognitive-behavioral, should be carefully monitored and frequently re-evaluated. Consideration of the effects of various pharmacologic agents on sleep is paramount.

Sleep and Common Medication Treatments for Chronic Pain

In patients with chronic pain, sleep improvement is complicated by the actions of commonly prescribed medications to manage pain (**Table 4**). Many directly disrupt the "restorative" nature of sleep, which is believed to depend predominantly on timing, duration, and continuity of sleep.

Table 4
Commonly prescribed pharmacologic agents in pain populations and sleep effects

Commonly Prescribed Analgesics	Summarized Drug Effects on Sleep
Non-Opioids NSAIDS (eg. aspirin, ibuprofen, acetaminophen)	No clear evidence that NSAIDs significantly affect sleep[77–79]
Opioids	↑light sleep (N2), ↓deep sleep (N3), ↓REM sleep in healthy individuals,[80,81] postoperative patients,[82] and opioid addicts[83] Increased prevalence of SBD[84] and OSA in patients with chronic pain[85] Low-dose opioids, coupled with naloxone, effective for RLS and sleep[86] Opioid-induced hyperalgesia observed[87]; underlying mechanisms unclear

Adjuvant Analgesics
Antidepressants (eg. TCAs, SNRIs, SSRIs)
Anticonvulsants (eg. carbamazepine, gabapentin, pregabalin)
	Comprehensive reviews[88,89] discussion on variable effects of the different antidepressants on sleep[90]
	TCAs: ↓↓REM sleep, ↑REM SL, ↑deep sleep, ↑TST[90,91]
	SSRIs: ↓↓REM sleep,[90] ↑WASO ↓TST[89,90]
	SNRIs: ↓↓ generally REM sleep[90]
	  Antidepressant use commonly associated with sleep disorders (eg, RLS, PLMs, OSA)[89]
	Comprehensive reviews on anticonvulsants and sleep[92,93]
	  Carbamazepine (short-term): ↓↓ and fragmented REM sleep, ↑sleep stage shifts in healthy volunteers and patients with epilepsy[94]
	Pregabalin, gabapentin: ↓pain-related subjective sleep disturbance in chronic pain populations, including diabetic neuropathy[95] and fibromyalgia[96,97]
	Pregabalin:
	  ↓WASO[98] in patients with epilepsy
	  ↑deep sleep (duration and percentage), ↓awakenings, ↑SE, ↑TST, ↓SL, ↓REM sleep duration in healthy individuals[99]
	  ↓WASO, ↓number of nocturnal awakenings, ↑TST, ↑SE, ↑SWS in patients with fibromyalgia[100]
	Gabapentin:
	  ↑REM sleep, ↑deep sleep, ↓WASO, ↓N1 sleep, in healthy adults and in epilepsy[101,102]

Abbreviations: NSAIDs, nonsteroidal anti-inflammatory drugs; OSA, obstructive sleep apnea; PLM, periodic leg movement; SBD, sleep-related breathing disorders; SE, sleep efficiency; SL, sleep latency; SNRI, serotonin and noradrenaline reuptake inhibitor; SSRI, selective serotonin reuptake inhibitor; SWS, slow wave sleep; TCA, tricyclic amine; TST, total sleep time; WASO, wakefulness after sleep onset.

Commonly prescribed analgesics, broadly categorized as nonopioids, opioids, and adjuvant analgesics, all have documented efficacy in patients with chronic pain.[16,73–75] However, they also affect sleep (see **Table 4**). As mentioned in treating CPP, when pain is described using words such as "burning, stabbing or shoorting" (ie, more typically considered to be neuropathicc pain), medications, such as gabapentin/pregalalin, should be considered for adjunct therapy.[16]

IMPLICATIONS FOR RESEARCH

So far, integration of the extant evidence about sleep quality, patterns, or impact across studies is a challenge (**Table 5**). Prominent is insufficient accounting for factors affecting sleep, such as insomnia and sleep-related disorders. For the studies reviewed, many were descriptive and lacked control subjects, weakening interpretation of results. Most descriptive studies were comparative with healthy control subjects (potentially insufficiently screened), individuals diagnosed with another painful or chronic condition, or groups within a disease having more or less severe disease or symptom activity. More probing using objectively recorded sleep measures is needed with larger groups of patients. As wearable monitoring devices continue to emerge with advanced biophysical and biochemical sensing, the ability

Table 5
Sleep research issues and suggestions for future studies

Sleep Research Issues	Suggestions for Future Research
Heterogeneity of methods and design	Comprehensive screening (pain and sleep) using common measures; appropriate comparisons and control for multiple mediating/modulating variables
Lack of differentiating sleep pattern markers	More PSG studies with larger, well-defined, more refined probing of brain mechanisms (eg, electroencephalogram power spectral analysis, topography mapping, brain imaging)
Reproductive hormone fluctuations for women	Control for female reproductive status (menstrual cycle, pregnancy, menopause transition)
Variety of outcomes and mismatch between reported and recorded sleep indicators	Complete assessment of sleep pattern indicators, preferably both self-report and physiologic detection, including brain function probing beyond PSG PSG allows expanded insight; however, subjective-objective mobile monitoring over time is needed as inexpensive, and less obtrusive option to evaluate impact of pain Concurrent measurements and correspondent analysis, such as for SL, time in bed, TST, frequency and duration of WASO, and SE; contributors to divergence or convergence
Few intervention studies aimed at discovering ways to relieve pain through improving sleep	Test interventions to deepen and consolidate sleep, such as combined mind and body (pharmacologic) treatments; slow wave sleep enhancement
Insufficient knowledge of stress-related outcomes of sleep and pain	More measures of stress-endocrine and systemic inflammation in context of chronic pain and sleep, or with sleep and/or pain manipulations
Insufficient knowledge of contributors to the pain-sleep relationship	Pursuing precursors, such as genetic, stress-immune activation profiles, personal style profiles, life events, lifestyle, early detection, and personalized (precision) treatments
Varied responses to interventions and complex person/lifestyle contributors to pain and insomnia	Testing of novel interventions tailored to subtypes using mechanistic outcome indicators (bio and behavioral markers)

Abbreviations: SE, sleep efficiency; SL, sleep latency; TST, total sleep time; WASO, wakefulness after sleep onset.

to link what is perceived to be important aspects of mind-body empirical function holds promise. Thus, women might be better helped with novel forms of biofeedback to reduce pain and improve coping.

Underlying contributors to the pain-sleep relationship in women could be better understood by knowing precursors and capturing data, perhaps clusters of symptoms, when they first appear. Similar to the conclusion arrived at in studying people with insomnia[76], people with chronic pain and poor sleep diverge on many factors. This supports the necessity of deriving sub-type profiles based on a variety of contributors.

SUMMARY

Chronic pain and poor sleep (primary insomnia) provoke persistent stress-immune activation. Given the evidential effects on quality of life and other medical and psychiatric manifestations that chronic pain and insomnia each have, and the notable pain-sleep connections, an exaggerated combined effect is not to be underestimated or ignored. Therefore, clinical assessment of pain and sleep impact is critical, along with effective treatment of these phenomena and consideration of the effects of medication on sleep. Along with medications, behavioral therapies that involve mindfulness for either pain or sleep may be complementary in alleviating chronic pain and insomnia or in counterbalancing some side effects of medications. Although not addressed in detail in this narrative review, it is important to determine how mood, cognitive-emotional propensities (personality), and environmental features (high strain) contribute to chronic pain and poor sleep. Generating evidence of commonalities across conditions, and not solely within one medical diagnosis, should be encouraged in future research.

REFERENCES

1. Shaver JL. Sleep disturbed by chronic pain in fibromyalgia, irritable bowel, and chronic pelvic pain syndromes. Sleep Med Clin 2008;3:47–60.
2. Ali T, Choe J, Awab A, et al. Sleep, immunity and inflammation in gastrointestinal disorders. World J Gastroenterol 2013;19(48):9231–9.
3. Faraut B, Boudjeltia KZ, Vanhamme L, et al. Immune, inflammatory and cardiovascular consequences of sleep restriction and recovery. Sleep Med Rev 2012;16(2):137–49.
4. Irwin MR, Olmstead R, Carroll JE. Sleep disturbance, sleep duration, and inflammation: a systematic review and meta-analysis of cohort studies and experimental sleep deprivation. Biol Psychiatry 2016;80(1):40–52.
5. Smith MT, Haythornthwaite JA. How do sleep disturbance and chronic pain inter-relate? Insights from the longitudinal and cognitive-behavioral clinical trials literature. Sleep Med Rev 2004;8(2):119–32.
6. Finan PH, Smith MT. The comorbidity of insomnia, chronic pain, and depression: dopamine as a putative mechanism. Sleep Med Rev 2013;17(3):173–83.
7. Iacovides SG, George K, Kamerman P, et al. Sleep fragmentatiopn hypersesitizes health young women to deep and superficial experimental pain. J Pain 2017;18(7):844–54.
8. Finan PH, Goodin BR, Smith MT. The association of sleep and pain: an update and a path forward. J Pain 2013;14(12):1539–52.
9. Lee KA. The need for longitudinal research on chronic pain and sleep disturbance. Sleep Med Rev 2016;26:108–10.
10. Covarrubias-Gomez A, Mendoza-Reyes JJ. Evaluation of sleep quality in subjects with chronic non-oncologic pain. J Pain Palliat Care Pharmacother 2013;27(3):220–4.
11. Baker TA, Whitfield KE. Sleep behaviors in older African American females reporting nonmalignant chronic pain: understanding the psychosocial implications of general sleep disturbance. J Women Aging 2014;26(2):113–26.
12. Menefee LA, Cohen MJ, Anderson WR, et al. Sleep disturbance and nonmalignant chronic pain: a comprehensive review of the literature. Pain Med 2000;1(2):156–72.
13. Aerenhouts D, Ickmans K, Clarys P, et al. Sleep characteristics, exercise capacity and physical activity in patients with chronic fatigue syndrome. Disabil Rehabil 2015;37(22):2044–50.
14. Mirbagher L, Gholamrezaei A, Hosseini N, et al. Sleep quality in women with systemic lupus erythematosus: contributing factors and effects on health-related quality of life. Int J Rheum Dis 2016;19(3):305–11.
15. Bjurstrom MF, Irwin MR. Polysomnographic characteristics in nonmalignant chronic pain populations: a review of controlled studies. Sleep Med Rev 2016;26:74–86.
16. Vincent K. Chronic pelvic pain in women. Postgrad Med J 2009;85(999):24–9.
17. Zondervan KT, Yudkin PL, Vessey MP, et al. The community prevalence of chronic pelvic pain in women and associated illness behaviour. Br J Gen Pract 2001;51(468):541–7.
18. Cosar E, Cakir Gungor A, Gencer M, et al. Sleep disturbance among women with chronic pelvic pain. Int J Gynaecol Obstet 2014;126(3):232–4.
19. Singh JK, Learman LA, Nakagawa S, et al. Sleep problems among women with noncancerous

gynecologic conditions. J Psychosom Obstet Gynaecol 2014;35(1):29–35.

20. Dunlap KT, Yu L, Fisch BJ, et al. Polysomnographic characteristics of sleep disorders in chronic pelvic pain. Prim Care Update Ob Gyns 1998;5(4):195.

21. Maggiore UL, Bizzarri N, Scala C, et al. Symptomatic endometriosis of the posterior cul-de-sac is associated with impaired sleep quality, excessive daytime sleepiness and insomnia: a case-control study. Eur J Obstet Gynecol Reprod Biol 2017; 209:39–43.

22. Nunes FR, Ferreira JM, Bahamondes L. Pain threshold and sleep quality in women with endometriosis. Eur J Pain 2015;19(1):15–20.

23. Schwertner A, Conceicao Dos Santos CC, Costa GD, et al. Efficacy of melatonin in the treatment of endometriosis: a phase II, randomized, double-blind, placebo-controlled trial. Pain 2013; 154(6):874–81.

24. Chen LC, Hsu JW, Huang KL, et al. Risk of developing major depression and anxiety disorders among women with endometriosis: a longitudinal follow-up study. J Affect Disord 2016;190:282–5.

25. Proctor M, Farquhar C. Diagnosis and management of dysmenorrhoea. BMJ 2006;332(7550): 1134–8.

26. Iacovides S, Avidon I, Baker FC. What we know about primary dysmenorrhea today: a critical review. Hum Reprod Update 2015;21(6):762–78.

27. Sahin S, Ozdemir K, Unsal A, et al. Review of frequency of dysmenorrhea and some associated factors and evaluation of the relationship between dysmenorrhea and sleep quality in university students. Gynecol Obstet Invest 2014; 78(3):179–85.

28. Baker FC, Driver HS, Rogers GG, et al. High nocturnal body temperatures and disturbed sleep in women with primary dysmenorrhea. Am J Physiol 1999;277(6 Pt 1):E1013–21.

29. Araujo P, Hachul H, Santos-Silva R, et al. Sleep pattern in women with menstrual pain. Sleep Med 2011;12(10):1028–30.

30. Iacovides S, Avidon I, Bentley A, et al. Diclofenac potassium restores objective and subjective measures of sleep quality in women with primary dysmenorrhea. Sleep 2009;32(8):1019–26.

31. Polat A, Celik H, Gurates B, et al. Prevalence of primary dysmenorrhea in young adult female university students. Arch Gynecol Obstet 2009;279(4): 527–32.

32. Woosley JA, Lichstein KL. Dysmenorrhea, the menstrual cycle, and sleep. Behav Med 2014;40(1): 14–21.

33. Gagua T, Tkeshelashvili B, Gagua D. Primary dysmenorrhea: prevalence in adolescent population of Tbilisi, Georgia and risk factors. J Turk Ger Gynecol Assoc 2012;13(3):162–8.

34. Mariman AN, Vogelaers DP, Tobback E, et al. Sleep in the chronic fatigue syndrome. Sleep Med Rev 2013;17(3):193–9.

35. Roth T, Bhadra-Brown P, Pitman VW, et al. Characteristics of disturbed sleep in patients with fibromyalgia compared with insomnia or with pain-free volunteers. Clin J Pain 2016;32(4):302–7.

36. Besteiro Gonzalez JL, Suarez Fernandez TV, Arboleya Rodriguez L, et al. Sleep architecture in patients with fibromyalgia. Psicothema 2011;23(3): 368–73.

37. Diaz-Piedra C, Catena A, Sanchez AI, et al. Sleep disturbances in fibromyalgia syndrome: the role of clinical and polysomnographic variables explaining poor sleep quality in patients. Sleep Med 2015;16(8):917–25.

38. Miro E, Martinez MP, Sanchez AI, et al. When is pain related to emotional distress and daily functioning in fibromyalgia syndrome? The mediating roles of self-efficacy and sleep quality. Br J Health Psychol 2011;16(4):799–814.

39. Munguia-Izquierdo D, Legaz-Arrese A. Determinants of sleep quality in middle-aged women with fibromyalgia syndrome. J Sleep Res 2012;21(1): 73–9.

40. Wu Y-L, Chang LY, Lee HC, et al. Sleep disturbances in fibromyalgia: a nmeta-analysis of case-control studies. J Psychosom Res 2017;96: 89–97.

41. Diaz-Piedra C, Di Stasi LL, Baldwin CM, et al. Sleep disturbances of adult women suffering from fibromyalgia: a systematic review of observational studies. Sleep Med Rev 2015;21:86–99.

42. Spitzer AR, Broadman M. A retrospective review of the sleep characteristics in patients with chronic fatigue syndrome and fibromyalgia. Pain Pract 2010; 10(4):294–300.

43. Mork PJ, Nilsen TI. Sleep problems and risk of fibromyalgia: longitudinal data on an adult female population in Norway. Arthritis Rheum 2012;64(1): 281–4.

44. Brooks L, Hadi J, Amber KT, et al. Assessing the prevalence of autoimmune, endocrine, gynecologic, and psychiatric comorbidities in an ethnically diverse cohort of female fibromyalgia patients: does the time from hysterectomy provide a clue? J Pain Res 2015;8:561–9.

45. Hsiao YH, Chen YT, Tseng CM, et al. Sleep disorders and increased risk of autoimmune diseases in individuals without sleep apnea. Sleep 2015; 38(4):581–6.

46. Palagini L, Mauri M, Faraguna U, et al. Insomnia symptoms, perceived stress and coping strategies in patients with systemic lupus erythematosus. Lupus 2016;25(9):988–96.

47. Kasitanon N, Achsavalertsak U, Maneeton B, et al. Associated factors and psychotherapy on sleep

disturbances in systemic lupus erythematosus. Lupus 2013;22(13):1353–60.

48. Vina ER, Green SL, Trivedi T, et al. Correlates of sleep abnormalities in systemic lupus: a cross-sectional survey in an urban, academic center. J Clin Rheumatol 2013;19(1):7–13.

49. Greenwood KM, Lederman L, Lindner HD. Self-reported sleep in systemic lupus erythematosus. Clin Rheumatol 2008;27(9):1147–51.

50. Palagini L, Tani C, Mauri M, et al. Sleep disorders and systemic lupus erythematosus. Lupus 2014; 23(2):115–23.

51. Iaboni A, Ibanez D, Gladman DD, et al. Fatigue in systemic lupus erythematosus: contributions of disordered sleep, sleepiness, and depression. J Rheumatol 2006;33(12):2453–7.

52. Valencia-Flores M, Resendiz M, Castano VA, et al. Objective and subjective sleep disturbances in patients with systemic lupus erythematosus. Arthritis Rheum 1999;42(10):2189–93.

53. Balderas-Diaz S, Martinez MP, Guerrero-Contreras G, et al. Using actigraphy and mHealth systems for an objective analysis of sleep quality on systemic lupus erythematosus patients. Methods Inf Med 2017;56(2):171–9.

54. Guo G, Fu T, Yin R, et al. Sleep quality in Chinese patients with rheumatoid arthritis: contributing factors and effects on health-related quality of life. Health Qual Life Outcomes 2016;14(1):151.

55. Løppenthin K, Esbensen BA, Jennum P, et al. Sleep quality and correlates of poor sleep in patients with rheumatoid arthritis. Clin Rheumatol 2015;34(12):2029–39.

56. Westhovens R, Van der Elst K, Matthys A, et al. Sleep problems in patients with rheumatoid arthritis. J Rheumatol 2014;41(1):31–40.

57. Gjevre JA, Taylor-Gjevre RM, Nair BV, et al. Do sleepy rheumatoid arthritis patients have a sleep disorder? Musculoskeletal Care 2012;10(4): 187–95.

58. Nociti V, Losavio FA, Gnoni V, et al. Sleep and fatigue in multiple sclerosis: a questionnaire-based, cross-sectional, cohort study. J Neurol Sci 2017; 372:387–92.

59. Vitkova M, Rosenberger J, Gdovinova Z, et al. Poor sleep quality in patients with multiple sclerosis: gender differences. Brain Behav 2016;6(11): e00553.

60. Braley TJ, Segal BM, Chervin RD. Obstructive sleep apnea and fatigue in patients with multiple sclerosis. J Clin Sleep Med 2014;10(2):155–62.

61. Brass SD, Li CS, Auerbach S. The underdiagnosis of sleep disorders in patients with multiple sclerosis. J Clin Sleep Med 2014;10(9):1025–31.

62. Leonavicius R, Adomaitiene V. Features of sleep disturbances in multiple sclerosis patients. Psychiatr Danub 2014;26(3):249–55.

63. Vitkova M, Gdovinova Z, Rosenberger J, et al. Factors associated with poor sleep quality in patients with multiple sclerosis differ by disease duration. Disabil Health J 2014;7(4):466–71.

64. Veauthier C, Gaede G, Radbruch H, et al. Treatment of sleep disorders may improve fatigue in multiple sclerosis. Clin Neurol Neurosurg 2013; 115(9):1826–30.

65. Li Y, Munger KL, Batool-Anwar S, et al. Association of multiple sclerosis with restless legs syndrome and other sleep disorders in women. Neurology 2012;78(19):1500–6.

66. Newland PK, Fearing A, Riley M, et al. Symptom clusters in women with relapsing-remitting multiple sclerosis. J Neurosci Nurs 2012;44(2):66–71.

67. Veauthier C, Radbruch H, Gaede G, et al. Fatigue in multiple sclerosis is closely related to sleep disorders: a polysomnographic cross-sectional study. Mult Scler J 2011;17(5):613–22.

68. Merlino G, Fratticci L, Lenchig C, et al. Prevalence of 'poor sleep' among patients with multiple sclerosis: an independent predictor of mental and physical status. Sleep Med 2009;10(1):26–34.

69. Veauthier C, Paul F. Sleep disorders in multiple sclerosis and their relationship to fatigue. Sleep Med 2014;15(1):5–14.

70. Mullington JM, Haack M, Toth M, et al. Cardiovascular, inflammatory, and metabolic consequences of sleep deprivation. Prog Cardiovasc Dis 2009; 51(4):294–302.

71. Aktas A, Walsh D, Rybicki L. Symptom clusters: myth or reality? Palliat Med 2010;24(4):373–85.

72. Davis LL, Kroenke K, Monahan P, et al. The SPADE symptom cluster in primary care patients with chronic pain. Clin J Pain 2016;32(5):388–93.

73. Moore RA, Straube S, Wiffen PJ, et al. Pregabalin for acute and chronic pain in adults. Cochrane Database Syst Rev 2009;(3):CD007076.

74. Moore RA, Wiffen PJ, Derry S, et al. Gabapentin for chronic neuropathic pain and fibromyalgia in adults. Cochrane Database Syst Rev 2014;(4): CD007938.

75. Brick N. Carbamazepine for acute and chronic pain in adults. Clin J Oncol Nurs 2011;15(3):335–6.

76. Benjamins JS, Migliorati F, Dekker K, et al. Insomnia heterogeneity: characteristics to consider for data-driven multivariate subtyping. Sleep Med Rev 2017;36:71–81.

77. Murphy PJ, Badia P, Myers BL, et al. Nonsteroidal anti-inflammatory drugs affect normal sleep patterns in humans. Physiol Behav 1994;55(6):1063–6.

78. Gengo F. Effects of ibuprofen on sleep quality as measured using polysomnography and subjective measures in healthy adults. Clin Ther 2006; 28(11):1820–6.

79. Lavie P, Nahir M, Lorber M, et al. Nonsteroidal anti-inflammatory drug therapy in rheumatoid arthritis

patients. Lack of association between clinical improvement and effects on sleep. Arthritis Rheum 1991;34(6):655–9.

80. Dimsdale JE, Norman D, DeJardin D, et al. The effect of opioids on sleep architecture. J Clin Sleep Med 2007;3(1):33–6.

81. Shaw IR, Lavigne G, Mayer P, et al. Acute intravenous administration of morphine perturbs sleep architecture in healthy pain-free young adults: a preliminary study. Sleep 2005;28(6):677–82.

82. Cronin AJ, Keifer JC, Davies MF, et al. Postoperative sleep disturbance: influences of opioids and pain in humans. Sleep 2001;24(1):39–44.

83. Kay DC, Pickworth WB, Neider GL. Morphine-like insomnia from heroin in nondependent human addicts. Br J Clin Pharmacol 1981;11(2):159–69.

84. Walker JM, Farney RJ. Are opioids associated with sleep apnea? A review of the evidence. Curr Pain Headache Rep 2009;13(2):120–6.

85. Webster LR, Choi Y, Desai H, et al. Sleep-disordered breathing and chronic opioid therapy. Pain Med 2008;9(4):425–32.

86. Silber MH, Becker PM, Buchfuhrer MJ, et al. The appropriate use of opioids in the treatment of refractory restless legs syndrome. Mayo Clin Proc 2018;93(1):59–67.

87. Lee M, Silverman SM, Hansen H, et al. A comprehensive review of opioid-induced hyperalgesia. Pain Physician 2011;14(2):145–61.

88. Wilson S, Argyropoulos S. Antidepressants and sleep: a qualitative review of the literature. Drugs 2005;65(7):927–47.

89. Bohra MH, Kaushik C, Temple D, et al. Weighing the balance: how analgesics used in chronic pain influence sleep? Br J Pain 2014;8(3):107–18.

90. Mayers AG, Baldwin DS. Antidepressants and their effect on sleep. Hum Psychopharmacol 2005;20(8):533–59.

91. Hartmann E, Cravens J. The effects of long term administration of psychotropic drugs on human sleep. 3. The effects of amitriptyline. Psychopharmacologia 1973;33(2):185–202.

92. Jain SV, Glauser TA. Effects of epilepsy treatments on sleep architecture and daytime sleepiness: an evidence-based review of objective sleep metrics. Epilepsia 2014;55(1):26–37.

93. Placidi F, Diomedi M, Scalise A, et al. Effect of anticonvulsants on nocturnal sleep in epilepsy. Neurology 2000;54(5 Suppl 1):S25–32.

94. Gigli GL, Placidi F, Diomedi M, et al. Nocturnal sleep and daytime somnolence in untreated patients with temporal lobe epilepsy: changes after treatment with controlled-release carbamazepine. Epilepsia 1997;38(6):696–701.

95. Roth T, van Seventer R, Murphy TK. The effect of pregabalin on pain-related sleep interference in diabetic peripheral neuropathy or postherpetic neuralgia: a review of nine clinical trials. Curr Med Res Opin 2010;26(10):2411–9.

96. Straube S, Derry S, Moore RA, et al. Pregabalin in fibromyalgia: meta-analysis of efficacy and safety from company clinical trial reports. Rheumatology (Oxford) 2010;49(4):706–15.

97. Prelle K, Igl BW, Obendorf M, et al. Endpoints of drug discovery for menopausal vasomotor symptoms: interpretation of data from a proxy of disease. Menopause 2012;19(8):909–15.

98. de Haas S, Otte A, de Weerd A, et al. Exploratory polysomnographic evaluation of pregabalin on sleep disturbance in patients with epilepsy. J Clin Sleep Med 2007;3(5):473–8.

99. Hindmarch I, Dawson J, Stanley N. A double-blind study in healthy volunteers to assess the effects on sleep of pregabalin compared with alprazolam and placebo. Sleep 2005;28(2):187–93.

100. Roth T, Lankford DA, Bhadra P, et al. Effect of pregabalin on sleep in patients with fibromyalgia and sleep maintenance disturbance: a randomized, placebo-controlled, 2-way crossover polysomnography study. Arthritis Care Res 2012;64(4):597–606.

101. Placidi F, Mattia D, Romigi A, et al. Gabapentin-induced modulation of interictal epileptiform activity related to different vigilance levels. Clin Neurophysiol 2000;111(9):1637–42.

102. Foldvary-Schaefer N, De Leon Sanchez I, Karafa M, et al. Gabapentin increases slow-wave sleep in normal adults. Epilepsia 2002;43(12):1493–7.

Effects of Exercise on Sleep in Women with Breast Cancer: A Systematic Review

Ellyn E. Matthews, PhD, RN, AOCNS, CBSM[a],*,
Dalton W. Janssen, BSN, RN[a],
Dilorom M. Djalilova, BA, BSN, RN[b],
Ann M. Berger, PhD, APRN, AOCNS[b]

KEYWORDS

- Sleep deficiency • Exercise • Intervention • Breast cancer • Systematic review

KEY POINTS

- Eleven of the 15 studies meeting inclusion criteria showed improvement in sleep; all walking interventions resulted in positive sleep outcomes but the exercise-based integrative interventions (eg, yoga) showed inconsistent sleep outcomes.
- Most exercise interventions designed to improve sleep in women with breast cancer were aerobic; most studies used only self-report measures and were conducted during treatment and in several countries.
- Exercise interventions varied in frequency and intensity as well as participant adherence.
- A synthesis of these review findings would suggest that sleep outcomes may be influenced more by the type and intensity of exercise than by the phase of cancer treatment.

INTRODUCTION

Women with breast cancer are at elevated risk for sleep deficiency, defined as the discrepancy in sleep duration and/or quality obtained compared with the amount needed for optimal health.[1,2] Sleep deficiency can occur at the time of breast cancer diagnosis or during primary treatment[3,4] and can persist for years after cancer treatment is completed.[5–7] For example, in adults with various types of cancer diagnoses (N = 962) at perioperative baseline, findings revealed high rates of sleep deficiency at baseline (59%) that declined but remained pervasive even at 18 months postsurgery (36%).[7] Nearly half of the sample were women with breast cancer (49%), in which the sleep deficiency rates were the highest compared with other types of cancer (69% at baseline and 42% at 18 months).[7] Sleep deficiency can negatively affect health outcomes, including cognitive functioning,[8] quality of life,[5] immune function, and survival.[9,10] Among women with breast cancer, sleep problems may affect self-care and help-seeking behaviors, as well as adherence to recommended therapeutic interventions such as hormonal therapy.[11–13] Other consequences include fatigue, psychological distress, and impaired functioning.[14]

EXERCISE INTERVENTIONS FOR WOMEN WITH BREAST CANCER

Pharmacologic interventions have been shown to improve sleep deficiency in patients with chronic

Disclosures: The authors have no financial disclosures to report.
[a] College of Nursing, University of Arkansas for Medical Sciences, 4301 West Markham Street # 529, Little Rock, AR 72205-7199, USA; [b] College of Nursing, University of Nebraska Medical Center, 985330 Nebraska Medical Center, Omaha, NE 68198-5330, USA
* Corresponding author.
E-mail address: eematthews@uams.edu

insomnia but may have adverse effects.[15] Cognitive behavioral therapy for insomnia has been effective in patients with cancer[16,17] but access to this therapy is often limited.[17] Physical activity and exercise, defined in **Box 1**,[18] are attractive options for managing sleep deficiency because of the favorable safety profile, availability, and positive impact on other health outcomes.[19,20] Proposed mechanisms by which exercise reduces sleep deficiency include improved body weight, fitness, mood, and positive effects on inflammation and circadian rhythms.[21–23] Yet, the question of whether exercise is effective in improving sleep in adults with cancer remains unanswered, particularly in breast cancer.

A recent systematic review of exercise interventions in adults with mixed cancers identified 21 trials, including 17 randomized controlled trials (RCT), involving more than 2077 patients with cancer who reported sleep quality as an endpoint.[24] Eight of the studies (38%) had sample sizes of 40 or less, 10 included only women with breast cancer (48%), and yoga was excluded as an exercise.[24] Although the overall findings suggest a beneficial effect of exercise interventions on sleep in several studies (48%), the meta-analysis for RCT studies showed no significant effect on subjective or objective sleep measures.[24] The investigators suggest that additional large, rigorous studies are needed to determine the type of exercise, timing, and dosage with the most benefit in patients with cancer, including subgroups such as women with breast cancer.[24]

Other reviews of exercise interventions on sleep outcomes during and after cancer treatments[25,26] included 20 trials with more than 1000 patients with cancer. Although the findings suggest that exercise has a modest beneficial effect on sleep quality during and after treatment, most of the trials were pilot studies with less than 100 participants who had various cancer diagnoses, or studies were focused on general quality of life outcomes. Other reviews have focused on exercise interventions in women with breast cancer only during adjuvant treatment[27] or in adults with hematological malignancies,[28] which limits the scope of the conclusions. Previous reviews have neither examined the impact of exercise on sleep in women with breast cancer across the phases of care, nor included exercise-based integrative interventions such as yoga, dance, qigong, and tai chi. A systematic review of the literature assessing the effect of exercise on sleep in women with breast cancer is needed to summarize the available evidence and to determine to what extent exercise is efficacious as a sleep-enhancing intervention.

OBJECTIVES

This article aims to (1) summarize and critically analyze current evidence regarding the effect of exercise on sleep deficiency in women with breast cancer at various phases of care, (2) identify gaps in this body of evidence, and (3) formulate recommendations for future research and adoption into practice.

METHODS
Eligibility Criteria

Preferred reporting items for systematic reviews and meta-analyses (PRISMA) guidelines for the conduct of systematic reviews and meta-analyses were followed.[29] To be included, English language studies had to include at least 40 women with nonmetastatic breast cancer with an exercise intervention and sleep outcomes and at least 20 per group at randomization (**Table 1**). The authors included only women with stage 0-III breast cancer because advanced stage IV disease may affect a participant's adherence to exercise interventions and the study outcomes.[24] Past reviews of sleep outcomes excluded yoga due to heterogeneity of yoga types and variability in intensity[24]; however, new evidence suggests that exercise-based integrative interventions such as yoga and tai chi have an aerobic component.[30] For example, studies that compared posture-based yoga with conventional exercise indicated that physiologic benefits were similar to conventional cycling or brisk walking[31] and concluded that yoga was as efficacious as exercise in health-related outcomes in a variety of conditions.[31,32]

Box 1
Definition of physical activity and exercise

Physical activity is body movement that is produced by the contraction of skeletal muscles, resulting in significantly increased energy expenditure.

Exercise is a subset of physical activity that is planned, structured, and repetitive. Its purpose is to improve or maintain at least one aspect of physical fitness (eg, muscular strength, muscular endurance, flexibility, cardiovascular endurance, body composition).

Data from Bernardo LM, Becker BJ. Exercise and physical activity for people living with cancer: nurses' edition. Pittsburgh (PA): Oncology Nursing Society; 2016.

Table 1
Study eligibility criteria

Inclusion Criteria	Exclusion Criteria
• Experimental design study published in English	• Systematic review, meta-analysis, or nonexperimental study design
• Examined various forms of exercise interventions, including aerobic, resistance, or a combination; exercise could be combined with other interventions (eg, flexibility, counselling).	• <40 women in total sample or <20 per group at randomization
	• Did not contain an established sleep measure or sleep subscale within an established instrument
• Included women ≥18 y with nonmetastatic breast cancer before, during, or after cancer treatment	• Rated as poor quality (<18.71 on the Yates quality scale[33])
• Any exercise frequency, intensity, or duration; could be home-based or supervised	
• Control groups could be usual care or an alternative intervention (eg, relaxation)	

Box 2
PubMed search strategy

The following search strategy was used: (breast neoplasms [mesh] OR "breast cancer"[tiab]) AND (sleep wake disorders/th [mesh] OR "sleep"[tiab]) AND ((Exercise Movement Techniques OR Breathing Exercises OR dance therapy OR tai ji OR exercise therapy OR motion therapy, continuous passive OR muscle stretching exercises OR plyometric exercise OR resistance training OR physical therapy modalities [Mesh:NoExp])) OR ("aerobic exercise" OR "resistance exercise" OR walking OR running OR jogging OR "motor activity" OR sports [mesh] OR bicycling OR golf OR gymnastics OR tennis OR "weight training").

Literature Search Strategy and Study Selection

PubMed, the Cochrane library, the Cumulative Index of Nursing, and Allied Health Literature (CINAHL) electronic databases were searched from the earliest date available through July, 2017. The main search terms included "breast cancer," "sleep," and "exercise." MeSH terms were individualized for each search database's vocabulary map. For example, the PubMed search is described in **Box 2**. After duplicates were removed, titles and abstracts were examined independently by 3 authors (EM, DJ, DD) to identify studies meeting the selection criteria. The full text of the selected studies was further assessed by all investigators to verify eligibility for final inclusion in the review. Disagreements were resolved by consensus. Manual searches (eg, hand-searching, perusing reference lists) were used to ensure that all relevant studies were included.

Study Quality

Methodological quality was assessed using the Yates Quality Rating Scale,[33] which has been

used to rate quality in other sleep-related reviews.[34] Total quality scores range from 0 to 35 using 2 subscales. The treatment quality subscale (0–9) evaluates rationale for treatment, manual use/adherence, therapist training, and patient engagement. The design and methods quality subscale (0–26) evaluates inclusion/exclusion criteria, attrition, sample description, bias (randomization method, allocation bias, blinding, and equality of treatment expectations), outcome selection, follow-up periods, analyses, and choice of control. Two teams (ie, EM & DJ, AB & DD) independently rated the included studies, and consensus was reached after the teams discussed initial comparison ratings.

RESULTS
Study Selection and Data Extraction

The initial search of electronic databases yielded 112 references. After reviewing titles and abstracts, 77 publications were excluded because they were duplicates or did not meet the inclusion criteria, leaving 35 studies. One additional study was found via hand search. Then 36 full text studies were reviewed in detail, and 15 met the inclusion criteria for the current review. A CONSORT-type flow diagram depicts the studies at each stage of review (**Fig. 1**). Data were systematically extracted from the eligible studies, and tables were created with investigators, year of publication, methods, participant characteristics, intervention details, and results (**Tables 2 and 3**).

Study Quality Results

The mean total Yates Quality Rating Scale score[33] for the 15 studies was 25 out of a possible 35 points, the mean treatment quality score was 5.9 out of a possible 9 points, and the mean

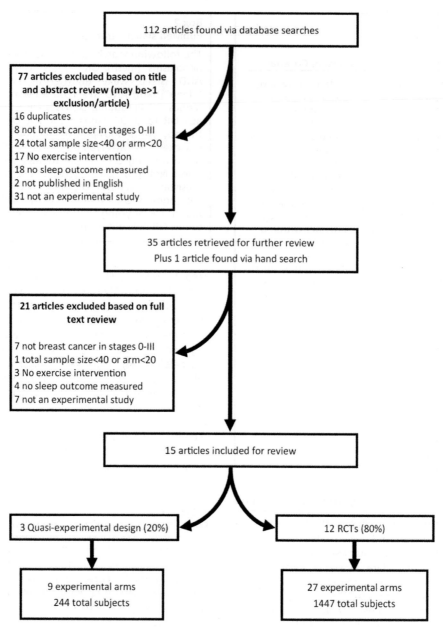

Fig. 1. Flowchart of study selection process.

design/method quality score was 19 out of a possible 26 points (**Table 4**). Supplemental publications[35–39] referenced in 5 studies[40–44] were used to obtain additional details for quality scores. No studies met all quality criteria, but this does not imply that the studies were of poor quality; rather, the reports were not complete and criteria were only determined from the available information. The original Yates validation study[33] did not identify cut-off scores for high-quality studies, but listed the average total quality scores for "excellent," "average," and "poor" studies as 22.7

(SD = 1.95), 18.71 (SD = 2.25), and 12.10 (SD = 3.17), respectively. Thus, the total score of 12 (80%) of the studies included in this review are considered "excellent" and 3 (20%; scored 19, 21, 22) are "average" quality.

Study Characteristics

Studies varied by geography, design, and sample characteristics (see **Table 2**). Six studies were conducted in the United States[43–48]; 3 in Germany[40,49,50]; 2 in China[51,52]; and 1 each in

Table 2
Study design and sample characteristics

First Author, Year	Study Location	Sample: N = Total Sample, M = Mean Age, Total (±SD), EX Intervention = xx, UC/Other Group = xx	Study Design	TX Status	Cancer Stage: %	Primary Cancer TX (%)
Chandwani et al,[45] 2014	USA	N = 163, M = 51.86, EX/Yoga = 53, EX/Stretching = 56, WLC = 54	3-group RCT	After breast surgery, awaiting 6 wks of XRT	0: 11%, I: 31%, II: 27%, III: 31%	Surgery: 100%, CTX: 64%
Chen et al,[51] 2013	China	N = 96, M = 45.01, EX/Qigong = 49, UC = 47	2-group RCT	After breast surgery, awaiting 5–6 wks of XRT	0: 4.3%, I: 17.4%, II: 34.7%, III: 34.7%	Lumpectomy: 36.7%, Mastectomy: 63.3%, XRT: 100%, 25 Fractions: 78.3%, 30 Fractions: 19.6%, 35 Fractions: 2.2%
Courneya et al,[42] 2014	Canada	N = 301, M = 50 ± 8.7, EX/all groups: STAN EX = 96, HIGH EX = 101, COMB = 104	3-group RCT (multicenter)	During CTX, beginning 1–2 wks before starting CTX and ending 3–4 wks after CTX	I–IIa: 68%, IIb–IIIa: 31.4%	Lumpectomy: 56.4%, Mastectomy: 43.6%, CTX: 100%
Ghavami & Akyolcu,[53] 2017	Turkey	N = 80, M = 48.99 (±9.42), EX/aerobic = 40, UC = 40	2-group RCT	Within 3–18 mo of completing primary TX (surgery, CTX, XRT)	Stage I–III: % not reported	Mastectomy: 96.3%, BCT: 3.8%, CTX: 100%, XRT: 100%
Ho et al,[52] 2016	China	N = 139, M = 48.9, EX/DMT = 69, UC = 70	2-group RCT (single-blind)	During XRT	0: 7%, I: 25%, II: 42%, III: 24%, Missing: 2%	Simple mastectomy: 8%, BCT surgery: 42%, MRM surgery: 50%

(continued on next page)

Table 2
(continued)

First Author, Year	Study Location	Sample N = Total Sample M = Mean Age, Total (±SD) EX Intervention = xx UC/Other Group = xx	Study Design	TX Status	Cancer Stage: %	Primary Cancer TX (%)
Kiecolt-Glaser et al,[46] 2014	USA	N = 200 M = 51.6 (±9.2) EX/Yoga = 100 UC = 100	2-group RCT	Within 2–36 mo of completing primary TX (surgery, CTX, XRT)	0: 9% I: 45% IIA: 26% IIB: 11% III: 9%	Surgery only: 13% Surgery + XRT: 26% Surgery + CTX: 23% Surgery + XRT + CTX: 38%
Kröz et al,[49] 2017	Germany	N = 126 M = 59.8 (±9.8) EX/AT = 28 MT = 44 EX/CT = 54	3-group pragmatic trial allocation by randomization or participant preference (multicenter)	≤45 mo from BC diagnosis and ≥36 mo after completing primary TX (surgery, CTX, XRT)	0: 2% I: 61% II: 21% III: 11% Missing: 5%	Surgery: 83% XRT: 64% CTX: 42%
Larkey et al,[47] 2015	USA	N = 87 M = 58.8 (±8.94) EX/QG-TCE = 42 SQG = 45	2-group RCT (double-blind)	Within 6–60 mo of completing primary TX (surgery, CTX, XRT)	I: 39.08% II: 45.98% III: 3.45%	Primary cancer TX not reported; estrogen suppressive therapy: 68.97%
Lötzke et al,[50] 2016	Germany	N = 92 M = 51.2 EX/Yoga = 45 EX/PEI = 47	2-group RCT	During (neo)adjuvant CTX and endocrine TX	Stage I–III (% not reported)	CTX only: 67% XRT only: 1% Endocrine TX only: 4% XRT + endocrine TX: 16% CTX + XRT + endocrine TX: 4.3%

Study	Country	Sample	Design	Timing	Stage	Treatment
Mock et al,[48] 1997	USA	N = 46 M = 49.24 EX/walking = 22 UC = 24	2-group, pre-, posttest, experimental design	After surgery, awaiting XRT	I: 72% II: 28%	BCT surgery: 100% XRT: 100%
Rogers et al,[44] 2009	USA	N = 41 M = 53 (±9) EX/walking = 21 UC = 20	2-group RCT	≥8 wks after surgery, currently taking aromatase inhibitor or estrogen receptor modulator	I: 29% II: 51% III: 20%	Surgery: 100% CTX: 83% XRT: 82% Hormonal TX: 100%
Rogers et al,[43] 2015	USA	N = 46 M = 56.2 (±7.7) EX/aerobic = 22 UC = 24	2-group RCT	≥4 wks after completing primary TX	DCIS: 18.2% I: 47.7% II: 34.1%	XRT: 63.6% CTX: 40.9% Hormonal TX: 52.3%
Roveda et al,[41] 2017	Italy	N = 42 M = 55.2 (±6.8) EX/walking = 21 Usual activity = 21	2-group RCT (multicenter)	Mastectomy or conservative surgery for primary BC, any type, within the previous 5 y	"Early-stage BC"	Surgery:100%
Steindorf et al,[40] 2017	Germany	N = 160 M = 55.6 (±9) EX = 80 Relaxation control = 80 EX/HW = 25	2-group RCT, with age-matched HW controls	After lumpectomy or mastectomy awaiting XRT	0: 9.4% I: 51.3% IIa: 22.5% IIb: 7.5% III: 9.2%	BCT surgery: 86.9% Mastectomy: 13.1% XRT (boost/3D/IMRT): 100% CTX: 35.6% Hormone therapy: 48.8%
Wang et al,[54] 2011	Taiwan	N = 72 M = 50.42 (±9.64) EX/walking = 35 UC = 37	2-group quasi-experimental, longitudinal RM design	After surgery and during CTX	I: 22.2% II: 77.8%	BCT surgery: 41.7% MRM surgery: 50% Simple mastectomy: 8.3%

Abbreviations: AT, aerobic training; BC, breast cancer; BCT, breast-conserving therapy; CG, control group; COMB, combined dose of aerobic and multimodal program together; CTX, chemotherapy; DCIS, ductal carcinoma in situ; DMT, dance movement therapy; EX, exercise group; HIGH EX, higher dose of aerobic exercise; HW EX, healthy women exercise group; IG, intervention group; IMRT, intensity-modulated radiation therapy; M, mean; MRM, modified radical mastectomy surgery; MT, multimodal program; N, number; PEI, physical exercise intervention; QG/TCE, qigong and tai chi easy; RCT, randomized controlled trial; RM, repeated measures; SQG, sham Qigong; STAN EX, "standard dose" of aerobic exercise; TX, treatment; UC, usual care; WL/WLC, waitlist/waitlist control; XRT, radiotherapy; YI, yoga intervention.

Table 3
Intervention characteristics and results

First Author, Year	Exercise and Control Groups	Components and Intensity (Description in Text)	Session Length (minutes)	Frequency/Week	Duration	Total Supervised Intervention Time = Session Length (min) × Frequency/wk × Duration (wk)	Adherence	Sleep and Other Measures	Effect on Sleep	Effect on Other Outcomes
Chandwani et al,[45] 2014	Yoga Stretching WLC	Yoga included: (1) preparatory warm-up synchronized with breathing; (2) selected postures (asana); (3) deep relaxation (supine posture); (4) alternate-nostril breathing (pranayama); (5) meditation. Stretching included standing, lying down, sitting positions with horizontal arm stretch, breast stroke, neck stretch, "throwing football" movements	Yoga and stretching: 60	Up to 3/wk	6 wks during XRT	60 × 3 × 6 = 1080 An audio CD and written manual was provided to encourage at-home practice; a practice log monitored length/frequency of practice	87% of yoga and 85% stretching groups attended ≥12 classes and at 1-, 3-, and 6-mo, 71%, 55%, and 45% of yoga and 53%, 69%, and 60% of stretching practice >2 times/week outside class	Sleep: PSQI QOL: FACT-G Fatigue: BFI Depression: CES-D	There were no significant group differences at any time point for PSQI scores	Compared with the WLC, the yoga and stretching groups had a reduction in fatigue (P<.05); the physical component of QOL increased in the yoga group at 1 and 3 mo; there was no group differences in depression.
Chen et al,[51] 2013	Qigong WLC	Intensity level not reported; Qigong exercise included shallow squatting movements, gentle arm movements, walk in a circle synchronizing breathing, arm movements, and steps focusing on body movement to calm one's mind, relax parts of the body and the mind, and revitalizing the qi (life-force); first done slowly and then fast using windlike breathing	Qigong: 40	1/wk	5 sessions over 5-6 wks during XRT	40 × 1 × 5 = 200 A DVD recording and written materials were provided to encourage practice qigong at home	30.4% of women attended 100% of the sessions, 65.2% attended ≥80%, 78.3% attended ≥50%, and ≥13.0% attended <20% of the sessions	Sleep: PSQI QOL: FACT-G Fatigue: BFI Depression: CES-D	No significant group difference was found for sleep disturbance.	Women in the qigong group reported less depressive symptoms over time than the control group (P = .05). Women with less depressive symptoms at the onset of XRT reported less fatigue (P<.01) and better overall QOL in the qigong compared to control group (P<.05).

Study	Intervention	Session duration (min)	Frequency	Duration	Total dose	Adherence	Outcome measures	Sleep results	Other results
Courneya et al.,[42] 2014	STAN: 25–30 min of aerobic exercise. HIGH: 50–60 min of aerobic exercise. COMB: 50–60 min of combined aerobic and resistance exercise	STAN: 25–30 HIGH: 50–60 COMB: 50–60	STAN: 3/wk HIGH: 3/wk COMB: 3/wk	The mean duration of CTX and intervention was 16.4 wk, resulting in an average of 49 possible exercise sessions.	STAN: 25–30 × 3 × 16.4 = 1230 to 1476 HIGH: 50–60 × 3 × 16.4 = 2460 to 2952 COMB: 50–60 × 3 × 16.4 = 2460 to 2952	STAN, HIGH, and COMB completed 88% (43/49), 82% (40/49), and 78% (39/50) of their supervised exercise sessions.	Sleep: PSQI (global and component scores, without the sleep disturbance component)	HIGH was superior to STAN group for global sleep quality (mean group difference = −0.90; 95% CI −0.05 to −1.76; $P = .039$), subjective sleep quality ($P = .028$; $d = 0.26$), and sleep latency ($P = .049$; $d = 0.18$). COMB was superior to STAN for sleep efficiency ($P = .040$; $d = 0.24$) and % of poor sleepers ($P = .045$; $d = 0.20$)	Not assessed
Ghavami & Akyolcu,[53] 2017	EX: supervised aerobic exercise + individualized weekly healthy eating advice. UC: continue usual routine	EX: moderate-intensity aerobic exercise including 10 min light aerobic warm-up, 30 min aerobic exercise at intensity of 70%–85% of heart rate reserve, and 10 min cool-down (10 + 30 + 10 = 50 total)	EX: 50	3–5/wk	24 wk	50 × 3–5 × 24 = 3600 to 6000	Adherence data not reported	Sleep: PSQI (Persian version) QOL: EORTC QLQ-BR23 Fatigue: CFS	From pre-post intervention, mean PSQI scores in the EX group decreased more than the UC group ($P<.001$)	From pre-post intervention, mean CFS scores in the EX group decreased more than the UC group ($P<.001$); also from pre-post intervention, QOL functional and symptom subscale scores in the EX group improved more than the UC group ($P<.001$)
Ho et al.,[52] 2016	DMT: dance movement therapy. UC	DMT: intensity level not reported; included tailored stretching, relaxation exercises, movement games and rhythmic body movement to exercise the upper extremities, improvisational dance and movement to explore positive emotions	EX: 90	2/wk	3 wk	90 × 2 × 3 = 540	Over 90% attended 5 or more sessions	Sleep: PSQI QOL: FACT-BC Fatigue: BFI Depression: HADS	No significant effect of DMT on sleep disturbance between groups ($P = .24$).	No significant effect of DMT on QOL, fatigue severity, fatigue interference, or depression between groups ($P = $ ns).

(continued on next page)

Table 3
(continued)

First Author, Year	Exercise and Control Groups	Components and Intensity (Description in Text)	Session Length (minutes)	Frequency/ Week	Duration	Total Supervised Intervention Time = Session Length (min) × Frequency/wk × Duration (wk)	Adherence	Sleep and Other Measures	Effect on Sleep	Effect on Other Outcomes
Kiecolt-Glaser et al,[46] 2014	Hatha yoga WLC	Intensity level not reported; Yoga included various poses on the floor, standing, seated, restorative, and breathing practices; investigators state that aerobic or resistance exercise was not included	90	2/wk	12 wk	90 × 2 × 12 = 2160 Home practice was encouraged, women recorded total home plus class practice in weekly logs.	Women in the yoga group attended a mean of 18.1/24 classes (75.4%) with a median of 19 (79.1%), and reported a mean of 24.69 min per day of total home plus class practice across 12 wk.	*Sleep: PSQI* Fatigue: MFSI-SF Depression: CES-D	After adjusting for baseline levels, the yoga group reported improved sleep compared with the control group ($P = .03$).	At 3-mo post-treatment, fatigue was lower in the yoga group ($P = .002$; Cohen's $d = 0.36$); there were no group differences in fatigue immediately post-intervention. Groups did not differ on depression at any time point.

			Supervised: / Home:	Frequency	Sessions	Dose calculation	Home practice	Outcomes	Sleep results	Fatigue results
Kröz et al,[49] 2017	AT: aerobic training alone MT: nonexercise multimodal therapy (sleep education, psycho-education, eurythmy and painting therapy) alone CT: combination of MT + AT	AT: intensity level not reported; aim was to improve endurance and physical performance and improve fatigue; initially, trainer evaluated performance by ergometric monitoring of heart rate as steps increased by 25 W every 2 min; during training, performance adjustments were made on the basis of heart rate monitor watches; specifics about types of exercise were not reported	Supervised: 45 Home: 30–45	Estimated 1/wk	8 sessions (over 10 wk)	AT: supervised sessions: 45 × 1 × 8 = 360 Home: 30–45 × 3–5 × 8 = 720 to 1800 (MT = 1450 and CT = 1810 minutes over a 10-week period as estimated by investigators)	AT group home practice averaged 223 ± 179 min/wk (low adherence rate of 67%); CT group home practice averaged 155 min/wk (low adherence rate of 52.3%).	*Sleep: PSQI* *Fatigue: CFS-D* (German versions)	The standardize effect sizes of PSQI scores for the AT, MT, and CT group for change from baseline to post-intervention (T1) were 0.29, 0.83, and 0.64, respectively; and 0.09, 0.69, and 0.79 for the change from baseline to 6 mo (T2), respectively. Compared to AT, the CT group had greater improvements at T2 in PSQI total score ($P = .007$), subjective sleep quality ($P = .041$), sleep latency ($P = .0296$), and sleep duration ($P = .036$). Compared to AT, the MT group had greater improvement in PSQI total score at T1 ($P = .044$) and T2 ($P = .047$) and at T1 in sleep latency ($P = .004$).	The effect sizes of the fatigue scores in the AT, MT, and CT group for change from baseline to post-intervention (T1) were 0.72, 1.16, and 0.98, respectively; and 0.39, 1.18, and 0.90 for the change from baseline to 6 mo (T2), respectively. Compared to AT, the MT group had greater improvements at T2 in CFS total score ($P = .004$), CFS physical subscale ($P = .003$), and in CFS affective subscale at both T1 ($P = .004$) and T2 ($P = .004$).
Larkey et al,[47] 2015	QG-TCE: Qigong and Tai Chi Easy Control: Sham Qigong (SQG; without breathing and meditative aspects of QG-TCE)	QG and TC moves and postures described as low-impact with a low-to-moderate level of aerobic exertion. Movements for the QG-TCE intervention and SQG control included reaching with the arms upward, outwards, sideways, and in arcs; swaying and circling shoulders and hips; and slow, relaxed dancelike flowing movements alternating with a few muscle-tightening, isometric movements	Supervised: 60 Home: 30	2/wk in wk 1–2; 1/wk in wk 3–12 Home: 5 sessions/wk	12 wk	Supervised: 60 × 2 × 2 + 60 × 1 × 10 = *840* Home practice: 30 × 5 × 12 = *1800* (A DVD with 10 core exercises and written instruction was provided to encourage home practice; a log monitored length/frequency of home practice and class times)	QG-TCE mean total minutes practiced = 1290 ± 1106; SQG = 1194 ± 617, $P = 613$	*Sleep: PSQI* *Fatigue: FSI* *Depression: BDI*	There was no difference in sleep improvement by group, but sleep improved over time for both interventions ($P<.05$)	Fatigue decreased significantly in the QG-TCE group compared to control at post-intervention ($P = .005$) and 3 mo follow-up ($P = .024$). There was no difference in depression by group, but improvement in depression occurred for both interventions over time ($P<.05$).

(continued on next page)

Table 3
(continued)

First Author, Year	Exercise and Control Groups	Components and Intensity (Description in Text)	Session Length (minutes)	Frequency/Week	Duration	Total Supervised Intervention Time = Session Length (min) × Frequency/wk × Duration (wk)	Adherence	Sleep and Other Measures	Effect on Sleep	Effect on Other Outcomes
Lötzke et al,[50] 2016	Yoga: Iyengar (Hatha) Yoga PEI: a physical exercise intervention	Yoga: intensity not reported; consisted of Iyengar (Hatha) yoga with traditional elements (positions and breath control) with use of props (eg, blocks) to keep positions PEI: intensity not reported; consisted of a 60-min physical exercise session	Yoga and PEI: Supervised: 60 Home: 20	Supervised: 1/wk Home: 2/wk	12 wk	Supervised: 60 × 1 × 12 = 720 Home: 20 × 2 × 12 = 480 (Written instructions provided; participants completed an exercise protocol for home practice)	Adherence not reported; high drop-out rate: 29 in yoga and 22 from PEI, total of 54 patients dropped out (59%)	*Sleep:* EORTC-QLQ-C30 sleep subscale *Fatigue:* CFS-D + EORTC-QLQ-C30 sleep subscale	No significant changes over time in sleep disturbance and no differences in sleep disturbance by group	Fatigue improved from baseline to 3 mo in PEI ($P < .05$) but not yoga group QOL (role and emotional functioning subscales) improved from baseline to post-intervention in yoga group ($P < .001$)
Mock et al,[48] 1997	EX: Walking UC	Walking: intensity not reported; self-paced, brisk 20–30 min walk, followed by 5 min slow (cool down) walking	25–35	4–5/wk	6 wk	25–35 × 4–5 × 6 = 600 to 1050	86% reported exercising	*Sleep:* SAS *Fatigue:* PFS *Depression:* SAS	Compared to UC, the walking group showed greater improvement in difficulty sleeping in the pre to post-test values ($P = .027$).	Compared to UC, the walking group showed greater improvement in total fatigue and fatigue level in the pre to post-test values ($P = .018$), but there were no group differences in depression pre- to post-test values.
Rogers et al,[44] 2009	EX: Walking UC	EX: behavior change intervention included group discussion, face-to-face counselling, home-based walking (moderate intensity); goal was to increase to 150 min of moderate walking in 12 wk UC: received physical activity materials from the American Cancer Society	Self-guided	Supervised: 3/wk in wk 1–2; 2/wk in wk 3–4; 1/wk in wk 5–6 Home: 2/wk in wk 3–4; 3/wk in wk 5–6; 5/wk in wk 7–12	12 wk	Session length variable or self-guided; goal was to reach 150/wk by week 12 (Physical activity was recorded in weekly exercise logs)	Intervention participants completed 100% (252/252) of the individual exercise sessions, 95% (60/63) of the individual update sessions, and 98% (123/126) of the group sessions for an overall 99% adherence to all possible intervention sessions (435/441).	*Sleep:* PSQI *QOL:* FACT-BC	No significant group, time, or group by time interaction was noted for sleep (total or subscales) with the exception of a significant group effect for sleep latency ($F = 4.17$; $P = .048$).	No significant group by time interactions were noted for overall QOL.

| Rogers et al,[43] 2015 | EX: aerobic and strength training Control: "maintain usual exercise behaviours" | EX: supervised, on-site treadmill aerobic walking of moderate intensity and resistance training, plus home-based aerobic walking, not necessarily on a treadmill (moderate intensity based on Karvonen method) | Not reported | Variable frequency; 26 planned supervised exercise sessions | 12 wk | Session lengths variable or self-guided; goal was to increase to 40 min of moderate intensity walking 4/wk by week 9 with supervised resistance training 2/wk; home exercise included 2/wk walking sessions in wk 3-12 | Adherence to supervised aerobic exercise sessions was 91% and adherence to the resistance exercise sessions was 93% (based on session record sheets). | *Sleep: PSQI, PROMIS® sleep, actigraphy,* PROMIS® Fatigue, Depression, | PSQI sleep duration (less sleep/night) demonstrated a difference between the intervention compared with control group (+0.2 versus-0.4. *d* = 0.73, *P*<.05). PSQI daytime somnolence (higher score indicate greater daytime somnolence) showed group difference for the intervention vs control group being −0.5 vs −0.1, *d* = −0.63, *P* = .05). No significance between groups differences were noted for other PSQI outcomes, PROMIS® sleep disturbance, actigraphic efficiency/latency. | Exercise intervention effect sizes for fatigue were: fatigue intensity *d* = 0.30 (*P* = .34), interference *d* = −0.38 (*P* = .22), and general fatigue *d* = −0.49 (*P* = .13) |

(continued on next page)

Table 3 (*continued*)

First Author, Year	Exercise and Control Groups	Components and Intensity (Description in Text)	Session Length (minutes)	Frequency/Week	Duration	Total Supervised Intervention Time = Session Length (min) × Frequency/wk × Duration (wk)	Adherence	Sleep and Other Measures	Effect on Sleep	Effect on Other Outcomes
Roveda et al,[41] 2017	EX: walking Control: recommended "30 min of daily physical activity"	Moderate (1-h brisk walking)	60 brisk walking + 10 cool-down static stretching	Supervised: 2/wk	12 wk	70 × 2 × 12 = 1680	The adherence to PA was 86.8 ± 4.9% of the total numbers of training sessions).	*Sleep: Actigraph actiwatch × 1 wk, sleep diary*	Overall, the CG showed a deterioration of sleep, whereas the EX group showed a stable pattern. From pre- to post-intervention, sleep efficiency decreased significantly in the CG (*P*<.01) but was unchanged in the EX group. Both groups showed a reduction in actual sleep time from pre- to post-intervention (*P* = .03), but no interaction between time and group. Compared to the CG, where sleep latency (*P* = .46) and sleep fragmentation (*P* = .02) increased from pre-to post-intervention, sleep latency in the EX group did not change and fragmentation showed a less pronounced change (*P* = .02).	Not assessed

Study	Intervention / Control	Exercise details		Frequency	Duration	Total dose	Adherence	Measures	Sleep results	Fatigue/QOL results
Steindorf et al,[40] 2017	EX: resistance strength training in BC and age-matched HW; Control: progressive muscle relaxation	EX: intensity not reported; 8 different machine-based progressive resistance exercises (3 sets of 8–12 repetitions at 60%–80% of one repetition maximum)	EX and relaxation control: 60	2/wk	12 wk	$60 \times 2 \times 12 = 1440$	Adherence was similar in both BC groups. Of 24 scheduled sessions, the median attended = 19 (range 13–23) in EX group and 19 (range 12–22) in BC CG.	Sleep: FAQ global sleep problem item, EORTC-QLQ-C30 insomnia subscale, and sleep characteristic items: sleep duration, awakenings, and prolonged sleep latency/wk (German versions)	Compared to the relaxation control, the BC EX group reported decreased global sleep problems from baseline to the end of XRT ($P = .03$) and to the end of the intervention ($P = .005$) even when adjusting for cofounders. There were no significant intervention effects on frequency of any sleep characteristics.	Physical fatigue showed a significant association with sleep problems ($P = .003$).
Wang et al,[54] 2011	EX: walking UC	EX: walking described as low-moderate as measured by a heart rate maximum	30	3–5/wk	6 wk	$30 \times 3{-}5 \times 6 = 540{-}900$ (Walking activity was recorded in weekly exercise logs by participants)	Study completion rate was 80.6% with good adherence (n = 58, 93.6%). The number and % of sample that were non-adherent was low for exercise intensity (1, 3.3%), frequency (2, 6.7%), and time (2, 6.7%)	Sleep: PSQI Fatigue: FACIT-F QOL: FACT-G version 4	Hierarchical linear model analysis indicated that the EX had less sleep disturbance than the UC group over the 4 time points (linear growth rate, $P<.001$) and (quadratic growth rate, $P = .006$).	The EX had a more improvement in and a stable pattern of QOL compared to the UC group (linear growth rate, $P<.001$) and (quadratic growth rate, $P = .011$). Participants in the EX had significantly less fatigue than the UC group after the exercise intervention ($P = .003$).

Abbreviations: AT, aerobic training; BCT, breast conserving therapy; BDI, beck depression inventory; BFI, brief fatigue inventory; CBT-I, cognitive behavioral therapy intervention; CES-D, center for epidemiologic studies depression scale; CFS-D, cancer fatigue scale; CG, control group; COMB, combined dose of aerobic and resistance; CT, aerobic training and multimodal program together; EX, exercise group; FACIT-F, functional assessment of chronic illness treatment-fatigue; FACT-BC, FACT-G, functional assessment of cancer therapy - breast cancer/general; FAQ, fatigue assessment questionnaire; FSI, fatigue symptom inventory; HADS, hospital anxiety and depression scale; HIGH, higher dose of aerobic exercise; HW, healthy women; IG, intervention group; IMRT, intensity modulated radiation therapy; MFSI-SF, multidimensional fatigue symptom inventory-short form; MRM, modified radical mastectomy surgery; MT, multimodal program; N, total sample size; PEI, physical exercise intervention; PFS, piper fatigue scale; PROMIS, patient reported outcomes measurement information system; PSQI, Pittsburgh sleep quality index; QG/TCE, qigong and tai chi easy; QOL, quality of life; RT, radiation therapy; SAS, symptom assessment scales; SQG, sham Qigong; STAN, "standard dose"; TCC, Tai chi chih; UC, usual care; WLC, waitlist control; YI, yoga intervention.

Table 4
Total and subscale quality ratings by study using Yates Quality Rating Scale

Author, Year	Treatment Quality Subscore	Quality of Design and Methods Subscore	Total Score
Chandwani et al,[45] 2014	7	22	29
Chen et al,[51] 2013	6	18	24
Courneya et al,[42] 2014	5	23	28
Ghavami & Akyolcu,[53] 2017	3	18	21
Ho et al,[52] 2016	5	21	26
Kiecolt-Glaser et al,[46] 2014	9	21	30
Kröz et al,[49] 2017	6	19	25
Larkey et al,[47] 2015	8	24	32
Lötzke et al,[50] 2016	4	18	22
Mock et al,[48] 1997	8	16	24
Rogers et al,[44] 2009	8	20	28
Rogers et al,[43] 2015	5	19	24
Roveda et al,[41] 2017	5	14	19
Steindorf et al,[40] 2017	5	22	27
Wang et al,[54] 2011	5	17	22

Data from Yates SL, Morley S, Eccleston C, et al. A scale for rating the quality of psychological trials for pain. Pain 2005;117(3):314–25.

Canada,[42] Turkey,[53] Italy,[41] and Taiwan.[54] Twelve of 15 studies were RCT (80%)[40–47,50–53] and 3 were nonrandomized experimental designs.[48,49,54] Most studies (n = 12) used a 2-group design whereas 2 RCT[42,45] and 1 pragmatic trial[49] used a 3-group design. One 3-group RCT included a stretching control group with exercises structurally similar to the gross movements used in the yoga intervention, plus a waitlist control group.[45] A second 3-group RCT assigned participants to the following: (1) a "standard" condition that followed the Physical Activity Guidelines for Americans[55] minimum of 75 min/wk of vigorous aerobic exercise spread over 3 d/wk, (2) a "high" group condition that doubled the minimum guidelines to 150 min/wk over 3 d/wk, or (3) a "combined" group that followed the standard guidelines plus a strength training program over 3 d/wk. A third 3-group pragmatic trial evaluated the effectiveness of a nonexercise multimodal therapy separately, and in combination with aerobic training, compared with aerobic training alone.[49]

Total sample sizes ranged from 41 to 301 participants. Four studies had samples of 40 to 50,[41,43,44,48] 5 studies had samples of 51 to 100,[47,50,51,53,54] and 6 had samples of 101 to 301.[40,42,45,46,49,52] All studies reported pre- and posttreatment assessments. Six studies[40,42,43,48,51,54] had additional assessments during the intervention phase and 8 studies

reported follow-up assessments at 1 month,[46] 3 months,[44,47,50,51] and 6 to 12 months[40,45,49] after the postintervention assessment.

The authors carefully noted control conditions because good quality control groups should be matched to the general structure of the intervention group,[33] and control conditions can pose threats to internal validity.[56] Only 4[42,45,47,50] of the included studies used a structurally matched control group with equal length to the intervention group. Of the remaining studies, 6 included only usual care as a control[43,44,48,52–54] and 3 had a wait list control group.[45,46,51] Participants in 2 control groups were instructed to either maintain usual exercise behaviors[43] or exercise 30 minutes a day.[41] One study used a group relaxation as the comparison.[40]

Participants

Participants ranged in age from 45 to 60 years, with a mean of 52 years across all studies (see **Table 2**). Given the inclusion criteria for this review, participants were women with stage 0–III breast cancer. As seen in **Fig. 2**, cancer stage was specified in 10 studies.[40,44–49,51,52,54] At the time of the study, 67% of participants in 10 studies were receiving cancer treatment[40,42,44,45,48,50–54], whereas some participants (27%) were undergoing treatment in 4 studies[41,43,47,49] and all participants had completed treatment in one study.[46]

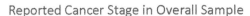

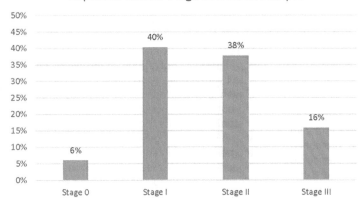

Fig. 2. Cancer stage (%) in combined study samples.

Of the 1691 participants included in this review, most underwent surgery (85%), more than half received chemotherapy (65%), and 68% received multiple, concurrent cancer treatments (**Fig. 3**).

Exercise Interventions

Interventions in this review varied in components, frequency, and intensity. In 6 studies, interventions were depicted as aerobic or included an aerobic component.[41–43,47,49,53] Two studies described interventions as moderate intensity walking[43] or aerobic walking.[41] Of the remaining studies, self-paced walking interventions not specifically described as aerobic were used in 3 studies.[44,48,54] Three studies tested the effects of yoga[45,46,50] and 2 studies examined qigong.[47,51] One study tested the effects of dance movement[52] and another study tested machine-based progressive resistance training to improve muscle strength.[40] Two studies integrated aerobic exercise with strength training.[37,47] Kröz and colleagues[49] combined aerobic exercise with multimodal therapy (ie, psychoeducation, sleep education, eurythmy therapy, and painting therapy), and Ghavami & Akyolcu[53] combined healthy eating education with aerobic exercise.

Exercise intensity was not reported in 8 studies.[40,45,46,48–52] Four studies identified the intervention as moderate intensity exercise[41,43,44,53] and 2 described low-moderate levels of intensity.[47,54] Only one study described vigorous aerobic exercise.[42] Intensity levels were not reported in any yoga studies,[45,46,50] but postures were included as the primary component combined with breathing.[5,46,50]

Exercise frequency ranged from one supervised session[49–51] to 3 to 5 sessions per week.[53] Three studies progressively lowered the frequency of supervised sessions from 2 to 3 per week to 1 to 2 per week supplemented by home-based exercise.[43,44,47] The most frequent number of weekly

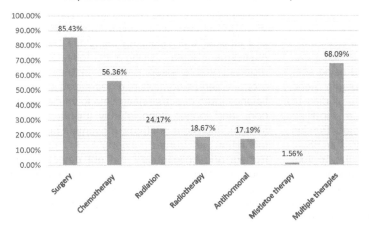

Fig. 3. Cancer treatments (%) in combined study samples.

sessions was 2[40,41,46,52] or 3.[42,45] The duration of the intervention ranged from 3 weeks[52] to 12 weeks, which was the most frequent duration (n = 7 studies).[40,41,43,44,46,47,50] Individual session lengths ranged from 25 to 35 minutes[42,48] to 90 minutes.[46,52]

Adherence to Exercise

The World Health Organization defines adherence as the extent to which an individual's health behavior correlates with health care provider's recommendations.[57] On average, adherence to treatments for chronic illness is estimated to be 50% in developed countries.[57] Adherence to exercise is reported typically as supervised session attendance or self-reported practice, but consensus about the best way to define and operationalize adherence has not been established.[58] In this review, the authors report adherence and attendance levels as described in the studies. Twelve studies provided some adherence data; but 3 studies did not report adherence data.[47,50,53] Adherence to interventions ranged from 52% for home-based exercise training[49] to 99% in a self-guided walking program.[44] Three studies reported greater than or equal to 90% adherence postintervention.[43,44,54] Four studies reported greater than or equal to 80% intervention adherence or attendance.[40,41,48,52] Chandwani and colleagues[45] initially had high class attendance (87% attended ≥12 yoga classes); yet home-based practice dropped from 71% at 1 month to 45% at 6 months. Chen and colleagues[51] categorized adherence as "high," with 30% of participants attending all sessions and 78% attending at least 50% of the 25 to 30 qigong sessions. One yoga study[46] had an average attendance of 75%, whereas a combined aerobic with resistance study[42] reported resistance session attendance of 66% and 98% for the prescribed weight, sets, and repetitions. Overall, adherence, measured as session attendance or reported practice, was usually more than 65%.

Sleep Outcomes

Most sleep outcomes were assessed using self-reported measurements. The Pittsburgh Sleep Quality Index (PSQI) was used in 11 studies to measure sleep quality, including a modified version of the PSQI,[42] and a validated Persian version of the PSQI.[53] In addition to the PSQI, Rogers and colleagues[43,44] included the 16-item Patient-Reported Outcomes Measurement Information System (PROMIS) sleep-wake disturbance scale in 2 studies. Only 2 studies used actigraph accelorometers,[41,43] where objective sleep data

were collected for 7 days at baseline and again at a 3-month follow-up. Key actigraphic parameters included sleep latency,[41,43] sleep efficiency,[41,43] actual awake time, immobility time, mean activity score, and movement and fragmentation index.[41] Actigraphy data were supplemented with a daily sleep diary.[41,43]

Eleven studies found that exercise improved sleep outcomes. Four of the integrative intervention studies, yoga,[45,50] qigong,[51] or dance movement[52] found no group differences in sleep outcomes at postintervention. Interventions with a moderate-vigorous aerobic component consistently improved sleep-related outcomes.[42,43,49,53] For example, vigorous aerobic exercise combined with strength training was superior to vigorous aerobic exercise alone (standard dose group) in improving sleep efficiency and reducing the number of poor sleepers ($P<.05$).[42] In addition, a vigorous aerobic exercise twice the duration of the standard aerobic exercise resulted in greater improvements in the modified global PSQI sleep quality score and sleep latency component score ($P<.05$).[42] Similarly, combined aerobic and strength training in another study improved the sleep duration component score ($P<.05$).[43] In yet another study, the combination of aerobic training and multimodal, nonexercise therapy resulted in greater improvements in the global PSQI sleep quality score and component scores of sleep quality, latency, and duration ($P<.05$) compared with aerobic training alone.[49] Compared with aerobic training alone, the nonexercise therapy alone improved the global PSQI score ($P<.05$), and sleep latency component score, but only at one time (after 10 weeks of intervention).[49] An RCT with a lifestyle intervention program that included supervised aerobic exercise sessions versus usual care showed that the exercise combined with nutrition counseling improved PSQI sleep quality score ($P<.001$).[53]

Among trials evaluating walking interventions, participants reported less sleep disturbances ($P<.01$),[54] shorter sleep onset latency ($P<.05$),[44] and less difficulty sleeping using the Symptom Assessment Scale.[48] Using actigraphy, Roveda[41] reported stable sleep patterns in the walking group, whereas controls had decreased sleep efficiency (ratio of actual sleep time to time spent in bed), and longer sleep latency (minutes to fall asleep), and more nocturnal movement and fragmentation (disrupted sleep).[41] In contrast, Rogers and colleagues[43] did not detect differences in actigraphic sleep latency and efficiency between the aerobic walking with resistance training group compared with controls (exercise avoidance).

Resistance training alone decreased global sleep problems assessed with a single item on the Fatigue Assessment Questionnaire (P<.05) from baseline to the end of radiotherapy treatment compared with group-based relaxation.[40] Yoga was efficacious in improving sleep as measured by the PSQI in only one study.[46] Both combined qigong and tai chi (QG-TCE) and sham qigong (without the breathing and meditative components of QG-TCE) improved sleep over time for both intervention and control groups (P<.05).[47] Similarly, no significant group differences in sleep parameters were found between qigong and wait list controls from baseline to 3 months follow-up.[51]

Co-occurring Fatigue and Depression

Because fatigue frequently co-occurs with sleep deficiency, particularly in those with cancer,[59] 12 studies reported fatigue outcomes. Seven of the 12 studies reported that exercise improved fatigue,[43,45–49,53,54] and 2 studies did not find a difference.[50,52] In 3 studies, fatigue was considered a contributing factor to sleep deficiency,[40] a baseline symptom for group differences,[51] or a mediator of daytime somnolence.[43] Two yoga studies reported lower fatigue postintervention,[45,46] and 1 of the 2 qigong/tai chi studies found a significant decrease in fatigue levels compared with sham qigong.[47] Overall, some studies indicated that walking and other exercises combined with mindfulness-based components,[49] supportive group membership,[48] phone calls,[54] or education[53] may be efficacious in reducing fatigue.

Depression was another frequently co-occurring symptom in 7 of the 15 studies.[43,45–48,51,52] Five studies reported no group differences in depression with exercise.[45–48,52] Rogers and colleagues[43] examined baseline depression scores as a mediating factor for fatigue scores, where higher baseline depression scores were more likely to have favorable fatigue outcome postintervention. Similarly, Chen at al.[51] found that women with higher depressive symptoms at the start of treatment reported lower fatigue and better overall quality of life postintervention. These 2 studies suggest that baseline depression levels moderate the fatigue outcomes.

DISCUSSION
Summary of Evidence

This systematic review summarizes the most current evidence from 12 RCT and 3 nonrandomized experimental trials containing data from 1691 middle-aged women with breast cancer. These studies focused on the effect of various exercise interventions on sleep outcomes across the cancer care continuum. Six studies were published between 2016 and 2017[40,41,49,50,52,53] and 80% of the 15 studies were judged to be of excellent or good quality. This is the first systematic review of exercise to focus exclusively on women with breast cancer, and the first to include exercise-based integrative interventions (eg, yoga). Despite high variability in exercise type, dose, and study methods, 11 (73%) of the studies showed improvement in sleep deficiency and all walking interventions resulted in positive sleep outcomes.

Ten studies reported positive sleep outcomes in the exercise group compared with a control group.[37,40,41,43,44,46,48,49,53,54] Of the 10 studies, 2 combined exercise with nonexercise components[49,53] and 1 qigong study reported sleep improvement over time but no difference between groups.[47] Walking was the most common aerobic intervention in studies showing a positive effect.[41,43,44,48,54] This observation is consistent with conclusions of the reviews of Langford and colleagues[60] and Mercier and colleagues[24] in which walking seemed to have a positive impact on sleep. Among the studies that offered aerobic exercise alternatives to walking, 2 had a positive impact on sleep outcomes.[42,53]

In contrast to the authors' prediction, exercise-based integrative interventions (eg, yoga) showed inconsistent sleep outcomes. Among the 6 studies that offered exercise-based integrative interventions, only 1 yoga and 1 qigong study had significant improvements for sleep.[46,47] It is unclear whether low intensity of these integrative interventions or other factors such as adherence explains the failure to demonstrate sleep improvement. Of note, most integrative interventions (yoga,[46,50] qigong,[51] and dance therapy[52]) failed to report intensity. Overall, it seems that positive sleep outcomes are associated with aerobic exercise and higher intensity exercise. However, the dosage of exercise required to improve sleep is uncertain because only one study compared a higher dose of aerobic exercise to a standard dose.[37]

Although poor sleep can be considered a subjective phenomenon, objective measures provide important additional data that strengthen the body of research on exercise and cancer-related sleep deficiency. Only 2 studies in the current review measured sleep objectively (actigraphy).[41,43] Eleven studies used the PSQI to measure sleep quality over the previous month, which facilitated comparison between studies. Self-report measures that elicit data over shorter periods (previous week), however, may reduce recall bias and improve reliability of subjective sleep data. Additional outcomes can be added to enhance understanding of the broader impact of exercise. For example, the mediation effects of exercise on sleep and long-term outcomes such as return to work and the effect on vehicular and occupational accidents were not evaluated in any studies but should be considered.

Although 5 studies conducted after completion of primary cancer treatment had positive outcomes, studies conducted during chemotherapy,[37,50,54] radiotherapy,[52] or immediately after surgery and before planned radiotherapy[40,45,48,51] also obtained positive sleep outcomes. The 4 studies conducted during treatment that failed to show positive outcomes examined yoga, qigong, and dance.[45,50–52] This finding suggests that outcomes may be influenced more by the type and intensity of exercise rather than the phase of cancer treatment. Exercise seems to be feasible and effective even during cancer treatment. However, replication of these findings is warranted.

Women's past history of sleep deficiency, or present sleep habits, were not evaluated in any studies. Therefore, it is possible that studies without significant sleep effects could be partially explained by a floor effect, with little room for sleep improvement. To avoid a "floor effect," participants in one study were included only if they reported average fatigue greater than or equal to 3 on a 1 to 10 Likert scale or reported sleep disturbance greater than or equal to 1 on a 0 to 3 Likert scale.[43] Two studies included only women with significant fatigue.[47,49] These studies with fatigue and sleep disturbance inclusion criteria reported positive sleep outcomes. Although the impact of menopausal status on sleep outcomes is well established,[61] reproductive stage was not addressed explicitly in any study. Participants in only 1 study were exclusively postmenopausal.[47] Only 4 studies used an active match control group, whereas 9 studies had a usual care or wait list condition. These control conditions can lead to a contamination effect if participants are told to remain physically active without receiving a study exercise intervention.

Exercise interventions varied in frequency and intensity as did participant adherence. Most studies included at least one supervised session and most had 2 to 3 supervised sessions initially or throughout the intervention. Session attendance and postintervention adherence were generally high. Adherence in the included studies did not seem to be related to the number of weekly supervised sessions. Exercise intensity was varied and reported inconsistently. Eight studies failed to describe intervention intensity, including one multimodal[49]; one walking[48]; intervention; and most yoga, qigong, and dance studies.

Researchers and fitness professionals are increasingly using a specific framework for frequency, intensity, time, and type of physical activity and exercise. This is known as the FITT (frequency, intensity, time, and type) principle.[18] Using the FITT principle for reporting, exercise study characteristics will advance the field of cancer-related sleep science and provide important information for clinicians regarding individual interventions. Also, the FITT framework may aid in determining the optimal exercise dose.

Study Strengths/Limitations

The number of current RCTs from multiple countries, the large sample sizes, and the uniform analytical procedures and quality of the studies are strengths of this review. Also, the reviewers followed best practice guidelines for systematic reviews and did not restrict studies by date. Selection bias was avoided with a priori inclusion criteria, systematic search by an experienced medical librarian, and independent evaluation of inclusion by 4 reviewers. However, limitations of this review should be noted. First, because only published English-language studies were included, there is the potential for publication and language bias. Second, although all studies met average or excellent quality criteria, information about exercise intensity, adherence, and contamination was limited, hampering the ability to check whether these features were similar across studies. Third, although all studies included at least one comparison group, only 4 used a structurally matched control group. Fourth, although the authors focused on the shorter postintervention outcomes, studies included multiple follow-up assessments that differed between studies making it difficult to summarize outcomes by time periods. Finally, only 15 studies were ultimately included. Given the low number, the authors did not perform a meta-analysis, which would have provided additional meaningful information.

FUTURE DIRECTIONS

Several implications for future research were identified in this systematic review. Large RCT studies testing the effects of exercise on sleep are needed in women with cancer who receive multimodal cancer treatments. Exercise frequency and intensity need to be examined in future investigations in order to discern the inconsistencies in the findings among the intervention studies. Most of the current evidence relies on self-reported measurements. Future exercise studies will benefit from the use of both objective and subjective sleep measures together with co-occurring symptoms of fatigue and depression. Objective measures, such as actigraphy movement counts and inflammatory biomarkers, will aid in understanding the underlying biological mechanisms of these interventions and provide a more robust explanation of their relationship to sleep outcomes.

Prospective, rigorous RCTs need to test the effects of both supervised and home-based aerobic exercise in multimodal interventions. Specifically, mindfulness-based therapies may have potential to affect sleep-related outcomes. In addition, education and psychological support are important components in future interventions with oncology patients. Not all of the studies collected data on co-occurring symptoms or reported on mediating effects of fatigue and depression on sleep. Concurrent data collection on fatigue and depression together with sleep outcomes can help extrapolate the compounding effects of the intervention on the woman's overall well-being. Future studies also need to include long-term economic benefits and cost analysis of these interventions when providing clinical recommendations.

New cases of cancer are projected to grow by about 70% globally in the next 2 decades.[62] To reduce the negative impact of cancer and its treatment on quality of life, effective, low-cost, non-pharmacological interventions that target sleep and associated symptoms are urgently needed. The overall benefits of regular physical activity are widely accepted and recommended for patients with cancer.[63] Walking and home-based exercises together with psychosocial strategies may be an especially accessible and cost-effective intervention for women with breast cancer and should be recommended routinely during visits with providers.

ACKNOWLEDGMENTS

The authors gratefully acknowledge Sheila Louise Thomas, MA (LS), Medical Research and Clinical Search Services Coordinator, Education & Reference Department, University of Arkansas for Medical Sciences Library, Little Rock, AR for her professional literature search guidance and assistance on the project.

REFERENCES

1. National Institutes of Health. National Institutes of Health Sleep Disorders Research Plan. 2011. Available at: https://www.nhlbi.nih.gov/health-pro/resources/sleep/nih-sleep-disorders-research-plan-2011. Accessed April 11, 2017.

2. Buxton OM, Marcelli E. Short and long sleep are positively associated with obesity, diabetes, hypertension, and cardiovascular disease among adults in the United States. Soc Sci Med 2010;71(5): 1027–36.

3. Palesh OG, Roscoe JA, Mustian KM, et al. Prevalence, demographics, and psychological associations of sleep disruption in patients with cancer: University of Rochester cancer center-community clinical oncology program. J Clin Oncol 2010; 28(2):292–8.

4. Beck SL, Berger AM, Barsevick AM, et al. Sleep quality after initial chemotherapy for breast cancer. Support Care Cancer 2010;18(6):679–89.

5. Lowery-Allison AE, Passik SD, Cribbet MR, et al. Sleep problems in breast cancer survivors 1-10 years posttreatment. Palliat Support Care 2017;1–10. https://doi.org/10.1017/S1478951517000311.

6. Fontes F, Severo M, Goncalves M, et al. Trajectories of sleep quality during the first three years after breast cancer diagnosis. Sleep Med 2017; 34:193–9.

7. Savard J, Ivers H, Villa J, et al. Natural course of insomnia comorbid with cancer: an 18-month longitudinal study. J Clin Oncol 2011;29(26):3580–6.

8. Von Ah D, Tallman EF. Perceived cognitive function in breast cancer survivors: evaluating relationships with objective cognitive performance and other symptoms using the functional assessment of cancer therapy-cognitive function instrument. J Pain Symptom Manage 2015;49(4):697–706.

9. Trudel-Fitzgerald C, Zhou ES, Poole EM, et al. Sleep and survival among women with breast cancer: 30 years of follow-up within the Nurses' Health Study. Br J Cancer 2017;116(9):1239–46.

10. Palesh OG, Aldridge-Gerry A, Zeitzer JM, et al. Actigraphy-measured sleep disruption as a predictor of survival among women with advanced breast cancer. Sleep 2014;37(5):837–42.

11. Kravitz HM, Joffe H. Sleep during the perimenopause: a SWAN story. Obstet Gynecol Clin North Am 2011;38(3):567–86.

12. van Nes JG, Fontein DB, Hille ET, et al. Quality of life in relation to tamoxifen or exemestane treatment in postmenopausal breast cancer patients: a tamoxifen exemestane adjuvant multinational (TEAM) trial side study. Breast Cancer Res Treat 2012;134(1): 267–76.

13. Couzi RJ, Helzlsouer KJ, Fetting JH. Prevalence of menopausal symptoms among women with a history of breast cancer and attitudes toward estrogen replacement therapy. J Clin Oncol 1995;13(11): 2737–44.

14. Palesh O, Scheiber C, Kesler S, et al. Management of side effects during and post-treatment in breast cancer survivors. Breast J 2017. https://doi.org/10.1111/tbj.12862.

15. Sateia MJ, Buysse DJ, Krystal AD, et al. Adverse Effects of Hypnotic Medications. Journal of Clinical Sleep Medicine: JCSM: Official Publication of the American Academy of Sleep Medicine 2017; 13(6):839.

16. Savard J, Ivers H, Savard MH, et al. Long-term effects of two formats of cognitive behavioral therapy for insomnia comorbid with breast cancer. Sleep 2016;39(4):813–23.

17. Garland SN, Johnson JA, Savard J, et al. Sleeping well with cancer: a systematic review of cognitive behavioral therapy for insomnia in cancer patients. Neuropsychiatr Dis Treat 2014;10:1113–24.

18. Bernardo LM, Becker BJ. Exercise and physical activity for people living with cancer: nurses' edition. Pittsburgh (PA): Oncology Nursing Society; 2016.

19. Mishra SI, Scherer RW, Snyder C, et al. Exercise interventions on health-related quality of life for people with cancer during active treatment. Cochrane Database Syst Rev 2012;(8):CD008465.

20. Mishra SI, Scherer RW, Geigle PM, et al. Exercise interventions on health-related quality of life for cancer survivors. Cochrane Database Syst Rev 2012;(8): CD007566.

21. Tang MF, Liou TH, Lin CC. Improving sleep quality for cancer patients: benefits of a home-based exercise intervention. Support Care Cancer 2010;18(10): 1329–39.

22. Coleman EA, Goodwin JA, Kennedy R, et al. Effects of exercise on fatigue, sleep, and performance: a randomized trial. Oncol Nurs Forum 2012;39(5): 468–77.

23. Nimmo MA, Leggate M, Viana JL, et al. The effect of physical activity on mediators of inflammation. Diabetes Obes Metab 2013;15(Suppl 3):51–60.

24. Mercier J, Savard J, Bernard P. Exercise interventions to improve sleep in cancer patients: a systematic review and meta-analysis. Sleep Med Rev 2016; 36:43–56.

25. Mishra SI, Scherer RW, Snyder C, et al. The effectiveness of exercise interventions for improving health-related quality of life from diagnosis through active cancer treatment. Oncol Nurs Forum 2015; 42(1):E33–53.

26. Mishra SI, Scherer RW, Snyder C, et al. Are exercise programs effective for improving health-related quality of life among cancer survivors? A systematic review and meta-analysis. Oncol Nurs Forum 2014; 41(6):E326–42.

27. Furmaniak AC, Menig M, Markes MH. Exercise for women receiving adjuvant therapy for breast cancer. Cochrane Database Syst Rev 2016;(9):CD005001.

28. Eckert R, Huberty J, Gowin K, et al. Physical activity as a nonpharmacological symptom management approach in myeloproliferative neoplasms: recommendations for future research. Integr Cancer Ther 2017;16(4):439–50.

29. Moher D, Liberati A, Tetzlaff J, et al. Preferred reporting items for systematic reviews and meta-analyses: the PRISMA statement. J Clin Epidemiol 2009; 62(10):1006–12.

30. Mustian KM, Cole CL, Lin PJ, et al. Exercise recommendations for the management of symptoms clusters resulting from cancer and cancer treatments. Semin Oncol Nurs 2016;32(4):383–93.

31. Chu P, Gotink RA, Yeh GY, et al. The effectiveness of yoga in modifying risk factors for cardiovascular disease and metabolic syndrome: a systematic review and meta-analysis of randomized controlled trials. Eur J Prev Cardiol 2016;23(3):291–307.

32. Ross A, Thomas S. The health benefits of yoga and exercise: a review of comparison studies. J Altern Complement Med 2010;16(1):3–12.

33. Yates SL, Morley S, Eccleston C, et al. A scale for rating the quality of psychological trials for pain. Pain 2005;117(3):314–25.

34. Johnson JA, Rash JA, Campbell TS, et al. A systematic review and meta-analysis of randomized controlled trials of cognitive behavior therapy for insomnia (CBT-I) in cancer survivors. Sleep Med Rev 2016;27:20–8.

35. Rogers LQ, Vicari S, Trammell R, et al. Biobehavioral factors mediate exercise effects on fatigue in breast cancer survivors. Med Sci Sports Exerc 2014;46(6): 1077–88.

36. Rogers LQ, Hopkins-Price P, Vicari S, et al. A randomized trial to increase physical activity in breast cancer survivors. Med Sci Sports Exerc 2009;41(4):935–46.

37. Courneya KS, McKenzie DC, Mackey JR, et al. Effects of exercise dose and type during breast cancer chemotherapy: multicenter randomized trial. J Natl Cancer Inst 2013;105(23):1821–32.

38. Villarini A, Pasanisi P, Traina A, et al. Lifestyle and breast cancer recurrences: the DIANA-5 trial. Tumori 2012;98(1):1–18.

39. Steindorf K, Schmidt ME, Klassen O, et al. Randomized, controlled trial of resistance training in breast cancer patients receiving adjuvant radiotherapy: results on cancer-related fatigue and quality of life. Ann Oncol 2014;25(11):2237–43.

40. Steindorf K, Wiskemann J, Ulrich CM, et al. Effects of exercise on sleep problems in breast cancer patients receiving radiotherapy: a randomized clinical trial. Breast Cancer Res Treat 2017;162(3):489–99.

41. Roveda E, Vitale JA, Bruno E, et al. Protective effect of aerobic physical activity on sleep behavior in breast cancer survivors. Integr Cancer Ther 2017; 16(1):21–31.

42. Courneya KS, Segal RJ, Mackey JR, et al. Effects of exercise dose and type on sleep quality in breast cancer patients receiving chemotherapy: a multicenter randomized trial. Breast Cancer Res Treat 2014;144(2):361–9.

43. Rogers LQ, Fogleman A, Trammell R, et al. Inflammation and psychosocial factors mediate exercise effects on sleep quality in breast cancer survivors: pilot randomized controlled trial. Psychooncology 2015;24(3):302–10.

44. Rogers LQ, Hopkins-Price P, Vicari S, et al. Physical activity and health outcomes three months after completing a physical activity behavior change intervention: persistent and delayed effects. Cancer Epidemiol Biomarkers Prev 2009;18(5):1410–8.

45. Chandwani KD, Perkins G, Nagendra HR, et al. Randomized, controlled trial of yoga in women with breast cancer undergoing radiotherapy. J Clin Oncol 2014;32(10):1058–65.

46. Kiecolt-Glaser JK, Bennett JM, Andridge R, et al. Yoga's impact on inflammation, mood, and fatigue in breast cancer survivors: a randomized controlled trial. J Clin Oncol 2014;32(10):1040–9.

47. Larkey LK, Roe DJ, Weihs KL, et al. Randomized controlled trial of Qigong/Tai Chi Easy on cancer-related fatigue in breast cancer survivors. Ann Behav Med 2015;49(2):165–76.

48. Mock V, Dow KH, Meares CJ, et al. Effects of exercise on fatigue, physical functioning, and emotional distress during radiation therapy for breast cancer. Oncol Nurs Forum 1997;24(6):991–1000.

49. Kröz M, Reif M, Glinz A, et al. Impact of a combined multimodal-aerobic and multimodal intervention compared to standard aerobic treatment in breast cancer survivors with chronic cancer-related fatigue - results of a three-armed pragmatic trial in a comprehensive cohort design. BMC Cancer 2017; 17(1):166.

50. Lötzke D, Wiedemann F, Rodrigues Recchia D, et al. Iyengar-yoga compared to exercise as a therapeutic intervention during (neo)adjuvant therapy in women with stage i-iii breast cancer: health-related quality of life, mindfulness, spirituality, life satisfaction, and cancer-related fatigue. Evid Based Complement Alternat Med 2016;2016:5931816.

51. Chen Z, Meng Z, Milbury K, et al. Qigong improves quality of life in women undergoing radiotherapy for breast cancer: results of a randomized controlled trial. Cancer 2013;119(9):1690–8.

52. Ho RT, Fong TC, Cheung IK, et al. Effects of a short-term dance movement therapy program on symptoms and stress in patients with breast cancer undergoing radiotherapy: a randomized, controlled, single-blind trial. J Pain Symptom Manage 2016; 51(5):824–31.

53. Ghavami H, Akyolcu N. The impact of lifestyle interventions in breast cancer women after completion of primary therapy: a randomized study. J Breast Health 2017;13:94–9.

54. Wang YJ, Boehmke M, Wu YW, et al. Effects of a 6-week walking program on Taiwanese women newly diagnosed with early-stage breast cancer. Cancer Nurs 2011;34(2):E1–13.

55. U.S. Department of Health and Human Services. 2008 physical activity guidelines for Americans. Washington, DC: U.S. Department of Health and Human Services; 2008.

56. Mohr DC, Spring B, Freedland KE, et al. The selection and design of control conditions for randomized controlled trials of psychological interventions. Psychother Psychosom 2009;78(5):275–84.

57. Sabate E, World Health Organization. Adherence to long-term therapies: evidence for action. Geneva (Switzerland): World Health Organization; 2003.

58. Hawley-Hague H, Horne M, Skelton DA, et al. Review of how we should define (and measure) adherence in studies examining older adults' participation in exercise classes. BMJ Open 2016;6(6):e011560.

59. Miaskowski C, Barsevick A, Berger A, et al. Advancing symptom science through symptom cluster research: expert panel proceedings and recommendations. J Natl Cancer Inst 2017;109(4) [pii: djw253].

60. Langford DJ, Lee K, Miaskowski C. Sleep disturbance interventions in oncology patients and family caregivers: a comprehensive review and meta-analysis. Sleep Med Rev 2012;16(5):397–414.

61. Chang HY, Jotwani AC, Lai YH, et al. Hot flashes in breast cancer survivors: frequency, severity and impact. Breast 2016;27:116–21.

62. World Health Organization. Cancer: fact sheet. 2017. Available at: http://www.who.int/mediacentre/factsheets/fs297/en/. Accessed December 8, 2017.

63. Schmitz KH, Courneya KS, Matthews C, et al. American College of Sports Medicine roundtable on exercise guidelines for cancer survivors. Med Sci Sports Exerc 2010;42(7):1409–26.

Impact of Traumatic Stress on Sleep and Management Options in Women

Ihori Kobayashi, PhD[a],*, Mary Katherine Howell, MS[b]

KEYWORDS

- Trauma • Posttraumatic stress disorder • Women • Insomnia • Nightmares • Pharmacotherapy
- Cognitive behavioral therapy • Imagery rehearsal therapy

KEY POINTS

- After exposure to traumatic stress, women are at greater risk than men for developing symptoms of some psychiatric disorders, including insomnia and nightmares.
- Individuals with posttraumatic stress disorder (PTSD) often experience residual sleep disturbance after completing cognitive behavioral therapies for PTSD.
- Cognitive behavioral therapy for insomnia, imagery rehearsal therapy, and combinations of these techniques are possibly effective in treating insomnia and nightmares in trauma-exposed women.
- Prazosin as an adjunct to other psychotropic medications or psychotherapy is a potentially efficacious strategy for treating nightmares in trauma-exposed women.

INTRODUCTION

Insomnia, including trouble falling and staying asleep, is one of the most commonly reported symptoms after trauma exposure.[1,2] These symptoms are often persistent and may affect trauma survivors long term, even for several decades.[3] After exposure to a traumatic event, women are at greater risk than men for developing symptoms of psychiatric disorders, including posttraumatic stress disorder (PTSD), depression, and anxiety disorders.[4,5] Insomnia and recurrent nightmares about trauma are symptoms of some of these disorders.[6] Women and adolescent girls are more likely than men and boys to report insomnia and nightmares in the general population[7–10] and also after trauma exposure.[11–13] Therefore, it is particularly important for women to be properly assessed and treated for sleep disturbances after trauma. Although women face unique sleep challenges after trauma, treatment studies focusing on trauma-related sleep disturbances in women are limited. The purpose of this article is to briefly review findings from studies about sleep disturbances in trauma-exposed women. This article then focuses on psychotherapy and pharmacotherapy clinical trials examining efficacy for treating sleep-related symptoms in trauma-exposed women and suggests areas for further research.

SUBJECTIVE AND OBJECTIVE SLEEP CHANGES IN TRAUMA-EXPOSED WOMEN

A large proportion of trauma-exposed women suffer from insomnia and/or trauma-related nightmares. Sleep disturbance is particularly pronounced in women with PTSD, the diagnostic criteria for which include insomnia and recurrent trauma nightmares along with other symptoms, such as intrusive trauma memories, hyperarousal,

Disclosure Statement: I. Kobayashi receives research funding from Merck & Co (MISP53678).
[a] Department of Psychiatry and Behavioral Sciences, Howard University, 530 College Street Northwest, Washington, DC 20060, USA; [b] Department of Psychology, Howard University, 2041 Georgia Avenue Northwest, 4-West, Washington, DC 20060, USA
* Corresponding author.
E-mail address: ihori.kobayashi@howard.edu

Sleep Med Clin 13 (2018) 419–431
https://doi.org/10.1016/j.jsmc.2018.04.009
1556-407X/18/© 2018 Elsevier Inc. All rights reserved.

and avoidance of trauma reminders.[6] In a sample of female Vietnam veterans, 73% veterans with PTSD and 62% of those without PTSD endorsed trouble initiating sleep; 91% of veterans with PTSD versus 59% without PTSD reported trouble maintaining sleep.[14] In male Vietnam veterans, 44% of veterans with PTSD and 6% of those without PTSD reported trouble initiating sleep, and 91% with PTSD versus 63% without PTSD endorsed trouble maintaining sleep.[15] Female veterans may be more vulnerable to sleep-onset insomnia compared with male counterparts. Nightmares were reported by 73% of female rape victims with PTSD and by 27% of those without PTSD 4 weeks after rape, and persisting nightmares were experienced at 12 weeks post-rape, especially in victims with PTSD (reported by 63% of victims with PTSD and by 12% of victims without PTSD).[2]

Despite significant sleep disturbances reported by trauma-exposed individuals of both genders, trauma-related or PTSD-related objective sleep alterations are subtle and often observed in measures of sleep depth (ie, amount of light N1 stage of sleep and deep slow-wave sleep) or rapid eye movement sleep.[16,17] Lipinska and Thomas[17] examined effects of PTSD and trauma exposure on subjectively and objectively measured sleep by comparing female sexual assault survivors with and without PTSD and non–trauma-exposed controls. Their analysis of laboratory polysomnographic sleep revealed that trauma exposure was associated with decreased deep sleep (stage N3 slow-wave sleep) and that PTSD was related to increased light sleep (sleep stage N1). They did not find, however, any other trauma-related or PTSD-related objective sleep alterations.

Perceived safety of the laboratory sleep environment has been suggested as a potential explanation for the discrepancy between laboratory polysomnography and self-report survey findings in trauma-exposed individuals.[18] Consistent with this hypothesis, female sexual assault survivors, in particular those with PTSD, in the study by Lipinska and Thomas,[17] reported perceiving the laboratory sleep environment as quieter, safer, and more comfortable than home. Individuals with PTSD endorsed worse subjective sleep quality compared with the other groups in the home, but this group difference was not found in the laboratory setting.[17] In addition, an actigraphy study captured longer sleep-onset latency and lower sleep efficiency in women exposed to mixed types of trauma with PTSD compared with women without PTSD, suggesting sleep initiation and maintenance difficulties in the home sleep environment in women with PTSD.[19]

It has been suggested that people who experienced trauma in situations associated with sleep (eg, in a bedroom or darkness) are vulnerable to sleep disturbances because they are likely to experience heightened vigilance in sleep environments and perform sleep-interfering safety behaviors, such as checking locks multiple times or leaving lights on.[20] Women are more likely than men to be exposed to traumatic events that often occur in sleep-related situations and carry increased risk for persistent psychological disturbances, such as sexual violence, childhood sexual abuse, and intimate partner violence.[4,21,22] It is important that clinicians assess possible associations between the trauma context and sleep-interfering behaviors while planning insomnia treatment strategies for women.

COGNITIVE BEHAVIORAL STRATEGIES

Sleep disturbance has been considered one of the most refractory symptoms of PTSD.[23,24] Cognitive behavioral therapies (CBTs) for PTSD, including cognitive processing therapy (CPT) and prolonged exposure (PE), are evidence-based treatments for PTSD and reduce symptoms of insomnia, but patients often report clinically significant residual sleep symptoms after completing the treatment. Zayfert and DeViva[24] found that in 27 civilian participants (89% female) who achieved remission of overall PTSD after CBT for PTSD, approximately half of participants continued to report residual insomnia. In 2 studies of female sexual assault survivors with PTSD,[23,25] both sleep quality and insomnia symptoms improved after CPT or PE; however, overall subjective sleep disturbance remained at clinical levels post-treatment. **Table 1** lists findings of these and other studies of psychological treatments for trauma-related sleep disturbances that included female participants.

One of the most used evidence-based treatments for insomnia is CBT for insomnia (CBT-I). CBT-I is multimodal treatment, typically lasting between 6 sessions and 8 sessions, that includes sleep hygiene education, sleep restriction, stimulus control, sleep compression, relaxation, and cognitive therapy.[26] Stimulus control works through the extinction of a conditioned arousal in bed and bedroom by breaking associations between a person's bed/bedroom and wakefulness and by strengthening associations of the bed/bedroom with sleep. To promote the ability to relax and fall asleep in bed, patients are instructed to

Table 1
Psychotherapy clinical trials for sleep disturbance in trauma-exposed women

Citation	Intervention	Sample	Trauma Type	Sleep Outcomes[a]
Studies with an all-female sample (k = 4)				
Gutner et al,[25] 2013	CPT, PE, or minimal attention	N = 171 100% PTSD	Sexual assault	↓ Insomnia ↓ Nightmares ↑ Subjective sleep quality
Krakow et al,[38] 2001	IRT or waitlist control	N = 168 95% PTSD	Sexual assault	↓ Nightmares ↑ Subjective sleep quality
Galovski et al,[23] 2009	CPT or PE	N = 108 100% PTSD	Sexual assault (childhood or adulthood)	= Subjective sleep quality (between CPT and PE) For both conditions, pretreatment to post-treatment changes: ↑ Subjective sleep quality ↓ Insomnia
Krakow et al,[68] 2001	IRT or no-treatment control	N = 19 Unknown % PTSD	Sexual assault	↓ Nightmares = Subjective sleep quality
Studies with a mixed gender sample (k = 10)				
Zayfert & DeViva,[24] 2004	CBT for PTSD	N = 25 89% Female 100% PTSD	Mixed civilian	Pretreatment to post-treatment changes (significance not reported): ↓ Insomnia (88% to 48%) ↓ Severe insomnia (64% to 30%)
Krakow et al,[39] 2001	CBT-I + IRT	N = 62 84% Female 100% PTSD	Violent crime	Pretreatment to post-treatment changes: ↓ Nightmares ↑ Subjective sleep quality ↓ Insomnia
Wagley et al,[29] 2013	2 sessions CBT-I or treatment as usual	N = 30 70% Female 23% PTSD	Mixed civilian	= Subjective sleep quality Pretreatment to 4-wk follow-up change: ↑ Subjective sleep quality
Belleville et al,[69] 2011	CBT for PTSD	N = 55 69% Female 100% PTSD	Mixed civilian	Pretreatment to post-treatment changes: ↑ Subjective sleep quality ↓ Subjective sleep latency Post-treatment to 6-mo follow-up changes: ↓ Subjective sleep quality ↑ Subjective sleep latency

(continued on next page)

Table 1
(continued)

Citation	Intervention	Sample	Trauma Type	Sleep Outcomes[a]
Talbot et al,[30] 2014	CBT-I or waitlist control	N = 45 69% Female 100% PTSD	Mixed civilian and military	↓ Diary insomnia symptoms ↑ Subjective sleep quality ↓ Questionnaire insomnia ↓ Nightmares and disruptive nocturnal behaviors ↑ Polysomnography total sleep time = Actigraphy wake after sleep onset, total sleep time
Germain et al,[36] 2007	1 session version of BBT-I	N = 7 57% Female 100% PTSD	Violent crime	Pretreatment to post-treatment changes: ↑ Subjective sleep quality = Diary sleep quality = Diary insomnia
Ulmer et al,[40] 2011	CBT-I + IRT or treatment as usual	N = 22 32% Female 100% PTSD	Mixed military	↓ Diary and questionnaire insomnia ↓ Nightmares ↑ Subjective sleep quality
Germain et al,[35] 2014	BBT-I or information only control	N = 40 15% Female 30% PTSD	Combat	= Rate of insomnia remission post-treatment ↓ Insomnia ↑ Subjective sleep quality
Germain et al,[34] 2012	BBT-I, prazosin, or placebo control	N = 50 10% Female 58% PTSD	Mixed military	BBT-I and prazosin, compared with control: ↓ Insomnia = Subjective sleep quality = Sleep disturbances No difference between prazosin and BBT-I
Margolies et al,[70] 2013	CBT-I/IRT or waitlist control	N = 37 10% Female 100% PTSD	Mixed military	↓ Diary and questionnaire insomnia ↑ Subjective sleep quality ↓ Nightmares

Abbreviation: k, number of studies; ↑ and ↓, greater increase or decrease, respectively, in a treatment group compared to a control group unless otherwise specified; =, no statistically significant difference between treatment and control groups unless otherwise specified.

[a] This column indicates findings of comparisons between treatment and control groups unless otherwise specified.

use their bed only for sleep and sexual activities and leave their bedroom when they are not able to fall asleep. In the sleep restriction technique, the amount of time a person spends in bed is initially reduced, to build up pressure for sleep, leading to the reduction of unwanted wakefulness throughout the night.[26] The cognitive therapy module primarily focuses on cognitive restructuring of dysfunctional, overly held beliefs about sleep. Cognitive restructuring often relies on a combination of 2 techniques. One technique, commonly called "thought-stopping," includes recognizing the occurrence of dysfunctional thoughts about sleep and implementing cognitive and/or behavioral strategies to stop the thought. The other technique, often called "challenging automatic thoughts," involves developing alternative thoughts to dysfunctional automatic thoughts. For example, a dysfunctional belief about sleep, such as, "Insomnia is ruining my ability to enjoy life and prevents me from doing what I want," may increase distress and arousal presleep, thus interfering with sleep. By challenging automatic thoughts, such a belief may be adjusted to a more helpful, balanced thought like, "I have been able to enjoy my day occasionally and accomplish some things I want, even on days when I slept poorly. I would like to sleep better to function better during the day."

CBT-I has a large body of research supporting its efficacy. In Morin and colleagues'[27] review of 37 psychological insomnia treatment studies, 5 of CBT-I individual modules met criteria for empirically supported treatments for insomnia: stimulus control therapy, relaxation, paradoxic intention, sleep restriction, and cognitive-behavioral therapy. The most recent meta-analysis of 14 randomized controlled trials (RCTs) of CBT-I for primary insomnia[28] reported medium to large mean effect sizes for between-treatment-and-control-group (0.24–1.09) and within-subject effects (0.67–1.09) on indices of sleep initiation and maintenance.

Although the efficacy of CBT-I has also been studied in individuals with insomnia and comorbid PTSD, only a small number of studies included a significant proportion of female participants. Two RCTs of CBT-I have been conducted with individuals (approximately 70% female) with PTSD (see **Table 1**).[29,30] One of the RCTs, conducted by Wagley and colleagues,[29] revealed significant therapeutic effects on sleep outcomes only in the analysis of within-subject changes but not in the analysis of between-group differences.

Recently, brief behavioral therapy for insomnia (BBT-I), a 1-session to 4-session treatment comprising only behavioral modules of CBT-I, was developed,[31] and its efficacy has been demonstrated in various types of insomnia patients, including individuals with trauma-related insomnia.[32–36] The only BBT-I trial with a large proportion of women (57%) examined effects of a 1-session version of BBT-I in a small sample (N = 7) of victims of violent crimes with PTSD.[36] From baseline to 6-week post-treatment, sleep quality significantly improved. Although the improvements in diary-measured sleep initiation and maintenance had effect sizes of moderate to large, the changes were not statistically significant probably because of the small sample size. The efficacy of BBT-I has been suggested in controlled trials of trauma-exposed veterans; however, these trials included small proportions (10%–15%) of women.[34,35]

Imagery rehearsal therapy (IRT), initially developed to treat nightmares, has been applied to treatment of trauma-related nightmares.[37,38] IRT normally takes place over 3 sessions and includes education about the development and function of nightmares, prompting viewing recurrent nightmares as habits or learned behaviors, rescripting of nightmares, and then practicing the positive and more comfortable rescripted dream imagery during the daytime. In the largest trial of IRT with only female participants (N = 168), sexual assault survivors who received IRT had greater reductions in nightmare frequency and improvement in sleep quality and PTSD symptoms compared with women on a waitlist.[38]

IRT has also been combined with CBT-I techniques. In a majority female (84%) sample of victims of violent crimes with PTSD, 62 participants completed a 10-hour group treatment combining IRT techniques with CBT-I modules, including sleep hygiene, stimulus control, and sleep restriction.[39] Participants demonstrated pretreatment to post-treatment improvements in nightmare frequency, sleep quality, and insomnia. In a study of 22 veterans with PTSD (32% female), IRT was abbreviated and presented as a dream rescripting technique in combination with CBT-I.[40] This combined intervention yielded greater improvement in nightmares and symptoms of insomnia and PTSD compared with usual care. These results suggest that IRT in combination with more traditional CBT-I techniques may deliver relief from trauma-related nightmares, but further research is needed to determine whether the combination of IRT and CBT-I is more effective than IRT alone.

There have been only a few studies on efficacy of cognitive behavioral strategies for sleep disturbance in trauma-exposed women. Studies with female-only or predominantly female samples have showed therapeutic effects of CBT-I, IRT, and combinations of these techniques on sleep quality and insomnia and nightmare severity in trauma-exposed individuals; however, methodological shortcomings, such as small sample sizes, within-subject comparisons, and use of waitlist controls, limit the conclusiveness of the study findings.

PHARMACOLOGIC STRATEGIES

A large number of clinical trials have been conducted to examine efficacy of pharmacologic treatment of PTSD; however, not many studies report results specific to sleep problems or specific to women. Two selective serotonin reuptake inhibitors (SSRIs), sertraline and paroxetine, are the only medications currently approved for treating PTSD by the US Food and Drug Administration. Although these SSRIs help reduce PTSD symptoms, clinical trials have shown limited efficacy. In RCTs with PTSD patients, only half of the patients treated with sertraline achieved responder criteria,[41,42] and 30% of patients treated with paroxetine achieved remission.[43] Effects of SSRIs or other antidepressants on sleep-related PTSD symptoms have been examined in a small number of clinical trials, and none of the trials demonstrated sufficient treatment effects. Moreover, 2 RCTs with a large proportion of women with PTSD suggested that sertraline may increase the risk of insomnia.[41,44] Effects of nefazodone, a serotoninergic antidepressant, on insomnia symptoms and nightmares were observed only in open label trials (in men-only and women-only trials).[45–47] **Table 2** summarizes sleep-related findings of pharmacologic studies that included trauma-exposed female participants.

Benzodiazepines and other hypnotics are commonly prescribed medications for patients with PTSD, and higher prescription rates of these medications were observed in women with PTSD treated in the US Veterans Affairs health care system compared with male counterparts.[48,49] Benzodiazepines, however, have been ineffective in treating or preventing PTSD,[50] and some treatment guidelines for PTSD recommend against use of benzodiazepines, because associated risks, such as dependence, may outweigh benefits.[51,52] Furthermore, benzodiazepines may interfere with extinction of conditioned fear, a learning process essential for recovery from PTSD, and compromise the benefit of exposure therapy.[53,54] Two crossover design studies with small samples (6 male veterans and 6 patients with unspecified gender) have examined effects of benzodiazepines on sleep symptoms in PTSD,[55,56] but neither study indicated benefit.

Nonbenzodiazepine hypnotics, such as zolpidem and eszopiclone, are among the most commonly prescribed medications for insomnia in the US general population as well as in veterans with PTSD.[49,57] Despite their popularity, evidence for their efficacy in treating sleep symptoms in PTSD is limited. The authors' literature search yielded only 1 double-blind RCT indicating potential benefits of nonbenzodiazepine hypnotics on trauma-related sleep disturbance. In this small RCT in civilians with PTSD (N = 24, 71% female), eszopiclone improved sleep quality and shortened sleep-onset latency compared with placebo.[58] In contrast, in a clinical trial of male combat veterans with PTSD comparing zolpidem and hypnotherapy as an adjunctive treatment to an SSRI, zolpidem was less effective than hypnotherapy in improving sleep quality and decreasing sleep disturbance.[59]

Prazosin, a centrally active α_1-adrenergic receptor antagonist, is the only agent that has demonstrated efficacy in treating PTSD-related sleep symptoms in multiple double-blind RCTs.[60] In these trials, prazosin was administered adjunctively with stable psychotropic medications and/or psychotherapy. Several RCTs with prazosin that included women (5%–85%) have shown therapeutic effects for PTSD-related nightmares and insomnia symptoms (see **Table 2**).[34,61–63] Some studies, however, did not find significant therapeutic effects. A recent multicenter Veterans Affairs clinical trial for combat-related sleep disturbance (N = 304, 2% female) found that prazosin did not significantly change either nightmares or sleep quality compared with placebo.[64] Furthermore, Germain and colleagues[34] found no differences between prazosin and BBT-I in treating nightmares and insomnia (N = 50, 10% female), although both prazosin and BBT-I were superior to placebo (see **Table 1**).

DRUG-ASSISTED PSYCHOTHERAPY

Recently, drug-assisted psychotherapy has begun to gain traction as a strategy to enhance therapeutic effects of psychotherapy for PTSD. The authors found only 1 study reporting effects of this approach on sleep symptoms in a sample that included women. D-cycloserine, a partial agonist at the N-methyl-D-aspartate receptor, has been hypothesized to augment effects of exposure therapy by enhancing extinction learning.[65] In the double-blind RCT of individuals exposed to the 9/11 attacks (N = 25, 24% female), D-cycloserine was administered 90 minutes before each exposure therapy session, and participants reported lower insomnia severity at 6-month follow-up compared with placebo.[65]

Table 2
Pharmacologic clinical trials for sleep disturbance in trauma-exposed women

Citation	Medication (mg/d)	Design Duration	Sample	Trauma Type	Sleep Outcomes[a]
SSRIs; serotonin and norepinephrine reuptake inhibitors (k = 4)					
Meltzer-Brody et al,[71] 2000	Fluoxetine (10–60)	RDBPC 12 wk	N = 53 91% female 100% PTSD	Mixed civilian	= Nightmares ↓ Insomnia (questionnaire) = Insomnia (clinician interview)
Davidson et al,[44] 2001	Sertraline[b] (25–200)	RDBPC 12 wk	N = 208 78% female 100% PTSD	Mixed civilian	= Subjective sleep quality ↑ Insomnia as adverse event (35% vs 22%)
Brady et al,[41] 2000	Sertraline[b] (25–200)	RDBPC 12 wk	N = 187 73% female 100% PTSD	Mixed civilian and combat	↑ Insomnia as adverse event (16% vs 4%)
Stein et al,[72] 2009	Venlafaxine ER (37.5–300)	Pooled analysis of 2 RDBPC trials 12 wk	N = 687 61% female 100% PTSD	Mixed civilian and combat	= Insomnia = Nightmares
Other antidepressants (k = 4)					
McRae et al,[73] 2004	Nefazodone (100–600)	Randomized double-blind comparison to sertraline 12 wk	N = 26 77% female 100% PTSD	Mixed civilian	↑ Subjective sleep quality pretreatment to post-treatment No difference from sertraline
Davidson et al,[45] 1998	Nefazodone (50–600)	Open label 12 wk	N = 17 76% female 100% PTSD	Mixed civilian	Pretreatment to post-treatment changes: ↓ Insomnia ↓ Nightmares
Schneier et al,[74] 2015	Mirtazapine adjunct to sertraline[c] (30–45)	RDBPC 24 wk	N = 36 64% female 100% PTSD	Mixed civilian	= Subjective sleep quality
Becker et al,[75] 2007	Bupropion SR[d] (100–300)	RDBPC 8 wk	N = 30 21% female 100% PTSD	Mixed civilian and military	= Subjective sleep quality

(continued on next page)

Table 2
(continued)

Citation	Medication (mg/d)	Design Duration	Sample	Trauma Type	Sleep Outcomes[a]
GABA receptor agonist; GABA reuptake inhibitor (k = 3)					
Pollack et al,[58] 2011	Eszopiclone[e] (3)	RDBPC crossover 3 wk	N = 24 71% female 100% PTSD	Mixed civilian and military	↑ Subjective sleep quality ↓ Subjective sleep latency
Connor et al,[76] 2006	Tiagabine (4–16)	Open-label phase 12 wk followed by RDBPC phase 12 wk for only responders to open-label treatment	Open label phase: N = 26, 73% female, 100% PTSD RDBPC phase: N = 19	Mixed civilian	Open-label phase pretreatment to post-treatment changes: ↑ Subjective sleep quality ↓ Insomnia ↓ Nightmares RDBPC phase: = Subjective sleep quality ↓ Insomnia
Davidson et al,[77] 2007	Tiagabine (4–16)	RDBPC 12 wk	N = 232 66% female 100% PTSD	Mixed civilian and combat	= Insomnia = Nightmares
Prazosin (k = 7)					
Taylor et al,[78] 2008	Prazosin[d] (1–6)	RDBPC crossover 7 wk	N = 13 85% female 100% PTSD	Mixed civilian	↑ Objective total sleep time ↓ Nightmares ↓ Distressed awakening
Simpson et al,[79] 2015	Prazosin[d] (1–8)	RDBPC 6 wk	N = 30 37% female 100% PTSD and alcohol dependence	Mixed civilian and combat	= Nightmares

Study	Intervention	Design/Duration	Sample	Population	Findings
Ahmad-panah et al,[61] 2014	Prazosin[d] (1–15)	RDBPC comparison to hydroxyzine 8 wk	N = 100, 28% female, 100% PTSD	Mixed civilian and war-related	Prozosin and hydroxyzine, compared with placebo: ↑ Subjective sleep quality, ↓ Subjective sleep latency. Prazosin compared with the other groups: ↑ Subjective sleep duration, ↓ Nightmares
Raskind et al,[62] 2013	Prazosin[e] (1–25 for men; 1–12 for women)	RDBPC 15 wk	N = 67, 15% female, 100% PTSD	Combat	↓ Nightmares, ↑ Subjective sleep quality
Petrakis et al,[80] 2016	Prazosin[e] (2–16)	RDBPC 13 wk	N = 96, 6% female, 100% PTSD and alcohol dependence	Mixed military	= Nightmares, = Insomnia
Raskind et al,[63] 2007	Prazosin[e] (1–15)	RDBPC 8 wk	N = 40, 5% female, 100% PTSD	Combat	↓ Nightmares, ↑ Subjective sleep quality
Raskind et al,[64] 2018	Prazosin[e] (1–20 for men; 1–12 for women)	RDBPC 26 wk	N = 304, 2% female, 100% PTSD	Combat	= Nightmares, = Subjective sleep quality
Drug-assisted psychotherapy (k = 1)					
Difede et al,[65] 2014	D-cycloserine[d] (100 mg before weekly exposure therapy sessions)	RDBPC 10 wk	N = 25, 24% female, 100% PTSD	9/11 World Trade Center attack	↓ Insomnia

Abbreviations: k, number of studies; RDBPC, randomized, double-blind, placebo-controlled; ↑ and ↓, greater increase or decrease, respectively, in a treatment group compared to a control group unless otherwise specified; =, no statistically significant difference between treatment and control groups unless otherwise specified.
a This column indicates findings of comparisons between treatment and control groups unless otherwise specified.
b Ongoing psychotherapy other than CBT was allowed.
c Ongoing psychotherapy was allowed.
d Ongoing stable psychotropic medications were allowed.
e Ongoing stable psychotropic medications or psychotherapy were allowed.

SUMMARY

After a traumatic experience, women are more likely than men to experience symptoms of psychiatric disorders, including insomnia and recurrent nightmares. Sleep disturbance is one of the most commonly reported and refractory symptoms of PTSD. Only a small number of psychological or pharmacologic clinical trials, however, have focused on sleep symptoms in trauma-exposed women. SSRIs, currently first-line pharmacologic treatments for PTSD, have not demonstrated sufficient evidence for their efficacy in treating trauma-related sleep disturbance. Among multiple pharmacologic agents tested, prazosin has the strongest evidence for improving nightmares and insomnia symptoms in trauma-exposed individuals. Limited evidence suggests that eszopiclone and D-cycloserine–assisted exposure therapy may be effective in treating insomnia symptoms in trauma-exposed individuals, but more studies are needed. CBT for PTSD, a first-line psychological treatment, improved insomnia symptoms; however, patients often experienced residual sleep symptoms. Clinical trials have indicated that certain cognitive behavioral strategies, such as CBT-I, IRT, or combinations of these strategies, may contribute to the improvement of sleep disturbances in trauma-exposed women. Further evidence from methodologically strong studies, however, is needed.

It has been increasingly recognized that sleep contributes to the maintenance of mental and physical health.[66,67] Therefore, properly treating sleep disturbances after trauma is important not only for relieving distress associated with sleep difficulties but also for promoting health and quality of life of trauma-exposed women.

ACKNOWLEDGMENTS

The preparation of this article was supported by National Institutes of Health grant K01MH110647 and TL1TR001431 from the National Center for Advancing Translational Science.

REFERENCES

1. Galea S, Resnick H, Ahern J, et al. Posttraumatic stress disorder in Manhattan, New York City, after the September 11th terrorist attacks. J Urban Health 2002;79:340–53.
2. Rothbaum BO, Foa EB, Riggs DS, et al. A prospective examination of post-traumatic stress disorder in rape victims. J Trauma Stress 1992;5: 455–75.
3. Rosen J, Reynold CF III, Yeager AL, et al. Sleep disturbances in survivors of the Nazi holocaust. Am J Psychiatry 1991;148:62–6.
4. Kessler RC, Sonnega A, Bromet E, et al. Posttraumatic stress disorder in the national comorbidity survey. Arch Gen Psychiatry 1995;52:1048–60.
5. Breslau N, Davis GC, Peterson EL, et al. A second look at comorbidity in victims of trauma: the posttraumatic stress disorder–major depression connection. Biol Psychiatry 2000;48:902–9.
6. American Psychiatric Association. Diagnostic and statistical manual of mental disorders. 5th edition. Washington, DC: American Psychiatric Association; 2013.
7. Groeger JA, Zijlstra FRH, Dijk DJ. Sleep quantity, sleep difficulties and their perceived consequences in a representative sample of some 2000 British adults. J Sleep Res 2004;13:359–71.
8. Schredl M, Reinhard I. Gender differences in nightmare frequency: a meta-analysis. Sleep Med Rev 2011;15:115–21.
9. Hysing M, Pallesen S, Stormark KM, et al. Sleep patterns and insomnia among adolescents: a population-based study. J Sleep Res 2013;22: 549–56.
10. Nielsen TA, Laberge L, Paquet J, et al. Development of disturbing dreams during adolescence and their relation to anxiety symptoms. Sleep 2000;23:1–10.
11. Kobayashi I, Delahanty DL. Gender differences in subjective sleep after trauma and the development of posttraumatic stress disorder symptoms: a pilot study. J Trauma Stress 2013;26:467–74.
12. Fullerton CS, Ursano RJ, Epstein RS, et al. Gender differences in posttraumatic stress disorder after motor vehicle accidents. Am J Psychiatry 2001; 158:1486–91.
13. Saul AL, Grant KE, Carter JS. Post-traumatic reactions in adolescents: how well do the DSM-IV PTSD criteria fit the real life experience of trauma exposed youth? J Abnorm Child Psychol 2008;36: 915–25.
14. Kimerling R, Clum GA, Wolfe J. Relationships among trauma exposure, chronic posttraumatic stress disorder symptoms, and self-reported health in women: Replication and extension. J Trauma Stress 2000;13:115–28.
15. Neylan TC, Marmar CR, Metzler TJ, et al. Sleep disturbances in the Vietnam generation: findings from a nationally representative sample of male Vietnam veterans. Am J Psychiatry 1998;155:929–33.
16. Kobayashi I, Boarts JM, Delahanty DL. Polysomnographically measured sleep abnormalities in PTSD: a meta-analytic review. Psychophysiology 2007;44: 660–9.
17. Lipinska G, Thomas KG. Better sleep in a strange bed? sleep quality in South African women with posttraumatic stress disorder. Front Psychol 2017; 8:1555.
18. Woodward SH, Bliwise DL, Friedman MJ, et al. Subjective versus objective sleep in Vietnam combat

veterans hospitalized for PTSD. J Trauma Stress 1996;9:137–43.

19. Calhoun PS, Wiley M, Dennis MF, et al. Objective evidence of sleep disturbance in women with posttraumatic stress disorder. J Trauma Stress 2007;20:1009–18.

20. DeViva JC, Zayfert C, Pigeon WR, et al. Treatment of residual insomnia after CBT for PTSD: case studies. J Trauma Stress 2005;18:155–9.

21. Liu H, Petukhova MV, Sampson NA, et al. Association of DSM-IV posttraumatic stress disorder with traumatic experience type and history in the world health organization world mental health surveys. JAMA Psychiatry 2017;74(3):270–81.

22. Tjaden PG, Thoennes N. Extent, nature, and consequences of intimate partner violence. Washington (DC): U.S Department of Justice; 2000.

23. Galovski TE, Monson C, Bruce SE, et al. Does cognitive behavioral therapy for PTSD improve perceived health and sleep impairment? J Trauma Stress 2009;22:197–204.

24. Zayfert C, DeViva JC. Residual insomnia following cognitive behavioral therapy for PTSD. J Trauma Stress 2004;17:69–73.

25. Gutner CA, Casement MD, Stavitsky Gilbert K, et al. Change in sleep symptoms across cognitive processing therapy and prolonged exposure: a longitudinal perspective. Behav Res Ther 2013;51:817–22.

26. Manber R, Friedman L, Siebern AT, et al. Cognitive behavioral therapy for insomnia in veterans: Therapist manual. Washington, DC: U.S. Department of Veterans Affairs; 2014.

27. Morin CM, Bootzin RR, Buysse DJ, et al. Psychological and behavioral treatment of insomnia: update of the recent evidence. Sleep 1998-2004;2006(29):1398–414.

28. Okajima I, Komada Y, Inoue Y. A meta-analysis on the treatment effectiveness of cognitive behavioral therapy for primary insomnia. Sleep Biol Rhythms 2011;9:24–34.

29. Wagley JN, Rybarczyk B, Nay WT, et al. Effectiveness of abbreviated CBT for insomnia in psychiatric outpatients: sleep and depression outcomes. J Clin Psychol 2013;69:1043–55.

30. Talbot LS, Maguen S, Metzler TJ, et al. Cognitive behavioral therapy for insomnia in posttraumatic stress disorder: a randomized controlled trial. Sleep 2014;37:327–41.

31. Troxel WM, Germain A, Buysse DJ. Clinical management of insomnia with brief behavioral treatment (BBTI). Behav Sleep Med 2012;10:266–79.

32. Buysse DJ, Germain A, Moul DE, et al. Efficacy of brief behavioral treatment for chronic insomnia in older adults. Arch Intern Med 2011;171:887–95.

33. Watanabe N, Furukawa TA, Shimodera S, et al. Brief behavioral therapy for refractory insomnia in residual depression: an assessor-blind, randomized controlled trial. J Clin Psychiatry 2011;72:1651–8.

34. Germain A, Richardson R, Moul DE, et al. Placebo-controlled comparison of prazosin and cognitive-behavioral treatments for sleep disturbances in US military veterans. J Psychosom Res 2012;72:89–96.

35. Germain A, Richardson R, Stocker R, et al. Treatment for insomnia in combat-exposed OEF/OIF/OND military veterans: preliminary randomized controlled trial. Behav Res Ther 2014;61:78–88.

36. Germain A, Shear MK, Hall M, et al. Effects of a brief behavioral treatment for PTSD-related sleep disturbances: a pilot study. Behav Res Ther 2007;45:627–32.

37. Marks I. Rehearsal relief of a nightmare. Br J Psychiatry 1978;133:461–5.

38. Krakow B, Hollifield M, Schrader R, et al. A controlled study of imagery rehearsal for chronic nightmares in sexual assault survivors with PTSD: a preliminary report. J Trauma Stress 2000;13:589–609.

39. Krakow B, Johnston L, Melendrez D, et al. An open-label trial of evidence-based cognitive behavior therapy for nightmares and insomnia in crime victims with PTSD. Am J Psychiatry 2001;158:2043–7.

40. Ulmer CS, Edinger JD, Calhoun PS. A multi-component cognitive-behavioral intervention for sleep disturbance in veterans with PTSD: a pilot study. J Clin Sleep Med 2011;7:57–68.

41. Brady K, Pearlstein T, Asnis GM, et al. Efficacy and safety of sertraline treatment of posttraumatic stress disorder: a randomized controlled trial. JAMA 2000;283:1837–44.

42. Zohar J, Amital D, Miodownik C, et al. Double-blind placebo-controlled pilot study of sertraline in military veterans with posttraumatic stress disorder. J Clin Psychopharmacol 2002;22:190–5.

43. Tucker P, Zaninelli R, Yehuda R, et al. Paroxetine in the treatment of chronic posttraumatic stress disorder: results of a placebo-controlled, flexible-dosage trial. J Clin Psychiatry 2001;62(1):860–8.

44. Davidson JR, Rothbaum BO, van der Kolk BA, et al. Multicenter, double-blind comparison of sertraline and placebo in the treatment of posttraumatic stress disorder. Arch Gen Psychiatry 2001;58:485–92.

45. Davidson JR, Weisler RH, Malik ML, et al. Treatment of posttraumatic stress disorder with nefazodone. Int Clin Psychopharmacol 1998;13:111–3.

46. Gillin JC, Smith-Vaniz A, Schnierow B, et al. An open-label, 12-week clinical and sleep EEG study of nefazodone in chronic combat-related posttraumatic stress disorder. J Clin Psychiatry 2001;62:789–96.

47. Neylan TC, Lenoci M, Maglione ML, et al. The effect of nefazodone on subjective and objective sleep quality in posttraumatic disorder. J Clin Psychiatry 2003;64:445–50.

48. Mellman TA, Clark RE, Peacock WJ. Prescribing patterns for patients with posttraumatic stress disorder. Psychiatr Serv 2003;54:1618–21.

49. Bernardy NC, Lund BC, Alexander B, et al. Gender differences in prescribing among veterans diagnosed with posttraumatic stress disorder. J Gen Intern Med 2013;28:542–8.

50. Guina J, Rossetter SR, Derhodes BJ, et al. Benzodiazepines for PTSD: a systematic review and meta-analysis. J Psychiatr Pract 2015;21:281–303.

51. US Department of Veterans Affairs, Department of Defense. VA/DOD clinical practice guideline for the management of posttraumatic stress disorder and acute stress disorder Washington (DC): U.S. Department of Veterans Affairs; 2017;3.0.

52. Friedman MJ, Davidson JR, Stein DJ. Psychopharmacotherapy for adults. In: Foa EB, Keane TM, Friedman MJ, et al, editors. Effective treatments for PTSD: practice guidelines from the international society for traumatic stress studies. 2nd edition. New York: Guilford; 2009. p. 245–68.

53. van Minnen A, Arntz A, Keijsers GPJ. Prolonged exposure in patients with chronic PTSD: Predictors of treatment outcome and dropout. Behav Res Ther 2002;40:439–57.

54. Bouton ME, Kenney FA, Rosengard C. State-dependent fear extinction with two benzodiazepine tranquilizers. Behav Neurosci 1990;104:44.

55. Braun P, Greenberg D, Dasberg H, et al. Core symptoms of posttraumatic stress disorder unimproved by alprazolam treatment. J Clin Psychiatry 1990;51:236–8.

56. Cates ME, Bishop MH, Davis LL, et al. Clonazepam for treatment of sleep disturbances associated with combat-related posttraumatic stress disorder. Ann Pharmacother 2004;38:1395–9.

57. Bertisch SM, Herzig SJ, Winkelman JW, et al. National use of prescription medications for insomnia: NHANES 1999-2010. Sleep 2014;37:343–9.

58. Pollack MH, Hoge EA, Worthington JJ, et al. Eszopiclone for the treatment of posttraumatic stress disorder and associated insomnia: a randomized, double-blind, placebo-controlled trial. J Clin Psychiatry 2011;72:892–7.

59. Abramowitz EG, Barak Y, Ben-Avi I, et al. Hypnotherapy in the treatment of chronic combat-related PTSD patients suffering from insomnia: a randomized, zolpidem-controlled clinical trial. Int J Clin Exp Hypn 2008;56:270–80.

60. Lipinska G, Baldwin DS, Thomas KGF. Pharmacology for sleep disturbance in PTSD. Hum Psychopharmacol 2016;31:156–63.

61. Ahmadpanah M, Sabzeiee P, Hosseini SM, et al. Comparing the effect of prazosin and hydroxyzine on sleep quality in patients suffering from posttraumatic stress disorder. Neuropsychobiology 2014; 69:235–42.

62. Raskind MA, Peterson K, Williams T, et al. A trial of prazosin for combat trauma PTSD with nightmares in active-duty soldiers returned from Iraq and Afghanistan. Am J Psychiatry 2013;170:1003–10.

63. Raskind MA, Peskind ER, Hoff DJ, et al. A parallel group placebo controlled study of prazosin for trauma nightmares and sleep disturbance in combat veterans with post-traumatic stress disorder. Biol Psychiatry 2007;61:928–34.

64. Raskind MA, Peskind ER, Chow B, et al. Trial of prazosin for post-traumatic stress disorder in military veterans. N Engl J Med 2018;378:507–17.

65. Difede J, Cukor J, Wyka K, et al. D-cycloserine augmentation of exposure therapy for posttraumatic stress disorder: a pilot randomized clinical trial. Neuropsychopharmacology 2014;39:1052–8.

66. Itani O, Jike M, Watanabe N, et al. Short sleep duration and health outcomes: a systematic review, meta-analysis, and meta-regression. Sleep Med 2017;32:246–56.

67. Zhai L, Zhang H, Zhang D. Sleep duration and depression among adults: a meta-analysis of prospective studies. Depress Anxiety 2015;32:664–70.

68. Krakow B, Sandoval D, Schrader R, et al. Treatment of chronic nightmares in adjudicated adolescent girls in a residential facility. J Adolesc Health 2001; 29:94–100.

69. Belleville G, Guay S, Marchand A. Persistence of sleep disturbances following cognitive-behavior therapy for posttraumatic stress disorder. J Psychosom Res 2011;70:318–32.

70. Margolies SO, Rybarczyk B, Vrana SR, et al. Efficacy of a cognitive-behavioral treatment for insomnia and nightmares in Afghanistan and Iraq veterans with PTSD. J Clin Psychol 2013;69:1026–42.

71. Meltzer-Brody S, Connor K, Churchill E, et al. Symptom-specific effects of fluoxetine in post-traumatic stress disorder. Int Clin Psychopharmacol 2000;15: 227–31.

72. Stein DJ, Pedersen R, Rothbaum BO, et al. Onset of activity and time to response on individual CAPS-SX17 items in patients treated for post-traumatic stress disorder with venlafaxine ER: a pooled analysis. Int J Neuropsychopharmacol 2009;12:23–31.

73. McRae AL, Brady KT, Mellman TA, et al. Comparison of nefazodone and sertraline for the treatment of posttraumatic stress disorder. Depress Anxiety 2004;19:190–6.

74. Schneier FR, Campeas R, Carcamo J, et al. Combined mirtazapine and SSRI treatment of PTSD: a placebo-controlled trial. Depress Anxiety 2015;32: 570–9.

75. Becker ME, Hertzberg MA, Moore SD, et al. A placebo-controlled trial of bupropion SR in the treatment of chronic posttraumatic stress disorder. J Clin Psychopharmacol 2007;27:193–7.

76. Connor KM, Davidson JR, Weisler RH, et al. Tiagabine for posttraumatic stress disorder: effects of open-label and double-blind discontinuation treatment. Psychopharmacology 2006;184:21–5.

77. Davidson JR, Brady K, Mellman TA, et al. The efficacy and tolerability of tiagabine in adult patients with post-traumatic stress disorder. J Clin Psychopharmacol 2007;27:85–8.

78. Taylor FB, Martin P, Thompson C, et al. Prazosin effects on objective sleep measures and clinical symptoms in civilian trauma posttraumatic stress disorder: a placebo-controlled study. Biol Psychiatry 2008;63:629–32.

79. Simpson TL, Malte CA, Dietel B, et al. A pilot trial of prazosin, an alpha-1 adrenergic antagonist, for comorbid alcohol dependence and posttraumatic stress disorder. Alcohol Clin Exp Res 2015;39: 808–17.

80. Petrakis IL, Desai N, Gueorguieva R, et al. Prazosin for veterans with posttraumatic stress disorder and comorbid alcohol dependence: a clinical trial. Alcohol Clin Exp Res 2016;40:178–86.

Sleep Disorders in Women Veterans

Jennifer L. Martin, PhD[a,b,*], M. Safwan Badr, MD, MBA[c], Salam Zeineddine, MD[d]

KEYWORDS

- Veterans • Women • Insomnia • Sleep-disordered breathing • Sleep apnea • Nightmares
- Posttraumatic stress disorder • Depression

KEY POINTS

- Sleep complaints are common among women veterans.
- Women veterans who are treated for sleep disorders are likely to benefit in terms of improved physical and psychological health.
- Insomnia disorder is common among women veterans, and evidence shows those with comorbid mental health conditions such as posttraumatic stress disorder have more severe insomnia.
- Sleep-disordered breathing is also common among women veterans, and studies on how to provide optimal treatment are lacking.
- Research is limited on insufficient sleep among women veterans; however, women veterans are at elevated risk for insufficient sleep due to medical, psychiatric, and psychosocial factors.

INTRODUCTION

The number of women veterans is increasing, necessitating a need to optimize health care delivery for this growing segment of the veteran population. It is estimated that by 2020, there will be 1.9 million women veterans in the United States, representing 10% of the total veteran population.[1] Sleep disturbances are common among women during military service. Among active duty military personnel, women are more likely to be diagnosed with insomnia[2–4] and a significant number also experience sleep-disordered breathing (SDB). Foster and colleagues[4] reported that women with sleep disorders were also more likely to suffer from depression, anxiety, and posttraumatic stress disorder (PTSD).

The National Veteran Sleep Disorder Study reported that sleep apnea and insomnia were the most common sleep disorders diagnosed among veterans seeking medical care through the Veterans Health Administration (VHA) between 2000 and 2010.[5] There is evidence that the rate of diagnosis and treatment of insomnia is increasing specifically among women veterans.[6] Both disorders exhibited more than a 7-fold relative increase in incidence over the 11-year study period, suggesting increased recognition of sleep problems in VHA for both men and women veterans. Across time points, insomnia was more common among women compared with men, and sleep apnea was more common among men compared with women, similar to sex differences in the general

Disclosure Statement: The authors have nothing to disclose.

[a] Department of Medicine, David Geffen School of Medicine, University of California, Los Angeles, Los Angeles, 16111 Plummer Street, North Hills, CA 91343, USA; [b] Geriatric Research, Education and Clinical Center, VA Greater Los Angeles Healthcare System, VA Sepulveda Ambulatory Care Center, 11E, 16111 Plummer Street, North Hills, CA 91343, USA; [c] Division of Pulmonary Critical Care and Sleep Medicine, Department of Internal Medicine, Wayne State University, University Health Center, 4201 St. Antoine, 2E, Detroit, MI 48201, USA; [d] Division of Pulmonary Critical Care and Sleep Medicine, Department of Internal Medicine, Wayne State University, Harper University Hospital, 3 Hudson, 3990 John R, Detroit, MI 48323, USA
* Corresponding author. VA Sepulveda Ambulatory Care Center, 11E, 16111 Plummer Street, North Hills, CA 91343.
E-mail address: Jennifer.Martin@va.gov

Sleep Med Clin 13 (2018) 433–441
https://doi.org/10.1016/j.jsmc.2018.04.010
1556-407X/18/Published by Elsevier Inc.

population. Women veterans constituted less than 7% of the included patients, which highlights an important limitation on research about sleep disorders among veterans; few studies have included a sufficiently large population of women veterans to make definitive claims about sleep in this unique patient group.

Despite increasing numbers, women veterans remain underrepresented in research exploring sleep disorders. The limited available literature does indicate that women veterans suffer from severe and chronic sleep disturbance, which is often comorbid with psychiatric conditions, and that delivery of evidence-based treatments will likely benefit women veterans with sleep disorders. This article reviews what is known about rates of sleep disorders in women veterans, focusing on insomnia, sleep apnea, restless legs syndrome and insufficient sleep syndrome, because these are likely the most common disorders faced by clinicians. Special considerations related to treatment of women are highlighted and recommendations for future research are discussed.

EVALUATION OF WOMEN VETERANS WITH SUSPECTED SLEEP DISORDERS

Evaluation of sleep complaints among women veterans should follow standard recommendations, starting with a review of presenting symptoms, history of sleep difficulties, and comorbid conditions and medications. Special attention should be given to whether sleep difficulties began before, during, or after military service or deployments because these can serve as triggers for long-standing sleep difficulties. In women veterans, sleep disorders are often comorbid with psychiatric disorders.[4] Careful attention to the relative contribution of each can facilitate treatment prescription and inform overall recommendations. Based on the woman veteran's clinical history, clinicians should evaluate risk factors and symptoms of common sleep disorders, including insomnia, SDB and sleep apnea, restless legs syndrome (RLS), and insufficient sleep.

Evaluation of Insomnia Disorder

The diagnosis of insomnia requires establishment of a sleep-related complaint (difficulty initiating sleep, difficulty maintaining sleep, or waking up earlier than desired) that affects how the patient feels or functions during the day, occurs at least 3 times per week for at least 3 months, and cannot be fully accounted for by factors such as physical or mental health conditions or medications.[7,8] Insomnia diagnosis does not require objective testing. Women veterans often experience

insomnia for years without seeking treatment.[9] Physical examination and laboratory tests should be used to rule out possible contributory factors.

Evaluation of Sleep-Disordered Breathing

SDB should be considered if the patient reports snoring or witnessed apneas, daytime hypersomnolence despite an adequate sleep opportunity, or has comorbid conditions exacerbated by SDB, such as hypertension. Women may also present with less typical symptoms such as depressed mood and fatigue. Menopausal status, body mass index (BMI), neck circumference, and airway anatomy should all be considered in identifying risk factors for SDB among women.

Women with suspected SDB should undergo laboratory polysomnography, or if appropriate, home sleep apnea testing.[10] One consideration among women veterans is that they may experience challenges in completing in-laboratory testing. For example, because of socioeconomic factors, women veterans may have difficulty arranging overnight childcare, and some may not feel comfortable sleeping in the sleep laboratory setting, particularly in the presence of male technicians, due to past sexual or interpersonal trauma.

Evaluation of Insufficient Sleep

Women veterans are at high risk for insufficient sleep (defined as <7 hour of sleep per night) because an estimated 35% of the general population does not obtain adequate sleep,[11] and insufficient sleep is typical during military service.[12,13] Women veterans have multiple additional risk factors including being middle aged or older, being unable to work due to disabilities, or being unmarried, all of which are associated with insufficient sleep in general.[11,14,15] A sleep history often identifies women with insufficient sleep; however, in some instances, wrist actigraphy may be useful in objectively determining habitual total sleep time.

INSOMNIA DISORDER IN WOMEN VETERANS
Prevalence of Insomnia

Military personnel are a young, healthy population at baseline who are then subjected to multiple stressors that can result in disturbed sleep and predispose them to insomnia. Potential stressors include deployments, family separation, shift work, and extended work hours.[4] Insomnia is more prevalent among women compared with men in the general population.[16] Foster and colleagues[4] published a study that aimed to assess gender differences in sleep disorders in the US military. Insomnia was significantly more prevalent in women, even after adjusting for age and BMI. This was consistent with a recent study by Capener and colleagues.[2]

In a survey study of women veterans receiving care in one large VA health care system, Martin and colleagues[17] found that 52.3% of women met diagnostic criteria for insomnia disorder.[18] The highest rates of insomnia were observed among women in their mid-40s rather than in the oldest age cohorts.

Factors Contributing to Insomnia Among Women Veterans

A theoretic model for insomnia disorder suggests that insomnia develops due to predisposing factors, precipitating events, and perpetuating factors.[19] In addition to factors contributing to the development and maintenance of insomnia in the general population, women veterans experience several unique risk factors and precipitating events that can evolve into a chronic insomnia disorder. For example, feeling unsafe at night during combat operations may contribute to hypervigilance at night and that may contribute to habits that negatively affect sleep, such as leaving room lights on overnight. **Table 1** depicts possible application of this theoretical model for women veterans.

Treatment of Insomnia Disorder in Women Veterans

The American College of Physicians recommends cognitive behavioral therapy (CBT) for insomnia (CBT-I) as first-line therapy,[20] and the Department of Veterans Affairs has established programs for training mental health providers to deliver this treatment.[21,22] Therefore, women who receive VA health care may have better access to CBT-I than women in the general population. Nevertheless, significant challenges remain in the delivery

of these treatments, even though the VA has initiated a national "roll out" of CBT-I to increase access to this treatment for all veterans.[21]

Cognitive behavioral therapy for insomnia and challenges in delivering cognitive behavioral therapy for insomnia to women veterans

CBT-I typically involves 2 core behavioral therapies: stimulus control therapy and sleep restriction therapy, in combination with other strategies such as sleep hygiene education, relaxation training, and cognitive therapy exercises (**Table 2**).[14,19]

The challenge of delivering CBT-I to women veterans reflects barriers women face in accessing treatment in general. However, women veterans prefer nonpharmacological treatments over medications,[23] and efforts to increase accessibility and availability of CBT-I for women veterans are likely to be well received. One challenge in delivering CBT-I to women veterans with significant psychiatric comorbidities is that some may find it difficult to tolerate the temporary increase in sleepiness resulting from sleep restriction therapy due to overall high symptom burden. Culver and colleagues[23] reported that women veterans find CBT-I more acceptable than medications, even in the context of comorbid psychiatric symptoms. Hughes and colleagues[9] found high rates of comorbid PTSD in women veterans with insomnia disorder, and nearly all women in the study (91%) with comorbid insomnia and PTSD identified a specific trigger for their sleep difficulties. Most commonly, women reported nonsexual military trauma (27%), interpersonal trauma (27%), and economic/occupational stressors (20%). Sixteen percent of women attributed their insomnia onset to military sexual trauma. Among women without PTSD, 29% identified interpersonal trauma as an insomnia trigger.

Table 1
Examples of predisposing, precipitating, and perpetuating factors for women veterans

Predisposing Factors	Precipitating Events	Perpetuating Factors
Factors that increase risk for insomnia disorder	*Events that lead to sleep disruption*	*Behavioral and cognitive factors that sustain poor sleep quality over time*
• History of childhood or interpersonal trauma • Chronic mental health conditions, such as depression, anxiety, or PTSD • History of shift work/irregular schedule during service or deployments	• Accidents during training or military deployments, resulting in injuries and pain • Traumas, such as combat trauma, military sexual trauma, or interpersonal trauma during military service • Discharge from military service and return to civilian life	• Poor sleep environment • Sleep as an avoidance strategy to escape physical or emotional pain • Fear of sleep and vulnerability at night • Anxiety about sleep loss

Table 2
Core components of CBT-I and rationale for each component

Component	Rationale for Treatment	Approach
Sleep restriction therapy	Many patients with insomnia extend time in bed, which leads to sleep fragmentation and extended time awake while in bed	Adjust time in bed to more closely match total sleep time
Stimulus control therapy	Classically conditioned arousal in the sleep environment is disruptive to sleep	Remove nonsleep activities from the sleep environment and discourage sleeping in other locations
Sleep hygiene education	Poor habits can contribute to sleep disruption at night, including poor environment, caffeine, alcohol, and other factors	Identify and address specific sleep hygiene behaviors that may lead to improved sleep
Relaxation	Insomnia can be associated with anxiety and hyperarousal	Teaching and practicing relaxation skills can improve the patient's ability to relax in bed at night
Cognitive therapy	Patients with insomnia develop maladaptive ways of thinking about sleep, insomnia, and the consequences of sleep loss	Addressing maladaptive thoughts about sleep can reduce sleep-related anxiety and facilitate motivation to adhere to behavioral recommendations

Pharmacologic treatment options and challenges to pharmacotherapy for insomnia with women veterans

Insomnia disorder is commonly treated with sedative hypnotic medications despite limited supporting evidence.[20] Women are more likely to take prescription hypnotic medications for sleep in the general population.[24] However, a study of veterans who returned from Iraq or Afghanistan found that rates of zolpidem use were similarly high in men and women.[25] Clinicians should consider medications as second-line therapy for insomnia disorder in women veterans and should use CBT-I first. When medications are needed, the lowest-effective dose should always be used because there is some evidence that women are more prone to side effects of some sleep medications (discussed later).

Published guidelines on the use of pharmacologic agents to improve sleep recommend avoidance of several medications commonly used off-label, including trazodone, tiagabine, diphenhydramine, melatonin, tryptophan and valerian, because there is limited evidence for effectiveness and/or safety concerns.[26] However, within the VA health care system, off-label use of medications for treatment of sleep disorders remains common.[27,28]

Outcomes and Potential Complications of Insomnia Treatments

Many women veterans with insomnia disorder suffer from significant comorbidities and experience insomnia for many years before seeking treatment.[9]

Given the chronic nature of insomnia, treatments are typically focused on long-term (rather than short-term) improvements. In general, there are more data to support the long-term efficacy of CBT-I compared with medications in the treatment of insomnia.[29]

Cognitive behavioral therapy for insomnia

One reason CBT-I is recommended as first-line therapy is the durability of treatment effects.[20,30] A recent study of older veterans (men and women) reported benefits of CBT-I in terms of improved sleep quality for up to 1 year posttreatment.[31] In one study of CBT-I among veterans with PTSD, which included a majority of women patients, benefits were maintained for up to 6 months posttreatment.[32]

CBTs are generally safe; however, one concern of CBT-I administration is the temporary increase in sleepiness during the initial weeks of sleep restriction therapy. Otherwise, there is no evidence for adverse effects of CBT-I. There is risk that patients will experience periods of insomnia after CBT-I, and there is limited evidence on how best to treat these patients. In clinical practice, patients are typically brought in for additional sessions and helped to reestablish the sleep habits that were helpful during their original course of CBT-I. In other instances, pharmacotherapy is added.

Pharmacotherapy

The Food and Drug Administration (FDA)–approved indication for most hypnotics is for short-term use, given the limited evidence of long-term efficacy and durability. Very few studies have explored chronic nightly dosing of hypnotics. Krystal and colleagues[33] explored use of zolpidem for 6 months of nightly use and found that benefits relative to placebo were sustained, with no evidence of tolerance and minimal side effects. More often, studies on long-term efficacy have focused on intermittent dosing in an attempted effort to minimize potential adverse effects.[34] It is worth noting that a large placebo response is often seen in studies of sleep medications.[35]

The potential harm caused by first-generation hypnotics likely contributed to the popular belief that "the cure is worse than the disease" when it comes to sedative-hypnotic medications.[36] This has resulted in the benzodiazepine receptor agonist (BzRA) hypnotics being classified as Schedule 4 medications by the FDA. In addition, among patients with current or past drug use or abuse (illicit or prescription) or alcohol dependence, health care providers must exercise extreme caution prescribing medications such as BzRAs to treat insomnia disorder.

Importantly, there may be differences in the safety profiles for hypnotic medications, and women may be at higher risk for adverse outcomes. In 2012, the FDA issued a safety communication specifically related to the dosing of zolpidem in women due to dose-related side effects. This resulted in changes to prescribing protocols; however, most women using zolpidem are still prescribed higher than the recommended dose.[37] In the veteran population, there is also significant concern about suicide risk. Studies from nonveteran populations suggest that benzodiazepine use increases risk for suicide.[38]

SLEEP-DISORDERED BREATHING

SDB is a broad term that covers a range of respiratory issues seen during sleep, from snoring to obstructive sleep apnea. SDB is associated with significant adverse health consequences, including increased accident risks, impaired quality of life, and increased cardiac disease; the latter remains the leading cause of death for women worldwide. SDB is more common in men than women; however, clinic-based prevalence studies likely overestimated gender difference because of differing clinical manifestations between men and women and/or referral bias.[39]

Although SDB is a well-studied condition with known treatments, the existing literature has not focused on understanding this disorder among women. Unfortunately, many women continue to suffer from SDB for years before a definitive diagnosis is made.

Epidemiology and Clinical Features of Sleep-Disordered Breathing

The consistent difference in prevalence between clinical and community-based studies indicates underdiagnosis of SDB in women, either because of differences in the clinical manifestations or because of failure to refer women with suspected SDB for treatment. Much like heart disease, women with SDB present differently. Symptoms include insomnia, fatigue, or depression. Men are more likely to present with excessive sleepiness, snoring, or hypertension.[39] Clinicians should be aware of gender differences in clinical manifestations as they evaluate symptoms such as fatigue, sleepiness, and poor-quality sleep.

Large epidemiologic studies investigating the prevalence of SDB in the community found a 3-fold difference in the prevalence of SDB (without or without symptoms) between men and women; however, there is evidence that the difference is only 2-fold when the definition includes daytime sleepiness.[40] In both men and women, there is evidence that rates of SDB are increasing over time, likely due to increasing rates of obesity in the US population.[41] Using data from the Women's Health Initiative study, Rissling and colleagues[42] found that postmenopausal women veterans were more likely than nonveteran women to have insomnia and SDB together, but not SDB alone. They suggest this pattern of results may be related to high rates of PTSD in women veterans.

Menopause is a risk factor for SDB, and as the number of postmenopausal women veterans increases, this will become a growing concern.[43,44] The menopausal progression is associated with increased likelihood of SDB and higher AHI, independent of aging and changes in BMI. In addition, menopause is associated with increased prevalence of central sleep apnea, and increased SDB prevalence with menopause is likely due to changes in female sex hormones and not to aging per se.

Treatment of Sleep-Disordered Breathing

The most widely used treatment for SDB is positive airway pressure (PAP) therapy. Although PAP has demonstrated benefits, such as reducing blood pressure and improving daytime sleepiness, patients encounter numerous barriers to using PAP. Studies in the United States show that women have lower PAP adherence rates than men.[45,46]

Options for patients with SDB who are intolerant of PAP therapy include oral appliances, hypoglossal nerve stimulation, or surgery. Gender does not seem to influence the selection or response to alternative therapies.

Outcomes and Challenges to Positive Airway Pressure Therapy Adherence for Women Veterans

There are no studies of PAP therapy among women veterans, and few studies have examined the benefits of treatment of sleep apnea specifically among women. Among veterans with PTSD, there is some evidence that treatment with PAP therapy is associated with a reduction in PTSD symptoms.[47] Although the mechanism is not fully elucidated, Orr and colleagues[47] advocated that PAP should be an integral component of PTSD treatment in patients with concomitant obstructive sleep apnea. These results were confirmed in a similar study by El-Solh and colleagues.[48] Neither study commented on a gender-related difference in treatment outcomes.

Adherence to PAP therapy remains a challenge. Rates of refusal of PAP after one night range from 15% to 30%.[49] Early (1–3 month) PAP adherence ranges from 48% to 57%,[45,50] whereas long-term adherence (6–12 months) ranges from 22% to 55%.[51,52] There are multiple reasons for high rates of nonadherence, including side effects, lack of understanding about SDB and PAP, and competing demands in health maintenance. Research into factors determining PAP adherence have yielded conflicting results, especially regarding gender differences in PAP acceptance and PAP use, with potentially lower PAP adherence rates in women.[45,46] Women veterans are at high risk for nonadherence due to high rates of comorbidities known to reduce PAP adherence (eg, depression, PTSD) and high rates of comorbid insomnia disorder, which is also known to adversely affect PAP use.[53,54]

INSUFFICIENT SLEEP (SHORT SLEEP DURATION)

Short sleep has been linked to a myriad of adverse health outcomes, such as depression, PTSD, accidents and injuries, cardiac disorders, suicide, and overall mortality.[55] Sleep disturbances are endemic in military personnel and cause severe decrements in cognitive functions, decision-making, mood, and moral reasoning.[56]

Insufficient sleep syndrome, or short sleep duration, manifests by chronic volitional sleep restriction, resulting in excessive daytime sleepiness and/or fatigue.[18] Military personnel are subjected to insufficient sleep secondary to a host of causes. Irregular sleep/wake schedules, physical and psychological consequences of deployment and combat experiences, frequent relocation, as well as the stress related to postdeployment social reintegration. All contribute to short sleep duration. Furthermore, short sleep duration is often overlooked and considered to be an integral component of the military culture. Transitioning back to civilian life does not automatically lead to restored sleep habits, and military veterans are at high risk for insufficient sleep.

Consistent with insufficient sleep duration, self-reported sleep duration in service members ranged between 5.8 and 6.5 hours nightly, independent of deployment status.[12,13] It is logical to assume that comorbid physical illness, mental illness, or insomnia contributed to these findings. In a recent study of men and women veterans, 45% reported sleeping 6 or fewer hours per night, with higher risk among those with socioeconomic challenges.[15]

NIGHTMARE DISORDER (POSTTRAUMATIC STRESS DISORDER-ASSOCIATED NIGHTMARES)

Nightmares are more common among women compared with men,[57] and given high rates of PTSD among women veterans, nightmares can lead to significant sleep disruption. The 2 most common treatments for nightmare disorder include imagery rehearsal therapy (IRT) and prazosin.

IRT is a brief psychotherapy designed to help patients "rescript" their nightmares and imagine more helpful dreams. Some versions of IRT incorporate additional strategies. Prazosin is an antihypertensive agent with alpha 1–adrenergic receptor agonist actions that cross the blood brain barrier. In a recent meta-analytic review, IRT and prazosin were both shown to reduce nightmare frequency and improve sleep quality, with additional benefits when CBT-I is added to IRT.[58]

Intervention studies in civilian populations included predominantly women patients, whereas studies in military or veteran populations included primarily men. Because very few women were included in trials of veterans, it is not clear whether they benefit in different ways compared with men. However, available evidence suggests either IRT or prazosin as a viable treatment option for women veterans.

RESTLESS LEGS SYNDROME

RLS is a chronic movement disorder with a circadian tendency that may interfere with sleep, leading to poor sleep quality or insomnia.[59] Typical symptoms include an unpleasant sensation in the lower extremities, accompanied by an irresistible urge to move, which attenuates the sensation.[18] RLS can be a primary disorder or secondary to several conditions including iron deficiency, renal failure, or pregnancy; the latter resolves following delivery (see Corrado Garbazza and Mauro Manconi's article, "Management Strategies for Restless Legs Syndrome/Willis-Ekbom Disease during Pregnancy," in this issue).

RLS is a common disorder with an estimated prevalence of 5% to 10%. The prevalence in women is 1.5- to 2-fold higher than that in men. A strong familial tendency is noted, because 63% of adults have at least one first-degree relative with the condition. The prevalence of RLS among women veterans is not established but one study showed 4% of women veterans are diagnosed with RLS.[5] Treatment of RLS includes dopamine agonists or iron supplements if serum ferritin is low. A combined approach may be required in severe or refractory RLS. More details about RLS and treatment options are included in Corrado Garbazza and Mauro Manconi's article, "Management Strategies for Restless Legs Syndrome/Willis-Ekbom Disease during Pregnancy," in this issue.

SUMMARY

Sleep disorders are common among women veterans, and there is some evidence that insomnia comorbid with sleep apnea is more common among women veterans than among nonveteran women. Studies show that insomnia is more frequent among women veterans compared with men veterans.

Further research is needed to evaluate differences between men and women veterans and between women veterans and nonveterans. Given the unique predisposing, precipitating, and perpetuating factors that can affect sleep in women veterans (see **Table 1**), including stressors, environmental factors, and high comorbidity of disorders such as PTSD, strongly linked with sleep disturbances, more studies are needed to understand sleep disturbances in this context. Most studies of sleep disorders in veteran populations have been representative of the population, with inclusion of only 5% to 10% women. Because of their underrepresentation in research, very little can be concluded about their unique needs in terms of managing sleep disorders. In order to adequately understand differences in sleep disorders facing men and women who are military veterans, future research should start using strategies to oversample women veterans and to increase representation of women in research on sleep disorders among veterans.

REFERENCES

1. Washington DL, Bean-Mayberry B, Hamilton AB, et al. Health profiles of U.S. women veterans by war cohort: findings from the National Survey of Women Veterans. J Gen Intern Med 2013; 28(Suppl. 2):S571–6.
2. Capener DC, Brock MS, Hansen SL, et al. An initial report of sleep disorders in women in the U.S. military. Mil Med 2018. [Epub ahead of print].
3. Mysliwiec V, McGraw L, Pierce R, et al. Sleep disorders and associated medical comorbidities in active duty military personnel. Sleep 2013;36(2):167–74.
4. Foster SN, Hansen SL, Capener DC, et al. Gender differences in sleep disorders in the US military. Sleep health 2017;3(5):336–41.
5. Alexander M, Ray MA, Hebert JR, et al. The national veteran sleep disorder study: descriptive epidemiology and secular trends, 2000-2010. Sleep 2016; 9(7):1399–410.
6. A Caldwell J, Knapik JJ, Lieberman HR. Trends and factors associated with insomnia and sleep apnea in all United States military service members from 2005 to 2014. J Sleep Res 2017;26(5): 665–70.
7. American Academy of Sleep Medicine. International classification of sleep disorders. 3rd edition. Darien (IL): American Academy of Sleep Medicine; 2014.
8. American Psychiatric Association. Diagnostic and statistical manual of mental disorders. 5th edition. Washington, DC: American Psychiatric Association; 2013.
9. Hughes JM, Jouldjian S, Washington DL, et al. Insomnia and symptoms of post-traumatic stress disorder among women Veterans. Behav Sleep Med 2013;11(4):258–74.
10. Kapur VK, Auckley DH, Chowdhuri S, et al. Clinical practice guideline for diagnostic testing for adult obstructive sleep apnea: an American Academy of Sleep Medicine clinical practice guideline. J Clin Sleep Med 2017;13:479–504.
11. Liu Y, Wheaton AG, Chapman DP, et al. Prevalence of healthy sleep duration among adults–United States, 2014. MMWR Morb Mort Wkly Rep 2016; 65(6):137–41.
12. Luxton DD, Greenburg D, Ryan J, et al. Prevalence and impact of short sleep duration in rededeployed OIF soldiers. Sleep 2011;34(9):1189–95.
13. Seelig AD, Jacobson IG, Smith B, et al. Sleep patterns before, during, and after deployment to Iraq and Afghanistan. Sleep 2011;33(12):1615–22.

14. Frayne SM, Phibbs CS, Saechao F, et al. Women veterans in the veterans health administration. Volume 3 Sociodemographics, Utilization, Costs Care Health Profile 2014.

15. Widome R, Jensen A, Fu SS. Socioeconomic disparities in sleep duration among veterans of the US Wars in Iraq and Afghanistan. Am J Public Health 2015;105(2):e70–4.

16. Zhang G, Wing YK. Sex differences in insomnia: a meta-analysis. Sleep 2006;29:85–93.

17. Martin JL, Schweizer A, Hughes JM, et al. Estimated rate of insomnia among women veterans: results of a postal survey. Women's Health Issues 2017;27(3): 366–73.

18. American Academy of Sleep Medicine. The international classification of sleep disorders. 2nd edition. Westchester (IL): American Academy of Sleep Medicine; 2005.

19. Spielman A, Glovinsky PB. The varied nature of insomnia. In: Hauri PJ, editor. Case studies in insomnia. New York: Plenum Press; 1991.

20. Qaseem A, Kansagara D, Forciea MA, et al, Clinical Guidelines Committee of the American College of Physicians. Management of chronic insomnia disorder in adults: a clinical practice guideline from the American College of Physicians. Ann Intern Med 2016;165(2):125–33.

21. Trockel M, Karlin BE, Taylor CB, et al. Cognitive behavioral therapy for insomnia with veterans: evaluation of effectiveness and correlates of treatment outcomes. Behav Res Ther 2014;53(41):46.

22. Manber R, Carney C, Edinger J, et al. Dissemination of CBTI to the non-sleep specialist: protocol development and training issues. J Clin Sleep Med 2012;8(2):209–18.

23. Culver NC, Song Y, McGowan SK, et al. Acceptability of medication and non-medication treatment for insomnia among women veterans: effects of age, insomnia severity, and psychiatric symptoms. Clin Ther 2016;38(11):2373–85.

24. Kaufmann CN, Spira AP, Alexander GC, et al. Trends in prescribing of sedative-hypnotic medications in the USA: 1993-2010. Pharmacoepidemiol Drug Saf 2016;25(6):637–45.

25. Shayegani R, Song K, Amuan ME, et al. Patterns of zolpidem use among Iraq and Afghanistan veterans: a retrospective cohort analysis. PLoS One 2018; 13(1):e0190022.

26. Sateia MJ, Buysse DJ, Krystal AD, et al. Clinical practice guideline for the pharmacologic treatment of chronic insomnia in adults: an American Academy of Sleep Medicine clinical practice guideline. J Clin Sleep Med 2017;13(2):307–49.

27. Hermes ED, Sernyak M, Rosenheck R. Use of second-generation antipsychotic agents for sleep and sedation: a provider survey. Sleep 2013;36(4): 597–600.

28. Greenbaum MA, Neylan TC, Rosen CS. Symptom presentation and prescription of sleep medications for veterans with posttraumatic stress disorder. J Nerv Ment Dis 2017;205(2):112–8.

29. Smith MT, Perlis ML, Park A, et al. Comparative meta-analysis of pharmacotherapy and behavior therapy for persistent insomnia. Am J Psychiatry 2002;159(1):5–11.

30. National Institutes of Health. Manifestations and management of chronic insomnia in adults. Sleep 2005;28(9):1049–57.

31. Alessi CA, Martin JL, Fiorentino L, et al. Cognitive behavioral therapy for insomnia in older veterans using non-clinician sleep coaches: a randomized controlled trial. J Am Geriatr Soc 2016;64(9):1830–8.

32. Talbot LS, Maguen S, Metzler TJ, et al. Cognitive behavioral therapy for insomnia in posttraumatic stress disorder: a randomized controlled trial. Sleep 2014;37(2):327–41.

33. Krystal AD, Walsh JK, Laska E, et al. Sustained efficacy of eszopiclone over 6 months of nightly treatment: results of a randomized, double-blind, placebo-controlled study in adults with chronic insomnia. Sleep 2003;26(7):793–9.

34. Perlis ML, McCall WV, Krystal AD, et al. Long-term, non-nightly administration of zolpidem in the treatment of patients with primary insomnia. J Clin Psychiatry 2004;65(8):1128–37.

35. Winkler A, Rief W. Effect of placebo conditions on polysomnographic parameters in primary insomnia: a meta-analysis. Sleep 2015;38(6):925–31.

36. Perlis M, Gehrman P, Riemann D. Intermittent and long-term use of sedative hypnotics. Curr Pharm Des 2008;14(32):3456–65.

37. Harward JL, Clinard VB, Jiroutek MR, et al. Impact of a US food and drug administration drug safety communication on zolpidem dosing: an observational retrospective cohort. Prim Care Companion CNS Disord 2015;17(2).

38. Dodds TJ. Prescribed benzodiazepines and suicide risk: a review of the literature. Prim Care Companion CNS Disord 2017;19(2).

39. Larsson LG, Lindberg A, Franklin KA, et al. Gender differences in symptoms related to sleep apnea in a general population and in relation to referral to sleep clinic. Chest 2003;124(1):204–11.

40. Young T, Peppard PE, Gottlieb DJ. Epidemiology of obstructive sleep apnea: a population health perspective. Am J Respir Crit Care Med 2002; 165(9):1217–39.

41. Peppard PE, Young T, Barnet JH, et al. Increased prevalence of sleep-disordered breathing in adults. Am J Epidemiol 2013;177(9):1006–14.

42. Rissling MB, Gray KE, Ulmer CS, et al. Sleep disturbance, diabetes and cardiovascular disease in postmenopausal veteran women. Gerontologist 2016;56(S1):S54–66.

43. Bixler EO, Vgontzas AN, Lin HM, et al. Prevalence of sleep-disordered breathing in women: effects of gender. Am J Respir Crit Care Med 2001;163(3 Pt 1):608–13.

44. Mirer AG, Young T, Palta M, et al. Sleep-disordered breathing and the menopausal transition among participants in the Sleep in Midlife Women Study. Menopause 2017;24(2):157–62.

45. Joo MJ, Herdegen JJ. Sleep apnea in an urban public hospital: assessment of severity and treatment adherence. J Clin Sleep Med 2007;15(3):285–8.

46. Lettieri CJ, Shah AA, Holley AB, et al, CPAP Promotion and Prognosis-The Army Sleep Apnea Program Trial. Effects of a short course of eszopiclone on continuous positive airway pressure adherence: a randomized trial. Ann Intern Med 2009;151(10): 696–702.

47. Orr JE, Smales C, Alexander TH, et al. Treatment of OSA with CPAP is associated with improvement in PTSD symptoms among veterans. J Clin Sleep Med 2017;13(1):57–63.

48. El-Solh AA, Ayyar L, Akinnusi M, et al. Positive airway pressure adherence in veterans with posttraumatic stress disorder. Sleep 2010;33(11): 1495–500.

49. Collard P, Pieters T, Aubert P, et al. Compliance with nasal CPAP in obstructive sleep apnea. Sleep Med Rev 1997;1(1):33–44.

50. Ye L, Pack AI, Maislin G, et al. Predictors of continuous positive airway pressure use during the first week of treatment. J Sleep Res 2012;21(4):419–26.

51. Schwartz SW, Sebastiao Y, Rosas J, et al. Racial disparity in adherence to positive airway pressure among US Veterans. Sleep Breath 2016;20(3): 947–55.

52. Wallace DM, Vargas SS, Schwartz SJ, et al. Determinants of continuous positive airway pressure adherence in a sleep clinic cohort of South Florida Hispanic veterans. Sleep and breathing 2013; 17(1):351–63.

53. Stepnowsky C, Bardwell WA, Moore P, et al. Psychological correlates of CPAP compliance with continuous positive airway pressure. Sleep 2002;25(7): 758–64.

54. Wickwire EM, Smith MT, Birnbaum S, et al. Sleep maintenance insomnia complaints predict poor CPAP adherence: a clinical case series. Sleep Med 2010;11(8):772–6.

55. Bramoweth AD, Germain A. Deployment-related insomnia in military personnel and veterans. Curr Psychiatry Rep 2013;15(10):401.

56. Seelig AD, Jacobson IG, Donoho CJ, et al. Sleep and health resilience metrics in a large military cohort. Sleep 2016;39(5):1111–20.

57. Schredl M. Explaining the gender difference in nightmare frequency. Am J Psychol 2014;127(2): 205–13.

58. Seda G, Sanchez-Ortuno MM, Welsh CH, et al. Comparative meta-analysis of prazosin and imagery rehearsal therapy for nightmare frequency, sleep quality, and posttraumatic stress. J Clin Sleep Med 2015;11(1):11–22.

59. Wijemanne S, Ondo W. Restless legs syndrome: clinical features, diagnosis and a practical approach to management. Pract Neurol 2017;17(6):444–52.

Sleep and Sleep Disorders in the Menopausal Transition

Fiona C. Baker, PhD[a,b,*], Laura Lampio, MD, PhD[c,d],
Tarja Saaresranta, MD, PhD[c,e], Päivi Polo-Kantola, MD, PhD[c,f]

KEYWORDS

- Menopause • Climacteric • Subjective sleep quality • Sleep architecture • Polysomnography
- Vasomotor symptoms • Depressive symptoms

KEY POINTS

- There is an increase in self-reported sleep disturbance, particularly nocturnal awakenings, across the menopausal transition. Symptoms are bothersome and impact quality of life, health, and productivity.
- Vasomotor symptoms (both self-reported and measured hot flashes and sweating) are critical symptoms associated with disrupted sleep in the menopausal transition.
- Associations between menopausal stage and/or hormone levels and polysomnographic measures are less consistent, and further longitudinal studies are required.
- Sleep disturbances may arise during the menopausal transition in association with primary sleep disorders (eg, sleep-disordered breathing). Women with sleep complaints should be evaluated and appropriately treated.
- Effective management strategies for menopausal sleep disturbances include hormone therapy, other pharmacologic treatments (eg, gabapentin), and cognitive behavioral therapy for insomnia.

INTRODUCTION

Sleep disturbances increase in prevalence during the menopausal transition, with the most common complaint being nighttime awakenings.[1,2] Sleep disturbances impact health-related quality of life, work productivity, and health care utilization[3] and can have long-term effects on health and well-being across several years of the menopausal transition. Here, the authors aim to provide an overview of sleep disturbances in the context of the menopausal transition, considering self-reported and objectively measured indicators of sleep. The authors also consider factors that could mediate sleep disturbance, including female sex steroids, vasomotor symptoms (eg, hot flashes and sweating), aging, and stressful life events. Finally, they provide an overview of potential treatment options and their efficacy and highlight the need for further research. Understanding the causes as well as effective

Disclosure statement: This work is supported by National Institutes of Health grant HL103688 (F.C. Baker). The content is solely the responsibility of the authors and does not necessarily represent the official views of the National Institutes of Health. F.C. Baker has received funding unrelated to this work from Ebb Therapeutics Inc, Fitbit Inc, and International Flavors & Fragrances Inc. The other authors have nothing to disclose.
[a] Human Sleep Research Program, SRI International, 333 Ravenswood Avenue, Menlo Park, CA 94025, USA; [b] Brain Function Research Group, School of Physiology, University of the Witwatersrand, Johannesburg, South Africa; [c] Department of Pulmonary Diseases and Clinical Allergology, Sleep Research Centre, University of Turku, Turku, Finland; [d] Department of Obstetrics and Gynecology, Helsinki University Hospital, Helsinki, Finland; [e] Division of Medicine, Department of Pulmonary Diseases, Turku University Hospital, Turku, Finland; [f] Department of Obstetrics and Gynecology, Turku University Hospital, University of Turku, Turku, Finland
* Corresponding author. Human Sleep Research Program, SRI International, 333 Ravenswood Avenue, Menlo Park, CA 94025.
E-mail address: Fiona.baker@sri.com

Sleep Med Clin 13 (2018) 443–456
https://doi.org/10.1016/j.jsmc.2018.04.011
1556-407X/18/© 2018 Elsevier Inc. All rights reserved.

preventative and treatment strategies for menopausal sleep disturbances is essential for better health, quality of life, and work ability.

DEFINITION AND PHYSIOLOGY OF MENOPAUSE

Menopause (defined as the time of the final menstrual period) is a natural process in normal female aging, resulting from depletion of ovarian follicles, and occurs at a median age of 51 years,[4] with the menopausal transition usually starting at about 47 years of age.[5] The Stages of Reproductive Aging Workshop (STRAW +10) standardizes the division of a woman's late reproductive life, broadly grouping women into 3 categories (reproductive, menopausal transition, and postmenopause) further subdivided according to menstrual cycle length and regularity.[6] Perimenopause encompasses the menopausal transition and the first year after the final menstrual period. The term *climacteric* may also be used to describe perimenopause and the part of the postmenopausal period in which climacteric symptoms occur.

Ovarian function begins to deteriorate, and function of the hypothalamic-pituitary-ovarian axis begins to change several years before menopause. These endocrinologic changes typically occur gradually and are not linear. Levels of follicle-stimulating hormone (FSH) increase overall and are typically 25 IU/L or greater in the late menopausal transition. In association with the fluctuation and gradual decline in estrogen (typically estradiol [E2]) across the menopausal transition, menopausal symptoms emerge and include vasomotor symptoms (hot flashes and sweating), sleep disturbances, and mood symptoms (**Table 1**).

Table 1
Typical menopausal symptoms and their prevalence in midlife women

Symptom	Prevalence (%)
Hot flashes and/or night sweats	36–87
Sleep problems	40–60
Mood symptoms	15–78
Weight gain	60–70
Muscle and/or joint pain	48–72
Palpitation	44–50
Headache	32–71
Memory impairment	41–44
Genitourinary symptoms	25–30
Sexual dysfunction	20–30

Data from Refs.[7,28,41,141–145]

SLEEP QUALITY DURING THE MENOPAUSAL TRANSITION
Self-Reported Sleep Quality

Among menopausal symptoms, sleep disturbances are one of the most bothersome symptoms and are reported by 40% to 60% of menopausal women.[7] There is convincing evidence from several cross-sectional[8–12] and longitudinal[13–16] studies that the prevalence of perceived sleep disturbances increases in the menopausal transition, even after controlling for age. A recent meta-analysis of cross-sectional data from 24 studies reported higher odds of experiencing sleep disturbance in perimenopause (1.60), postmenopause (1.67), and surgical menopause (2.17) relative to women who are premenopausal.[17]

The most common sleep-related complaint is nighttime awakenings.[8,11,14,16] In their 7-year follow-up of 3045 women, the Study of Women's Health Across the Nation (SWAN) reported an increase in odds ratios (ORs) for difficulty staying asleep across the menopausal transition after adjusting for demographics and health-related factors.[14] ORs also increased for difficulty falling asleep across the transition but decreased for early morning awakening from late perimenopause to postmenopause. Although most studies examined associations between sleep and menopausal stages based on bleeding patterns, some studies have investigated the association between FSH concentrations and self-reported sleep.[14,16] Increasing FSH was associated with greater odds of waking up several times, whereas decreasing estrogen was associated with higher odds of difficulty falling and staying asleep in SWAN.[14]

Polysomnographic Studies

Even though the evidence for declining self-reported sleep quality across the menopausal transition is strong, polysomnographic (PSG) studies have generally not found a corresponding negative change in sleep architecture. PSG-derived measures of sleep do not necessarily reflect self-report sleep quality ratings,[18] and the psychological state may influence sleep quality judgments by affecting the sleep appraisal process rather than sleep itself.[19] Also, most PSG studies have been cross-sectional and included small samples, with few exceptions.[12,20] Further, studies have varied in methodology, including definitions of menopausal stages, age ranges, assessment of the presence of sleep disorders like obstructive sleep apnea, and inclusion of an adaptation night, leading to contradictory results and challenges when trying to make study comparisons.

Some studies have found no differences in sleep architecture between premenopausal and postmenopausal women,[21–23] whereas a few studies have reported more slow wave sleep (SWS) in perimenopausal and postmenopausal women than premenopausal women.[12,20,24] More SWS could be interpreted as reflecting a better sleep pattern, on the one hand, but alternatively could reflect a recovery response to sleep deprivation; further studies are needed to better understand potential changes in SWS after menopause. Postmenopausal women had a higher apnea-hypopnea index (AHI) and lower arterial oxyhemoglobin saturation.[20] Finally, SWAN investigators found no differences in PSG measures according to menopausal status.[21] However, late perimenopausal and postmenopausal women had more high-frequency beta electroencephalography (EEG) activity, suggesting greater cortical hyperarousal, during sleep than premenopausal and early perimenopausal women, an effect partially explained by a higher frequency of self-reported hot flashes.[21]

A limited number of studies have investigated the association between FSH, as an endocrine marker of transitioning menopause, with PSG measures. SWAN investigators found that a more rapid rate of FSH change over the previous few years was associated with a higher amount of SWS and longer total sleep time (TST) during

a subsequent sleep study.[25] Another cross-sectional study of women mostly in the early menopausal transition (aged 43–52 years) without sleep complaints found that higher FSH concentrations were associated with more wakefulness after sleep onset (WASO), awakenings, and arousals, after adjusting for age and body mass index (BMI).[26] However, in women with menopausal insomnia, PSG measures did not correlate with FSH and instead were associated with anxiety and depression symptoms.[26] In a small study that evaluated associations of sleep and hypothalamic-pituitary-ovarian axis hormones in a group of premenopausal and postmenopausal women with diagnoses of depression, FSH level was positively associated with WASO and negatively associated with SWS.[27]

In the only longitudinal study of changes in PSG measures across the menopausal transition, Lampio and colleagues[24] studied 60 midlife women at a premenopausal baseline visit and again 6 years later. At the follow-up, women had less TST and more WASO after adjusting for vasomotor symptoms, BMI, and mood (**Fig. 1** showing the PSG changes in a representative participant). These changes in sleep were linked with advancing age rather than increased FSH levels. Increasing FSH was associated with a greater proportion of SWS (although not with slow wave EEG activity), which the investigators proposed as reflecting an adaptive change to counteract the age-related sleep fragmentation.[24]

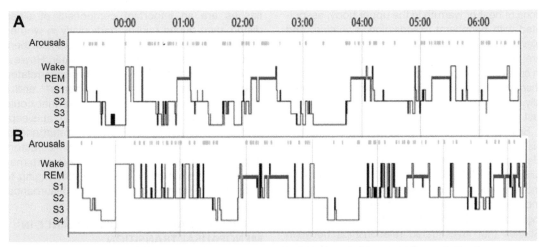

Fig. 1. Hypnograms derived from the polysomnograms of one representative participant during her premenopausal baseline visit (*A*) and at a follow-up visit 6 years later (*B*), when she was perimenopausal. REM, rapid eye movement. (*Data from* Lampio L, Polo-Kantola P, Himanen SL, et al. Sleep during menopausal transition: a 6-year follow-up. Sleep 2017;40(7).)

In summary, PSG studies have shown few consistent effects of menopausal stage on sleep architecture independent of age. All but one study were cross-sectional and, therefore, unable to track changes in sleep across the transition; few studies have used more complex indicators of sleep disruption, like quantitative EEG analysis. Given between-women variability in hormone trajectories, speed of transitioning menopause, and life experiences as they transition menopause, all of which can interact with sleep, further longitudinal studies are needed in midlife women to establish if PSG measures fluctuate in association with the changing hormone environment in the menopausal transition. Also, as discussed next, subgroups of women might be more susceptible to sleep disturbances, particularly women with severe vasomotor symptoms or insomnia disorder.

VASOMOTOR SYMPTOMS (HOT FLASHES AND SWEATING) AND SLEEP DISTURBANCE

Vasomotor symptoms, an umbrella term used to describe hot flashes and sweating, affect up to 80% of women during menopause transition.[28] Data from SWAN show a median duration for vasomotor symptoms of 7.4 years[29]; but the temporal pattern based on symptom onset and persistence varies,[30,31] with symptoms persisting more than 10 years in some women.[29,32]

The precise mechanism of vasomotor symptoms is poorly understood but is hypothesized to result from disturbance of the temperature-regulating system in the hypothalamus, triggered by a decline in E_2.[28] Vasomotor symptoms may occur at any time and usually begin with sensations of heat or warmth in the upper body, associated with peripheral vasodilation, sweating, and elevated skin blood flow.[33] Vasomotor symptoms are proposed to be triggered by small elevations in core body temperature acting within a narrowed thermoneutral zone.[33] The duration of a flash usually ranges from 1 to 5 minutes, but some flashes last up to 60 minutes.[28,33]

Self-reported vasomotor symptoms are consistently associated with poorer self-reported sleep quality and chronic insomnia.[10,14,34,35] Longitudinal SWAN data show that women with moderate-severe hot flashes are almost 3 times more likely to report frequent nocturnal awakenings compared with women without hot flashes.[36] Studies that investigated relationships between reported vasomotor symptoms and objectively measured sleep (with actigraphy or PSG) have produced conflicting results, with early studies showing no relationship[12,22] and more recent studies finding an association between hot flashes and disrupted sleep.[37–39]

Vasomotor symptoms can be measured objectively using sternal skin conductance.[40] Objectively detected vasomotor symptoms have been linked to sleep disruption in some[37,38,41,42] but not all studies.[22,39,43] Differences between studies might relate to the classification of hot flashes in association with awakenings[37] as well as between-women variability in the impact of hot flashes on sleep. In an experimental model of new-onset hot flashes in young premenopausal women treated with a gonadotropin-releasing hormone agonist that simulates menopause, hot flashes were linked with more PSG awakenings, more WASO, and more stage 1 sleep.[44] Thus, these data provide support for a link between hot flashes and disturbed sleep. In an analysis of the overall impact of hot flashes on sleep architecture, de Zambotti and colleagues[37] reported that wake time attributed to hot flashes was responsible for, on average, 27% of objective WASO, although there was wide variability in hot flash impact between women. They also reported that an awakening occurred coincident with most (69%) hot flashes.

In summary, although not all hot flashes are associated with disturbed sleep, they are a strong correlate of poor sleep; many nocturnal hot flash events are closely linked with periods of PSG wake. The strong overlap in timing between hot flash onset and awakenings suggests that these events may be driven by a common mechanism within the central nervous system in response to fluctuating estrogen levels, although sweating triggered by a hot flash may still contribute to, or extend, the interval of waking.[37] Nocturnal hot flashes are an important component of sleep disturbance during midlife, particularly in women with severe sleep difficulties that qualifies them for insomnia disorder, as discussed later. However, not all women who have menopause-related sleep problems complain of hot flashes[41] and it is important to consider other factors that could disturb sleep, including the presence of sleep-disordered breathing (SDB), mood disturbances, medical conditions, and socioeconomic factors (**Fig. 2**). Importantly, several of these factors may interact with each other, making it challenging to determine the primary cause of sleep disturbance.

DEPRESSION AND SLEEP DISTURBANCE IN MENOPAUSAL TRANSITION

The risk for depression increases during the menopausal transition, independently of other factors.[45–48] In SWAN, women were 2 to 4 times more

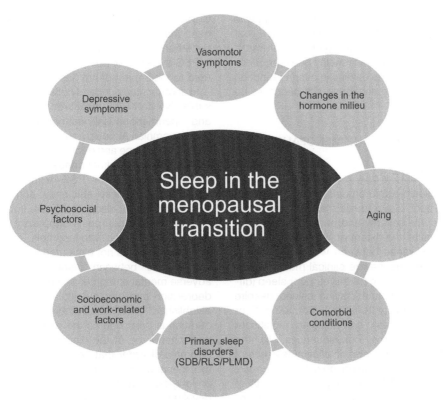

Fig. 2. Many factors are associated with sleep disturbances in the context of the menopausal transition. Some factors may also interact to worsen sleep quality. PLMD, periodic limb movement disorder; RLS, restless legs syndrome.

likely to develop major depressive disorder in menopausal transition and early postmenopause compared with premenopause, after adjusting for confounding factors.[46] It is hypothesized that fluctuation and an eventual drop in estrogen is responsible for impaired mood,[49,50] and women vulnerable to developing mood symptoms during other reproductive transitions (eg, premenstrual phase of the menstrual cycle or postpartum) are at greater risk for developing depressive symptoms in menopausal transition.[51]

There is a bidirectional relationship between mood and sleep disturbances.[52,53] The relationship between depressive symptoms and subjective sleep disturbances has also been documented in women in the menopausal transition.[54–56] In a longitudinal analysis of 309 women transitioning to menopause, Avis and colleagues[57] reported that depressive symptoms were unrelated to menopausal status or annual change in E_2 but were associated with hot flashes and sleep disturbance. Further, in a longitudinal analysis of SWAN data, Bromberger and colleagues[58] found that the presence of subjective sleep problems at baseline was a significant predictor of persistent/recurrent major depressive disorder at follow-up.

Researchers have also investigated the association of sleep architecture with depressive symptoms, although findings are conflicting. In one study, more depressive symptoms were associated with lower sleep efficiency and shorter TST in perimenopausal women and with a higher percentage of rapid eye movement sleep in postmenopausal women.[56] In contrast, a substudy of SWAN found that mood symptoms were not independently related to sleep architecture; anxiety symptoms were related to longer sleep-onset latency and lower sleep efficiency; however, this was found only in women who also reported vasomotor symptoms.[59]

The domino theory, which predicts that vasomotor symptoms lead to insomnia, which then leads to the development of mood symptoms,[60] currently has only partial support.[1] Recent data showed that hot flashes and depressive symptoms were associated with different sleep disturbance patterns, hot flashes being uniquely associated with frequent awakenings and depression uniquely associated with difficulty falling asleep and waking up earlier than desired.[61] Further, an intervention study of perimenopausal women with depressive symptoms found that, in adjusted models, improvement in depression was predicted by improved sleep and increasing E_2 but not by reduction of vasomotor symptoms.[62] Therefore, the causal directionality between these factors in relation to the decline in ovarian function in the approach to menopause still needs to be clarified.

SLEEP DISORDERS IN THE MENOPAUSAL TRANSITION
Insomnia Disorder

Although epidemiologic studies show a clear increase in poor sleep quality as women enter menopause, the severity and persistence of poor sleep, as well as the extent of impairment in daytime function, varies between women. Insomnia disorder is the most severe clinical manifestation of recurrent and chronic perceived poor sleep (difficulty falling asleep and staying asleep despite adequate opportunity to sleep), occurring 3 or more times per week and causing significant distress and daytime consequences. In the context of menopause, classic clinical features of insomnia, such as rumination, anxiety, and generalized hyperarousal,[63,64] overlap with aspects of insomnia specific to menopause, such as vasomotor symptoms.

Based on a structured phone interview of almost 1000 women, Ohayon[35] reported that 26% of perimenopausal women qualified for a *Diagnostic and Statistical Manual of Mental Disorders*, Fourth Edition diagnosis of insomnia, with difficulty maintaining sleep the most common symptom. The likelihood of having chronic insomnia symptoms increased with the severity of hot flashes.[35] Other factors that are associated with an increased risk for insomnia disorder in the context of the menopausal transition include personality factors such as neuroticism, past depression, a history of severe premenstrual symptoms, and chronic stress.[65–67]

There are limited data on PSG measures for insomnia disorder in the menopausal transition. One study found significant objective sleep disruption, with shorter TST, more WASO, and poorer sleep efficiency; the disruption matching subjective reports of poor sleep quality in this group relative to women without insomnia who were also in menopausal transition.[68] In fact, almost 50% of the insomnia group had short sleep duration (<6 hours). These data matched sleep diary data collected over a 2-week period.[68] Women with insomnia were more likely to have objectively measured hot flashes, and the presence of hot flashes predicted the number of PSG-awakenings per hour of sleep.[68] Although data

were only available from one study, findings suggest that in cases of severe subjective sleep disturbance qualifying for insomnia disorder, there is PSG evidence of poor sleep that is partly attributed to the impact of hot flashes.

In another study, Xu and colleagues[69] compared subjective and PSG measures in premenopausal and perimenopausal/postmenopausal women with insomnia. Although subjective measures of sleep disturbance and depression were similar between groups, perimenopausal/postmenopausal women had a longer PSG-defined total wake time and lower sleep efficiency, suggesting that PSG measures of sleep quality are impacted to a greater extent in peri/postmenopausal than in premenopausal women with insomnia. The presence of hot flashes was not evaluated in this study.

The links between insomnia disorder and adverse mental and physical conditions, including depression and cardiovascular disease, are well established[70]; insomnia combined with short sleep duration is proposed as the most biologically severe phenotype of the disorder.[71] It is unclear if insomnia disorder that develops in the context of the menopausal transition has a similar impact on long-term health compared with insomnia that develops in other circumstances and how comorbid features, such as hot flashes or depression, might interact with sleep difficulties to contribute to impairment. Emerging data show an association between menopausal insomnia and unfavorable nocturnal blood pressure[72] and heart rate[73] profiles; however, the causes and long-term consequences of this altered blood pressure profile remain to be determined.

Primary Sleep Disorders and Other Medical Disorders

Sleep disturbances may arise during the menopausal transition and postmenopause in association with primary sleep disorders, such as SDB, restless legs syndrome (RLS), and periodic limb movement disorder (PLMD).[2,74]

Sleep-disordered breathing
SDB is characterized by snoring, upper airway obstruction, inspiratory flow limitation, and excessive daytime sleepiness.[75] An AHI of 5 or more per hour of sleep is usually considered abnormal and indicates SDB.[75] The prevalence of SDB is higher in men than in women before menopause[76]; however, the prevalence increases in women following menopausal transition.[77–81]

In the Wisconsin Sleep Cohort, postmenopausal women were 2.6 times more likely to have an AHI of 5 or more per hour and 3.5 times more likely to have an AHI of 15 or more per hour, compared with premenopausal women, after adjusting for confounding factors (age, BMI, and smoking).[80] In the recent longitudinal analyses of that dataset, AHI increased from premenopause to perimenopause and postmenopause, independent of age and changes in body habitus, although these factors were also associated with AHI.[77] The greater prevalence of SDB after menopause might be due in part to loss of protective effects of female reproductive steroid hormones, especially progesterone,[80,81] as well as changes in fat distribution after menopause.[78]

The clinical picture of SDB in women usually differs from that of men. Women are more symptomatic with lower AHI compared with men, and they have more prolonged partial upper airway obstruction and report insomnia as a symptom of SDB more frequently.[82,83] Of importance, patients with SDB and insomnia-like symptoms have a higher burden of cardiovascular, pulmonary, and psychiatric comorbidity compared with patients with traditional sleepy phenotype despite less severe SDB in terms of AHI.[83] Further, patients with SDB and insomnia symptoms have lower adherence to continuous positive airway pressure treatment[83,84] and may benefit from concomitant cognitive behavioral therapy for insomnia (CBT-I).[85] Perhaps as a consequence of these differences in clinical presentation, women with SDB are more often underdiagnosed as well as undertreated compared with men.[86]

Restless legs syndrome and periodic limb movement disorder

The prevalence of RLS and PLMD increases with age, and RLS is more common in women.[87] Freedman and Roehrs[43] found periodic limb movements and apneas to be the best predictors for poorer sleep efficiency in perimenopausal and postmenopausal women reporting sleep disturbances. However, in a group of asymptomatic postmenopausal women, the incidence of periodic limb movements was unrelated to E_2 or FSH levels,[88] suggesting that the increase in prevalence of RLS and PLMD after menopause may be related more to aging than to hormonal changes.

Other medical disorders and use of medications

In addition to primary sleep disorders, other medical disorders, as well as the use of medications, become more common with advancing age and may affect sleep in midlife women.[89–91] In one of the few prospective studies assessing predictors for menopausal sleep disturbances, medical diseases and the use of prescribed medication predicted future sleep disturbances.[92] In another prospective study of depressive symptoms, personal crises, use of medications affecting the central nervous system, and perceived impaired general health already 5 years before menopause predicted various sleep disturbances in menopausal transition.[67]

DEMOGRAPHIC AND PSYCHOSOCIAL FACTORS AND SLEEP IN MENOPAUSAL TRANSITION

Women face multiple challenges and personal life stressors in midlife, including changing family roles, loss of significant others, changes and increasing demands at work, health concerns, and worries about retiring and getting old.[93] Perimenopausal women have higher levels of psychological distress compared with premenopausal women[94]; employment, depressed mood, and poor perceived health are among the most significant factors causing stress in midlife women.[95] Life stressors and experiencing stress could contribute to sleep disturbances.[93,96,97] Indeed, perceived stress and poor perceived health have been associated with sleep disturbances in midlife women.[16,90] Further, Hall and colleagues[66] found that midlife women with more chronic stress exposure over a 9-year period had greater PSG-assessed WASO and were more likely to have insomnia at follow-up than participants with moderate stress exposure.

A limited number of studies have investigated the relationship between work stresses specifically and menopausal symptoms including sleep disturbances. An Australian study of 476 perimenopausal and postmenopausal women working in the higher education sector found that higher supervisor support, being used on a full-time basis, and having control over workplace temperature were independently associated with lower menopausal symptom reporting.[98] This study did not specifically assess sleep disturbances. However, there is good evidence that job strain and high work demands are associated with increased prevalence of sleep disturbances in the general population.[99–101] A recent Finnish prospective study with more than 24,000 participants (82% women, mean age 44 years) showed that the disappearance of job strain was associated with lower odds of insomnia symptoms.[101] In addition, according to a sleep diary study, postmenopausal women had worse sleep than premenopausal women during working days, but few differences during leisure days, showing an existing coping mechanism of work stress after menopause and the necessity of enough rest.[102]

Some socioeconomic factors are protective against the development of sleep disturbances in the menopausal transition; higher educational level,[34] lower financial strain,[103] and satisfactory marriage[104,105] are all associated with less sleep disturbance. Further, the prevalence of menopausal sleep disturbance is influenced by race and ethnicity: Caucasian women have higher rates, whereas Hispanic women have lower rates of sleep disturbance.[14]

There is a bidirectional relationship between psychosocial factors and menopausal symptoms, including sleep disturbance. Just as psychological distress, stressors, and poor health can lead to sleep disturbances, sleep disturbances can also lead to poorer health and quality of life, depressed mood, and reduced work productivity. For example, in a study of 131 Egyptian teachers in the menopausal transition (aged 46–59 years), the most important menopausal symptoms that affected their work capacity and performance were tiredness (83%) and sleep disturbances (64%).[106] A larger study of 961 midlife women found that insomnia symptoms were the most problematic menopausal symptoms to affect daily life and working performance.[107]

Recent studies have demonstrated that the presence of menopausal symptoms increases health care utilization and costs as well as sick leave days.[3,108–110] In one study that assessed the burden of menopausal sleep disturbances on societal costs, Bolge and colleagues[3] concluded that menopausal chronic insomnia, characterized by nighttime awakenings, was linked with increased health care utilization and associated costs, decreased work productivity, and decreased health-related quality of life after adjustment for demographics and comorbidity.

MANAGEMENT OF SLEEP DISTURBANCES IN THE CONTEXT OF MENOPAUSE

As discussed in the earlier sections, there are potentially multiple, and sometimes overlapping, causes of sleep disturbances in midlife women as they approach and pass menopause. For some women, the sleep disturbances may be transient and without associated distress and, therefore, do not require active treatment. However, others may experience severe sleep disturbances with a significant impact on functioning and quality of life, necessitating treatment. In some cases, combined treatments may be required, such as for women who have depression in addition to severe vasomotor symptoms and sleep problems.

During evaluation of sleep problems with a sleep history assessment[111] or sleep diary,[112] women should be questioned about the timing of sleep difficulties in relation to menopausal symptoms, changes in bleeding patterns, and presence and severity of menopausal symptoms like hot flashes and night sweats, in addition to screening for sleep breathing and movement disorders. Treatment options include hormone therapy (HT), nonhormonal pharmacologic medications, and nonpharmacologic and self-management strategies.

Cognitive Behavioral Therapy for Insomnia

CBT-I is considered the primary intervention for patients with chronic insomnia[113] and is superior to sleep medication alone in the long-term.[114] CBT-I has recently been evaluated for insomnia during the menopausal transition in a randomized clinical trial of perimenopausal and postmenopausal women with insomnia symptoms as well as daily hot flashes.[115] Compared with a menopause education control condition, 8 weeks of CBT-I led to a greater reduction in insomnia symptoms, with improvements maintained at 6 months posttreatment.[115] Preliminary data from an open trial of CBT-I in women with menopausal sleep problems also indicated a reduction in insomnia (and depression) symptoms posttreatment.[116] Although further trials are needed, initial findings provide support for the effectiveness of CBT-I in women with insomnia during the menopausal transition.

Other nonpharmacologic approaches for treating menopausal insomnia, including acupuncture, yoga, massage, exercise, and nutritional supplements containing soy isoflavones, have been tried, with mixed effects (reviewed in Attarian and colleagues,[117] 2015).

Hormone Therapy and Sleep

HT, composed of estrogen combined with progestin or estrogen alone for women with a history of hysterectomy, is the most effective treatment of menopausal symptoms.[118] HT has other beneficial effects, including prevention of bone loss and osteoporosis-related fractures.[119,120] However, HT may also have negative effects. Oral (but not transdermal) administration of HT increases the risk for venous thromboembolism.[119,121] In addition, there is a slightly elevated risk for breast cancer that seems to be primarily, but not exclusively, related to the progestin used in combined therapy.[119,122,123] According to current opinion, therefore, the indications and possible contraindications (eg, history of breast or gynecologic cancer, venous thromboembolism, or severe cardiovascular diseases) should be evaluated before initiating HT. HT should be considered when the balance of potential benefits and risks is favorable for a woman[124] at the lowest effective dose, using transdermal administration when appropriate. The duration should be individualized based on the duration of menopausal symptoms, age, and possible risk factors.[119]

Several studies have evaluated the effect of HT on sleep; however, findings are mixed and difficult to compare, given the heterogeneity in study populations, tools to evaluate sleep, and various HT preparations (formulation, dose, and type of administration). According to a recent meta-analysis, HT modestly improves subjectively evaluated sleep disturbance.[125] In most studies, improved sleep quality has co-occurred with improvement in vasomotor symptoms.[125–129] However, there are also data on enhanced sleep quality with HT without the report of vasomotor symptoms.[127] PSG studies examining the effect of HT on sleep architecture in menopausal women share the same problems with study design as the studies evaluating subjective sleep quality and HT. Those studies are rare, and their results are conflicting. Some studies have observed positive changes in sleep architecture with HT,[130–133] mainly decreasing WASO, although other studies found no improvement.[134–136]

In cases whereby HT is contraindicated or not preferred, nonhormonal pharmacologic options for treating hot flashes and associated insomnia symptoms are available.[117] Low-dose selective serotonin/serotonin norepinephrine reuptake inhibitors reduce hot flashes to some extent and modestly reduce insomnia symptoms in women with hot flashes,[137–139] although the adverse-effect profiles of these medications need to be carefully considered before use. Evidence from a single trial shows that gabapentin improves sleep quality in perimenopausal women with hot flashes and insomnia.[140]

SUMMARY

Sleep difficulties increase as women approach menopause. For some women, sleep problems are severe and, thus, impact daytime functioning and quality of life, having long-term consequences for mental and physical health. Menopausal vasomotor symptoms typically interfere with sleep and are strongly associated with self-reports of sleep disturbances as well as PSG-measured wakefulness. However, when evaluating the causes of sleep disturbance during menopause, other factors directly related to the menopausal transition (eg, instability/changes in the hormone environment with progressive decreases in estradiol and increases in FSH) and factors coincident with the transition (eg, SDB or movement disorders, mood disturbance, presence of medical conditions, or life stressors) also need to be considered. Given the presence of unique sleep-disruptive factors (eg, hot flashes) and the multifactorial nature of sleep difficulties in women approaching menopause, often with many interacting factors, treatment options need to be tailored to the individual woman.

REFERENCES

1. Shaver JL, Woods NF. Sleep and menopause: a narrative review. Menopause 2015;22(8):899–915.
2. Polo-Kantola P. Sleep problems in midlife and beyond. Maturitas 2011;68(3):224–32.
3. Bolge SC, Balkrishnan R, Kannan H, et al. Burden associated with chronic sleep maintenance insomnia characterized by nighttime awakenings among women with menopausal symptoms. Menopause 2010;17(1):80–6.
4. Luoto R, Kaprio J, Uutela A. Age at natural menopause and sociodemographic status in Finland. Am J Epidemiol 1994;139(1):64–76.
5. Roberts H, Hickey M. Managing the menopause: an update. Maturitas 2016;86:53–8.
6. Harlow SD, Gass M, Hall JE, et al. Executive summary of the stages of reproductive aging workshop + 10: addressing the unfinished agenda of staging reproductive aging. J Clin Endocrinol Metab 2012;97(4):1159–68.
7. Nelson HD. Menopause. Lancet 2008;371(9614): 760–70.
8. Cheng MH, Hsu CY, Wang SJ, et al. The relationship of self-reported sleep disturbance, mood, and menopause in a community study. Menopause 2008;15(5):958–62.
9. Hung HC, Lu FH, Ou HY, et al. Menopause is associated with self-reported poor sleep quality in women without vasomotor symptoms. Menopause 2014;21(8):834–9.
10. Kravitz HM, Ganz PA, Bromberger J, et al. Sleep difficulty in women at midlife: a community survey of sleep and the menopausal transition. Menopause 2003;10(1):19–28.
11. Shin C, Lee S, Lee T, et al. Prevalence of insomnia and its relationship to menopausal status in middle-aged Korean women. Psychiatry Clin Neurosci 2005;59(4):395–402.
12. Young T, Rabago D, Zgierska A, et al. Objective and subjective sleep quality in premenopausal, perimenopausal, and postmenopausal women in the Wisconsin Sleep Cohort Study. Sleep 2003; 26(6):667–72.
13. Berecki-Gisolf J, Begum N, Dobson AJ. Symptoms reported by women in midlife: menopausal transition or aging? Menopause 2009;16(5):1021–9.

14. Kravitz HM, Zhao X, Bromberger JT, et al. Sleep disturbance during the menopausal transition in a multi-ethnic community sample of women. Sleep 2008;31(7):979–90.

15. Tom SE, Kuh D, Guralnik JM, et al. Self-reported sleep difficulty during the menopausal transition: results from a prospective cohort study. Menopause 2010;17(6):1128–35.

16. Woods NF, Mitchell ES. Sleep symptoms during the menopausal transition and early postmenopause: observations from the Seattle Midlife Women's Health Study. Sleep 2010;33(4):539–49.

17. Xu Q, Lang CP. Examining the relationship between subjective sleep disturbance and menopause: a systematic review and meta-analysis. Menopause 2014;21(12):1301–18.

18. Kaplan KA, Hardas PP, Redline S, et al, Sleep Heart Health Study Research Group. Correlates of sleep quality in midlife and beyond: a machine learning analysis. Sleep Med 2017;34:162–7.

19. Krystal AD, Edinger JD. Measuring sleep quality. Sleep Med 2008;9(Suppl 1):S10–7.

20. Hachul H, Frange C, Bezerra AG, et al. The effect of menopause on objective sleep parameters: data from an epidemiologic study in Sao Paulo, Brazil. Maturitas 2015;80(2):170–8.

21. Campbell IG, Bromberger JT, Buysse DJ, et al. Evaluation of the association of menopausal status with delta and beta EEG activity during sleep. Sleep 2011;34(11):1561–8.

22. Freedman RR, Roehrs TA. Lack of sleep disturbance from menopausal hot flashes. Fertil Steril 2004;82(1):138–44.

23. Kalleinen N, Polo-Kantola P, Himanen SL, et al. Sleep and the menopause - do postmenopausal women experience worse sleep than premenopausal women? Menopause Int 2008;14(3):97–104.

24. Lampio L, Polo-Kantola P, Himanen SL, et al. Sleep during menopausal transition: a 6-year follow-up. Sleep 2017;40(7).

25. Sowers MF, Zheng H, Kravitz HM, et al. Sex steroid hormone profiles are related to sleep measures from polysomnography and the Pittsburgh Sleep Quality Index. Sleep 2008;31(10):1339–49.

26. de Zambotti M, Colrain IM, Baker FC. Interaction between reproductive hormones and physiological sleep in women. J Clin Endocrinol Metab 2015; 100(4):1426–33.

27. Antonijevic IA, Murck H, Frieboes RM, et al. On the role of menopause for sleep-endocrine alterations associated with major depression. Psychoneuroendocrinology 2003;28(3):401–18.

28. Archer DF, Sturdee DW, Baber R, et al. Menopausal hot flushes and night sweats: where are we now? Climacteric 2011;14(5):515–28.

29. Avis NE, Crawford SL, Greendale G, et al. Duration of menopausal vasomotor symptoms over the menopause transition. JAMA Intern Med 2015; 175(4):531–9.

30. Mishra GD, Kuh D. Health symptoms during midlife in relation to menopausal transition: British prospective cohort study. BMJ 2012;344:e402.

31. Tepper PG, Brooks MM, Randolph JF Jr, et al. Characterizing the trajectories of vasomotor symptoms across the menopausal transition. Menopause 2016;23(10):1067–74.

32. Freeman EW, Sammel MD, Lin H, et al. Duration of menopausal hot flushes and associated risk factors. Obstet Gynecol 2011;117(5):1095–104.

33. Freedman RR. Menopausal hot flashes: mechanisms, endocrinology, treatment. J Steroid Biochem Mol Biol 2014;142:115–20.

34. Blümel JE, Cano A, Mezones-Holguin E, et al. A multinational study of sleep disorders during female mid-life. Maturitas 2012;72(4):359–66.

35. Ohayon MM. Severe hot flashes are associated with chronic insomnia. Arch Intern Med 2006; 166(12):1262–8.

36. Kravitz HM, Joffe H. Sleep during the perimenopause: a SWAN story. Obstet Gynecol Clin North Am 2011;38(3):567–86.

37. de Zambotti M, Colrain IM, Javitz HS, et al. Magnitude of the impact of hot flashes on sleep in perimenopausal women. Fertil Steril 2014;102(6): 1708–15.e1.

38. Joffe H, White DP, Crawford SL, et al. Adverse effects of induced hot flashes on objectively recorded and subjectively reported sleep: results of a gonadotropin-releasing hormone agonist experimental protocol. Menopause 2013;20(9):905–14.

39. Thurston RC, Santoro N, Matthews KA. Are vasomotor symptoms associated with sleep characteristics among symptomatic midlife women? Comparisons of self-report and objective measures. Menopause 2012;19(7):742–8.

40. Mann E, Hunter MS. Concordance between self-reported and sternal skin conductance measures of hot flushes in symptomatic perimenopausal and postmenopausal women: a systematic review. Menopause 2011;18(6):709–22.

41. Joffe H, Massler A, Sharkey KM. Evaluation and management of sleep disturbance during the menopause transition. Semin Reprod Med 2010; 28(5):404–21.

42. Savard MH, Savard J, Caplette-Gingras A, et al. Relationship between objectively recorded hot flashes and sleep disturbances among breast cancer patients: investigating hot flash characteristics other than frequency. Menopause 2013;20(10): 997–1005.

43. Freedman RR, Roehrs TA. Sleep disturbance in menopause. Menopause 2007;14(5):826–9.

44. Joffe H, Crawford S, Economou N, et al. A gonadotropin-releasing hormone agonist model

demonstrates that nocturnal hot flashes interrupt objective sleep. Sleep 2013;36(12):1977–85.

45. Bromberger JT, Matthews KA, Schott LL, et al. Depressive symptoms during the menopausal transition: the Study of Women's Health Across the Nation (SWAN). J Affect Disord 2007;103(1–3): 267–72.

46. Bromberger JT, Kravitz HM. Mood and menopause: findings from the Study of Women's Health Across the Nation (SWAN) over 10 years. Obstet Gynecol Clin North Am 2011;38(3):609–25.

47. Cohen LS, Soares CN, Vitonis AF, et al. Risk for new onset of depression during the menopausal transition: the Harvard study of moods and cycles. Arch Gen Psychiatry 2006;63(4):385–90.

48. Steinberg EM, Rubinow DR, Bartko JJ, et al. A cross-sectional evaluation of perimenopausal depression. J Clin Psychiatry 2008;69(6):973–80.

49. Soares CN. Mood disorders in midlife women: understanding the critical window and its clinical implications. Menopause 2014;21(2):198–206.

50. Borrow AP, Cameron NM. Estrogenic mediation of serotonergic and neurotrophic systems: implications for female mood disorders. Prog Neuropsychopharmacol Biol Psychiatry 2014;54:13–25.

51. Studd JW. A guide to the treatment of depression in women by estrogens. Climacteric 2011;14(6): 637–42.

52. Kahn M, Sheppes G, Sadeh A. Sleep and emotions: bidirectional links and underlying mechanisms. Int J Psychophysiol 2013;89(2):218–28.

53. Sivertsen B, Salo P, Mykletun A, et al. The bidirectional association between depression and insomnia: the HUNT study. Psychosom Med 2012; 74(7):758–65.

54. Burleson MH, Todd M, Trevathan WR. Daily vasomotor symptoms, sleep problems, and mood: using daily data to evaluate the domino hypothesis in middle-aged women. Menopause 2010;17(1): 87–95.

55. Pien GW, Sammel MD, Freeman EW, et al. Predictors of sleep quality in women in the menopausal transition. Sleep 2008;31(7):991–9.

56. Toffol E, Kalleinen N, Urrila AS, et al. The relationship between mood and sleep in different female reproductive states. BMC Psychiatry 2014;14:177.

57. Avis NE, Crawford S, Stellato R, et al. Longitudinal study of hormone levels and depression among women transitioning through menopause. Climacteric 2001;4(3):243–9.

58. Bromberger JT, Kravitz HM, Youk A, et al. Patterns of depressive disorders across 13 years and their determinants among midlife women: SWAN mental health study. J Affect Disord 2016;206: 31–40.

59. Kravitz HM, Avery E, Sowers M, et al. Relationships between menopausal and mood symptoms and EEG sleep measures in a multi-ethnic sample of middle-aged women: the SWAN Sleep Study. Sleep 2011;34(9):1221–32.

60. Eichling PS, Sahni J. Menopause related sleep disorders. J Clin Sleep Med 2005;1(3):291–300.

61. Vousoura E, Spyropoulou AC, Koundi KL, et al. Vasomotor and depression symptoms may be associated with different sleep disturbance patterns in postmenopausal women. Menopause 2015;22(10):1053–7.

62. Joffe H, Petrillo LF, Koukopoulos A, et al. Increased estradiol and improved sleep, but not hot flashes, predict enhanced mood during the menopausal transition. J Clin Endocrinol Metab 2011;96(7): E1044–54.

63. Riemann D, Nissen C, Palagini L, et al. The neurobiology, investigation, and treatment of chronic insomnia. Lancet Neurol 2015;14(5):547–58.

64. Shaver JL, Johnston SK, Lentz MJ, et al. Stress exposure, psychological distress, and physiological stress activation in midlife women with insomnia. Psychosom Med 2002;64(5):793–802.

65. Sassoon SA, de Zambotti M, Colrain IM, et al. Association between personality traits and DSM-IV diagnosis of insomnia in peri- and postmenopausal women. Menopause 2014;21(6):602–11.

66. Hall MH, Casement MD, Troxel WM, et al. Chronic stress is prospectively associated with sleep in midlife women: the SWAN sleep study. Sleep 2015;38(10):1645–54.

67. Lampio L, Saaresranta T, Engblom J, et al. Predictors of sleep disturbance in menopausal transition. Maturitas 2016;94:137–42.

68. Baker FC, Willoughby AR, Sassoon SA, et al. Insomnia in women approaching menopause: beyond perception. Psychoneuroendocrinology 2015;60:96–104.

69. Xu M, Belanger L, Ivers H, et al. Comparison of subjective and objective sleep quality in menopausal and non-menopausal women with insomnia. Sleep Med 2011;12(1):65–9.

70. Buysse DJ. Insomnia. JAMA 2013;309(7):706–16.

71. Vgontzas AN, Fernandez-Mendoza J, Liao D, et al. Insomnia with objective short sleep duration: the most biologically severe phenotype of the disorder. Sleep Med Rev 2013;17(4):241–54.

72. de Zambotti M, Trinder J, Javitz H, et al. Altered nocturnal blood pressure profiles in women with insomnia disorder in the menopausal transition. Menopause 2017;24(3):278–87.

73. de Zambotti M, Trinder J, Colrain IM, et al. Menstrual cycle-related variation in autonomic nervous system functioning in women in the early menopausal transition with and without insomnia disorder. Psychoneuroendocrinology 2017;75:44–51.

74. Guidozzi F. Sleep and sleep disorders in menopausal women. Climacteric 2013;16(2):214–9.

75. Shneerson JM. Obstructive sleep apnoeas and snoring. In: Shneerson JM, editor. Handbook of sleep medicine. 1st edition. Oxford (United Kingdom): Blackwell Science; 2000. p. 194–218.

76. Peppard PE, Young T, Barnet JH, et al. Increased prevalence of sleep-disordered breathing in adults. Am J Epidemiol 2013;177(9):1006–14.

77. Mirer AG, Young T, Palta M, et al. Sleep-disordered breathing and the menopausal transition among participants in the Sleep in Midlife Women Study. Menopause 2017;24(2):157–62.

78. Polesel DN, Hirotsu C, Nozoe KT, et al. Waist circumference and postmenopause stages as the main associated factors for sleep apnea in women: a cross-sectional population-based study. Menopause 2015;22(8):835–44.

79. Anttalainen U, Saaresranta T, Aittokallio J, et al. Impact of menopause on the manifestation and severity of sleep-disordered breathing. Acta Obstet Gynecol Scand 2006;85(11):1381–8.

80. Young T, Finn L, Austin D, et al. Menopausal status and sleep-disordered breathing in the Wisconsin Sleep Cohort Study. Am J Respir Crit Care Med 2003;167(9):1181–5.

81. Bixler EO, Vgontzas AN, Lin HM, et al. Prevalence of sleep-disordered breathing in women: effects of gender. Am J Respir Crit Care Med 2001;163(3 Pt 1):608–13.

82. Anttalainen U, Tenhunen M, Rimpilä V, et al. Prolonged partial upper airway obstruction during sleep - an underdiagnosed phenotype of sleep-disordered breathing. Eur Clin Respir J 2016;3:31806.

83. Saaresranta T, Hedner J, Bonsignore MR, et al. Clinical phenotypes and comorbidity in European sleep apnoea patients. PLoS One 2016;11(10):e0163439.

84. Pien GW, Ye L, Keenan BT, et al. Changing faces of obstructive sleep apnea: treatment effects by cluster designation in the Icelandic sleep apnea cohort. Sleep 2018;41(3).

85. Lack L, Sweetman A. Diagnosis and treatment of insomnia comorbid with obstructive sleep apnea. Sleep Med Clin 2016;11(3):379–88.

86. Lindberg E, Benediktsdottir B, Franklin KA, et al. Women with symptoms of sleep-disordered breathing are less likely to be diagnosed and treated for sleep apnea than men. Sleep Med 2017;35:17–22.

87. Harmell A, Ancoli-Israel S. Diagnosis and treatment of sleep disorders in older adults. In: Avidan AY, editor. Handbook of sleep medicine. 2nd edition. Philadelphia: Wolters Kluwer Health/Lippincott Williams & Wilkins; 2011. p. 261–73.

88. Polo-Kantola P, Rauhala E, Erkkola R, et al. Estrogen replacement therapy and nocturnal periodic limb movements: a randomized controlled trial. Obstet Gynecol 2001;97(4):548–54.

89. Polo-Kantola P, Laine A, Aromaa M, et al. A population-based survey of sleep disturbances in middle-aged women–associations with health, health related quality of life and health behavior. Maturitas 2014;77(3):255–62.

90. Vaari T, Engblom J, Helenius H, et al. Survey of sleep problems in 3421 women aged 41-55 years. Menopause Int 2008;14(2):78–82.

91. Plotkin K. Insomnia caused by medical disorders. In: Attarian HP, Schuman C, editors. Clinical handbook of insomnia. 2nd edition. Totowa (NJ): Humana; 2010. p. 195–208.

92. Tom SE, Kuh D, Guralnik JM, et al. Patterns in trouble sleeping among women at mid-life: results from a British prospective cohort study. J Epidemiol Community Health 2009;63(12):974–9.

93. Darling CA, Coccia C, Senatore N. Women in midlife: stress, health and life satisfaction. Stress Health 2012;28(1):31–40.

94. Bromberger JT, Meyer PM, Kravitz HM, et al. Psychologic distress and natural menopause: a multiethnic community study. Am J Public Health 2001;91(9):1435–42.

95. Woods NF, Mitchell ES, Percival DB, et al. Is the menopausal transition stressful? Observations of perceived stress from the Seattle Midlife Women's Health Study. Menopause 2009;16(1):90–7.

96. Saaresranta T, Polo-Kantola P, Polo O. Practical approach to the diagnosis and management of menopausal insomnia. In: Attarian HP, Viola-Saltzman Mari, editors. Sleep disorders in women: a guide to practical management. 2nd edition. New York: Humana Press/Springer; 2013. p. 293–324.

97. Cuadros JL, Fernandez-Alonso AM, Cuadros-Celorrio AM, et al. Perceived stress, insomnia and related factors in women around the menopause. Maturitas 2012;72(4):367–72.

98. Bariola E, Jack G, Pitts M, et al. Employment conditions and work-related stressors are associated with menopausal symptom reporting among perimenopausal and postmenopausal women. Menopause 2017;24(3):247–51.

99. Åkerstedt T, Garefelt J, Richter A, et al. Work and sleep–a prospective study of psychosocial work factors, physical work factors, and work scheduling. Sleep 2015;38(7):1129–36.

100. Chazelle E, Chastang JF, Niedhammer I. Psychosocial work factors and sleep problems: findings from the French national SIP survey. Int Arch Occup Environ Health 2016;89(3):485–95.

101. Halonen JI, Lallukka T, Pentti J, et al. Change in job strain as a predictor of change in insomnia symptoms: analyzing observational data as a non-randomized pseudo-trial. Sleep 2017;40(1). https://doi.org/10.1093/sleep/zsw007.

102. Lampio L, Saaresranta T, Polo O, et al. Subjective sleep in premenopausal and postmenopausal

women during workdays and leisure days: a sleep diary study. Menopause 2013;20(6):655–60.

103. Hall MH, Matthews KA, Kravitz HM, et al. Race and financial strain are independent correlates of sleep in midlife women: the SWAN sleep study. Sleep 2009;32(1):73–82.

104. Troxel WM, Buysse DJ, Matthews KA, et al. Marital/cohabitation status and history in relation to sleep in midlife women. Sleep 2010;33(7):973–81.

105. Troxel WM, Buysse DJ, Hall M, et al. Marital happiness and sleep disturbances in a multi-ethnic sample of middle-aged women. Behav Sleep Med 2009;7(1):2–19.

106. Hammam RA, Abbas RA, Hunter MS. Menopause and work–the experience of middle-aged female teaching staff in an Egyptian governmental faculty of medicine. Maturitas 2012;71(3):294–300.

107. Simon JA, Reape KZ. Understanding the menopausal experiences of professional women. Menopause 2009;16(1):73–6.

108. Kleinman NL, Rohrbacker NJ, Bushmakin AG, et al. Direct and indirect costs of women diagnosed with menopause symptoms. J Occup Environ Med 2013;55(4):465–70.

109. Whiteley J, DiBonaventura M, Wagner JS, et al. The impact of menopausal symptoms on quality of life, productivity, and economic outcomes. J Womens Health (Larchmt) 2013;22(11):983–90.

110. Whiteley J, Wagner JS, Bushmakin A, et al. Impact of the severity of vasomotor symptoms on health status, resource use, and productivity. Menopause 2013;20(5):518–24.

111. Morin CM, Espie CA. Insomnia: a clinical guide to assessment and treatment. New York: Kluwer Academic/Plenum Publishers; 2003.

112. Carney CE, Buysse DJ, Ancoli-Israel S, et al. The consensus sleep diary: standardizing prospective sleep self-monitoring. Sleep 2012; 35(2):287–302.

113. Sateia MJ, Buysse DJ, Krystal AD, et al. Clinical practice guideline for the pharmacologic treatment of chronic insomnia in adults: an American Academy of Sleep Medicine Clinical Practice Guideline. J Clin Sleep Med 2017;13(2):307–49.

114. Sivertsen B, Omvik S, Pallesen S, et al. Cognitive behavioral therapy vs zopiclone for treatment of chronic primary insomnia in older adults: a randomized controlled trial. JAMA 2006;295(24): 2851–8.

115. McCurry SM, Guthrie KA, Morin CM, et al. Telephone-based cognitive behavioral therapy for insomnia in perimenopausal and postmenopausal women with vasomotor symptoms: a MsFLASH randomized clinical trial. JAMA Intern Med 2016; 176(7):913–20.

116. Hall MH, Kline CE, Nowakowski S. Insomnia and sleep apnea in midlife women: prevalence and consequences to health and functioning. F1000Prime Rep 2015;7:63.

117. Attarian H, Hachul H, Guttuso T, et al. Treatment of chronic insomnia disorder in menopause: evaluation of literature. Menopause 2015;22(6):674–84.

118. Maclennan AH, Broadbent JL, Lester S, et al. Oral oestrogen and combined oestrogen/progestogen therapy versus placebo for hot flushes. Cochrane Database Syst Rev 2004;(4):CD002978.

119. de Villiers TJ, Hall JE, Pinkerton JV, et al. Revised global consensus statement on menopausal hormone therapy. Maturitas 2016;91:153–5.

120. Cauley JA, Robbins J, Chen Z, et al. Effects of estrogen plus progestin on risk of fracture and bone mineral density: the Women's Health Initiative randomized trial. JAMA 2003;290(13):1729–38.

121. Canonico M, Oger E, Plu-Bureau G, et al. Hormone therapy and venous thromboembolism among postmenopausal women: impact of the route of estrogen administration and progestogens: the ESTHER study. Circulation 2007;115(7):840–5.

122. Chlebowski RT, Anderson GL. Menopausal hormone therapy and cancer: changing clinical observations of target site specificity. Steroids 2014;90: 53–9.

123. Manson JE, Chlebowski RT, Stefanick ML, et al. Menopausal hormone therapy and health outcomes during the intervention and extended post-stopping phases of the Women's Health Initiative randomized trials. JAMA 2013;310(13):1353–68.

124. The NAMS 2017 Hormone Therapy Position Statement Advisory Panel. The 2017 hormone therapy position statement of the North American Menopause Society. Menopause 2017;24(7):728–53.

125. Cintron D, Lipford M, Larrea-Mantilla L, et al. Efficacy of menopausal hormone therapy on sleep quality: systematic review and meta-analysis. Endocrine 2017;55(3):702–11.

126. Hays J, Ockene JK, Brunner RL, et al. Effects of estrogen plus progestin on health-related quality of life. N Engl J Med 2003;348(19):1839–54.

127. Polo-Kantola P, Erkkola R, Helenius H, et al. When does estrogen replacement therapy improve sleep quality? Am J Obstet Gynecol 1998;178(5):1002–9.

128. Savolainen-Peltonen H, Hautamäki H, Tuomikoski P, et al. Health-related quality of life in women with or without hot flashes: a randomized placebo-controlled trial with hormone therapy. Menopause 2014;21(7):732–9.

129. Welton AJ, Vickers MR, Kim J, et al. Health related quality of life after combined hormone replacement therapy: randomised controlled trial. BMJ 2008; 337:a1190.

130. Parry BL, Meliska CJ, Martinez LF, et al. Menopause: neuroendocrine changes and hormone replacement therapy. J Am Med Womens Assoc (1972) 2004;59(2):135–45.

131. Montplaisir J, Lorrain J, Denesle R, et al. Sleep in menopause: differential effects of two forms of hormone replacement therapy. Menopause 2001;8(1): 10–6.

132. Polo-Kantola P, Erkkola R, Irjala K, et al. Effect of short-term transdermal estrogen replacement therapy on sleep: a randomized, double-blind crossover trial in postmenopausal women. Fertil Steril 1999;71(5):873–80.

133. Scharf MB, McDannold MD, Stover R, et al. Effects of estrogen replacement therapy on rates of cyclic alternating patterns and hot-flush events during sleep in postmenopausal women: a pilot study. Clin Ther 1997;19(2):304–11.

134. Tansupswatdikul   P,   Chaikittisilpa   S, Jaimchariyatam N, et al. Effects of estrogen therapy on postmenopausal sleep quality regardless of vasomotor symptoms: a randomized trial. Climacteric 2015;18(2):198–204.

135. Kalleinen N, Polo O, Himanen SL, et al. The effect of estrogen plus progestin treatment on sleep: a randomized, placebo-controlled, double-blind trial in premenopausal and late postmenopausal women. Climacteric 2008;11(3):233–43.

136. Purdie DW, Empson JA, Crichton C, et al. Hormone replacement therapy, sleep quality and psychological wellbeing. Br J Obstet Gynaecol 1995;102(9): 735–9.

137. Ensrud KE, Joffe H, Guthrie KA, et al. Effect of escitalopram on insomnia symptoms and subjective sleep quality in healthy perimenopausal and postmenopausal women with hot flashes: a randomized controlled trial. Menopause 2012; 19(8):848–55.

138. Ensrud KE, Guthrie KA, Hohensee C, et al. Effects of estradiol and venlafaxine on insomnia symptoms and sleep quality in women with hot flashes. Sleep 2015;38(1):97–108.

139. Pinkerton JV, Joffe H, Kazempour K, et al. Low-dose paroxetine (7.5 mg) improves sleep in women with vasomotor symptoms associated with menopause. Menopause 2015;22(1):50–8.

140. Yurcheshen ME, Guttuso T Jr, McDermott M, et al. Effects of gabapentin on sleep in menopausal women with hot flashes as measured by a Pittsburgh Sleep Quality Index factor scoring model. J Womens Health (Larchmt) 2009;18(9): 1355–60.

141. Brincat M, Studd JW. Menopause–a multi system disease. Baillieres Clin Obstet Gynaecol 1988; 2(2):289–316.

142. Kronenberg F. Hot flashes: epidemiology and physiology. Ann N Y Acad Sci 1990;592:52–86 [discussion: 123–33].

143. Erkkola R, Holma P, Järvi T, et al. Transdermal oestrogen replacement therapy in a Finnish population. Maturitas 1991;13(4):275–81.

144. Gold EB, Sternfeld B, Kelsey JL, et al. Relation of demographic and lifestyle factors to symptoms in a multi-racial/ethnic population of women 40-55 years of age. Am J Epidemiol 2000;152(5):463–73.

145. Santoro N. Perimenopause: from research to practice. J Womens Health (Larchmt) 2016;25(4): 332–9.

Impact of Poor Sleep on Physical and Mental Health in Older Women

Katie L. Stone, PhD[a],*, Qian Xiao, PhD[b,c,1]

KEYWORDS

- Sleep deficiency • Circadian rhythms • Cardiometabolic disorders • Older women
- Metabolic syndrome • Physical health • Mental health • Falls

KEY POINTS

- The prevalence of sleep disorders and disturbances increases with age and older women may be more sensitive to the impact of aging on sleep.
- Short sleep duration, poor sleep quality, insomnia, sleep-disordered breathing, and weakened rest–activity rhythms are associated with adverse cardiometabolic outcomes, including obesity, metabolic disorders, and cardiovascular disease.
- Sleep disorders and disturbances, and weakened rest–activity rhythms, are associated with adverse mental health outcomes, including increased risk of depressive symptoms, dementia, and cognitive decline.
- Disturbances in sleep and treatments for sleep contribute to other outcomes, such as falls, disability, and chronic pain.
- Clinicians should consider special needs of older women in the diagnosis and treatment of sleep problems.

INTRODUCTION

Sleep is an important determinant of human health, and healthy sleep is crucial for healthy aging. In a recent joint consensus statement of the American Academy of Sleep Medicine and Sleep Research Society, healthy sleep was defined as "adequate duration, good quality, appropriate timing and regularity, and the absence of sleep disturbances or disorders."[1] The prevalence of sleep disorders and disturbances increases dramatically with advancing age.[2] There is growing evidence that sleep disturbances may accelerate the aging process and contribute to a wide range of chronic diseases. Despite these health consequences, sleep problems frequently are undiagnosed and untreated, particularly in the elderly.[3]

Previous studies have suggested that, compared with men, women may be more sensitive to the impact of aging on sleep and older women are more likely to report sleep problems.[4,5] As the older population continues to grow in many parts of the world, it is important to understand the health effects of sleep disruption in the context of aging. This review synthesizes and presents epidemiologic and clinical evidence on the relationships between sleep deficiency and various health conditions that are highly prevalent in older

Disclosure Statement: The authors declare no conflict of interest.
[a] California Pacific Medical Center Research Institute, San Francisco, CA 94158, USA; [b] Department of Health and Human Physiology, University of Iowa, Iowa City, IA 52242, USA; [c] Department of Epidemiology, University of Iowa, Iowa City, IA 52242, USA
[1] Present address: 225 South Grand Avenue, E118 Field House, Iowa City, IA 52242.
* Corresponding author. Mission Hall, Second Floor, 550 16th Street, San Francisco, CA 94158.
E-mail address: kstone@psg.ucsf.edu

Sleep Med Clin 13 (2018) 457–465
https://doi.org/10.1016/j.jsmc.2018.04.012

women, explores potential mechanisms underlying such relationships, points out gaps in the literature that warrant future investigations, and considers implications for the clinical and public health settings.

SLEEP IN OLDER ADULTS

Many aspects of sleep change as people age. A 2004 meta-analysis by Ohayon and colleagues[6] synthesized findings from 65 studies with objective measurement of sleep using polysomnography (PSG) or actigraphy. They found that older age was associated with decreases in total sleep time, sleep efficiency and percentage of slow-wave sleep and rapid eye movement sleep; whereas sleep latency, percentage of light sleep, and minutes of wake after sleep onset significantly increased with age. Such changes in sleep architecture are consistent with an increase in sleep complaints in the older population. In more than 9000 people aged 65 years or older, Foley and colleagues[7] assessed the frequencies of reporting common sleep disturbances, including trouble falling asleep, waking up, waking too early, and nonrestorative sleep. In this study, half of the participants reported at least 1 complaint as frequently occurring, and up to a third of the population showed symptoms of insomnia.[7] Similarly high prevalence (15%–25%) of insomnia symptoms has also been reported in the Sleep Heart Health Study (SHHS).[8] Sleep-disordered breathing (SDB), another common sleep disorder, is estimated to affect from 30% to 60% of older adults, depending on the definition used and specific population.[9–13] Moreover, aging coincides with altered circadian activity rhythms, including decreased amplitude (height of rhythm),[14] fragmentation or loss of rhythms (weakening of rhythmic pattern),[15,16] and altered timing of peak rhythm activity. Timing changes in older adults frequently result in earlier onset of sleepiness in the evening and an earlier morning waking time.[16]

Interestingly, a growing body of evidence suggests that there are sex differences both in sleep and age-related changes in sleep.[4] In general, although women tend to have better objectively measured sleep quality, paradoxically, they are more likely than men to report subjective sleep problems, including shorter sleep and poorer sleep quality.[17] A meta-analysis of sex differences in insomnia showed that not only is the risk of insomnia higher in women than in men across all age groups, the difference in insomnia risk between women and men widens with age.[18]

SLEEP AND CARDIOMETABOLIC HEALTH

Sleep plays a vital role in numerous physiologic processes, including the regulation of metabolic, hormonal, and immune function, all of which are essential for cardiometabolic health. Numerous studies have linked disorders and disturbances of sleep to cardiometabolic outcomes, including obesity, hypertension, dyslipidemia, diabetes, and cardiovascular disease (CVD).

Sleep Duration

Short sleep duration is associated with obesity in children and younger adults; however, such a relationship in older adults remains less clear.[19–21] The mixed findings in the elderly may be partially due to the high prevalence of chronic conditions in this population, which may both confound and modify the effect of sleep on weight. In a study of more than 80,000 healthy men and women aged 51 to 72 years, those with self-reported short sleep (<7 hours) at baseline were more likely to experience substantial weight gain ($\geq$5 kg) and risk of developing obesity over 10 years of follow-up.[22] Interestingly, this association may be stronger in older women than in men. Two studies of middle-to-old-aged subjects in Finland and Spain reported an association between short sleep and higher weight gain in women but not in men.[23,24]

Short sleep duration has also been associated with other cardiometabolic consequences. Two meta-analyses showed that short sleep duration was associated with a 23% increase in hypertension risk,[25] a 48% increase in coronary heart disease, and a 15% increase in stroke,[26] and these associations were stronger in women. Another meta-analysis demonstrated that each 1-hour decrease in sleep duration was associated with a significant 9% increase in the risk of type 2 diabetes.[27]

Several studies have also reported an association between long sleep duration and obesity, diabetes, and CVD risk and mortality.[26,28] In a large observational study of older women, Stone and colleagues[29] found that those who reported 10 or more hours of sleep per 24 hours had a 77% increase in risk of cardiovascular-related mortality compared with older women who reported 8 to 9 hours of sleep. Several lines of evidence suggest that these associations with adverse health outcomes related to long sleep duration may be partially explained by comorbidities.[30–32]

Studies using objectively measured sleep duration in the older population are still limited and their findings are mixed. For example, a cross-sectional relationship between objectively measured short sleep and higher adiposity was observed in both the Multi-Ethnic Study of Atherosclerosis and the Study of Osteoporotic Fractures (SOF).[33,34] However, thus far, prospective analyses in younger adults have found no relationship between actigraphy-measured short sleep duration and weight gain.[35,36]

Insomnia and Poor Sleep Quality

Several studies reported greater adiposity associated with various measures of sleep quality, such as wakefulness, sleep fragmentation, daytime sleepiness, and overall poor sleep quality.[37–40] van den Berg and colleagues[39] found that greater objectively measured sleep fragmentation was associated with higher body mass index and greater risk of obesity in older adults. In addition, the association between short sleep duration and obesity was no longer significant after adjustment for sleep fragmentation. This suggests that, in older adults, the quality of sleep may be more important than the quantity in relation to cardiometabolic outcomes. Poor sleep quality, measured both subjectively and objectively, has also been linked to several markers of subclinical CVD,[41] as well as poorer glycemic control measured by increased hemoglobin A_{1c} in patients with type 2 diabetes.[42] However, Phillips and colleagues[43] found no association of insomnia symptoms with incident hypertension in older women.

Finally, some studies have suggested that objectively measured short sleep duration and insomnia symptoms together increase risk of CVD more strongly than either condition alone. For example, Bertisch and colleagues[44] examined short sleep (objectively measured based on PSG), insomnia, or poor sleep quality, and the interaction of these sleep problems for prediction of incident CVD in middle-aged to older adults. Although neither condition alone was significantly associated with incident CVD, those with both short sleep and insomnia or poor sleep quality had a significant 30% increase in risk of incident CVD over 11 years of follow-up. These results were similar in both women and men. This finding highlights the importance of considering sleep health as a multidimensional exposure in terms of the affect on health in aging.

Snoring and Sleep-Disordered Breathing

There is a well-established association between SDB and obesity, as well as obesity-related health outcomes.[45] In addition, several studies also showed that even occasional snoring may be a risk factor for obesity, metabolic syndrome, and diabetes in middle-to-old aged women.[46,47]

Among middle-aged women in the Nurses' Health Study, those who reported occasional snoring were 40% more likely to develop diabetes during 10 years of follow-up than those who reported never snoring.[46]

Epidemiologic studies have also established that SDB increases the risk for incident hypertension, heart failure, coronary heart disease, and stroke in men and younger adults.[48–50] However, effects of SDB on cardiovascular outcomes in older women are uncertain. Early findings from the SHHS showed associations with CVD only in men, whereas more recent data from the SHHS and Atherosclerotic Risk in Communities cohorts showed that SDB severity predicted higher troponin levels and increased risk for left ventricular hypertrophy, heart failure, and CVD-related mortality among elderly women compared with men.[51] These data, which focused on an older sample for a longer period of time than earlier analyses, underscore the importance of examining this risk in older women.

Weakened Rest–Activity Rhythms

Circadian rhythms are intrinsic physiologic cycles of approximately 24 hours that are critically involved in control of sleep–wake cycles and numerous physiologic processes. Circadian and sleep–wake rhythm abnormalities have been observed among those with a wide variety of medical conditions. However, it is not clear whether sleep–wake rhythms directly influence morbidity and mortality in aging, or are biomarkers of advanced physiologic age. Indeed, van Hilten and colleagues[52] studied the relationship of age with nocturnal behavior in 100 healthy older adults and found that, in the absence of illness, age itself has only marginal effects on sleep and wake.

Using actigraphy, a previous study of older women in the SOF found that lower amplitude, extreme timing (early or late) of peak activity, and weaker strength in the overall rhythmicity predicted higher cardiovascular mortality.[53] Similarly, a more fragmented and less stable rhythm of rest and activity was associated with total mortality in the Rotterdam Study, although the study did not specifically examine cardiovascular deaths.[54]

SLEEP AND DEPRESSION

Although the prevalence of major depression in older adults is relatively low at 1% to 2%, an increasing number of older adults experience clinically significant depressive symptoms[55] that are linked to greater risk of functional impairment, disability, and illness.[56] Furthermore, late-life depression disproportionately affects older women. Some evidence suggests that this is because older women tend to experience more persistent depressive symptoms over time and have longer survival compared with men.[55,57]

Sleep Duration

Cross-sectional studies have reported greater prevalence of depressive symptoms in older adults with both short and long sleep duration.[30,57,58] Although a protective role for sleep deprivation or short sleep in risk of depression has been reported in younger adults, these findings have not been confirmed in older adults.[59,60] Using data from the Nurses' Health Study, Patel and colleagues[30] found that depressive symptoms were strongly correlated with self-reported long sleep duration. Another study reported that an association between self-reported long sleep duration and depressive symptoms was significant in older men but not older women.[57]

Fewer studies have examined the association of sleep duration and the risk of developing depressive symptoms over time. A few longitudinal studies using both objective and subjective assessment of sleep in older adults have reported no significant association of sleep duration (either short or long) and risk of incident depressive symptoms.[61,62] However, Fernandez-Mendoza and colleagues[61] studied a cohort of adults (mean age 52 years) and found that those with insomnia and objectively measured short sleep duration had the highest risk of developing depressive symptoms over 7.5 years of follow-up. This finding further underscores the importance of considering sleep health more comprehensively rather than focusing on a single domain.

Insomnia and Poor Sleep Quality

Insomnia is common in older adults with depression but recent evidence suggests that this is a bidirectional association and that insomnia and poor sleep quality may also lead to incident depressive symptoms over time. For example, Maglione and colleagues[62] studied 952 women aged 70 years and older with minimal depressive symptoms at baseline. Sleep was assessed objectively using actigraphy and subjectively using the Pittsburgh Sleep Quality Index (PSQI). Higher PSQI scores (indicating more sleep disturbance) were associated with greater risk of developing depressive symptoms, with stronger associations for the sleep quality (OR 1.41, CI 1.13–1.77) and sleep latency (OR 1.21, CI 1.03–1.41) subscales. Objectively, prolonged minutes of wake after sleep onset emerged as a risk factor for incident

depressive symptoms, whereas sleep duration was not a significant predictor. These findings suggest that sleep quality, rather than the absolute quantity of sleep, may be more important for mental health in older women.

The effects of poor sleep on risk of depressive symptoms may not be limited to a single domain of sleep (eg, sleep duration). Furihata and colleagues[63] tested the association of an index of sleep health in relation to risk of incident depressive symptoms in older women. The 0 to 5 index was created by summing across 5 dimensions classified as poor, based on self-reported sleep, including satisfaction with sleep duration, daytime sleepiness, midsleep time, sleep onset latency, and sleep duration. Results showed a strong gradient of increasing risk of developing incident depressive symptoms with increasing number of poor sleep dimensions. Despite these intriguing findings, the body of evidence linking sleep to depression has tended to focus on 1 dimension at a time.

Weakened Rest–Activity Rhythms

Although aging promotes disruption in circadian rhythms, the relationship between depression and circadian rhythm disruption in older adults remains largely unexplored. Maglione and colleagues[64] examined the relationship between depressive symptoms and circadian activity rhythms in older adults among 3020 women (mean age 84 years). Greater levels of depressive symptoms were associated with greater desynchronization of circadian activity rhythms, as well as later average time becoming active in the morning; however, there was no association with acrophase. Further evidence of an association between circadian activity rhythms and risk of depression was reported in a longitudinal analysis by Smagula and colleagues.[65] Among 2124 older men with minimal depressive symptoms at baseline, those in the lowest quartile of rhythm robustness were 2.5 times more likely to develop clinically significant depressive symptoms during a 5-year follow-up (odds ratio [OR] 2.58, 95% CI 1.11–5.59). Rhythm timing and amplitude did not significantly predict development of depression. These associations have not been examined in older women.

SLEEP, COGNITIVE DECLINE, AND RISK OF DEMENTIA

Sleep disturbance is common in older adults with dementia, and evidence suggests that disturbed sleep may contribute to development of cognitive problems and risk of dementia.[66] Although the mechanisms are not completely understood, experimental studies suggest that even a single night of sleep deprivation leads to accumulation of beta-amyloid in the human brain.[67] Beta-amyloid is a metabolic waste product that may form plaques over time, contributing to Alzheimer disease. Sleep may, therefore, play a critical role in the prevention of cognitive decline and risk for Alzheimer disease. Evidence also suggests that SDB may pose a risk for development of cognitive problems in older women.

Sleep Duration and Poor Sleep Quality

Overall, there is little prospective evidence of an association between sleep duration and cognitive decline or risk of incident dementia. Chen and colleagues[68] studied 7444 community-dwelling older women to test whether self-reported sleep duration predicted incident mild cognitive impairment (MCI) or dementia during follow-up. They found a V-shaped association between sleep duration and risk of MCI or dementia, with both short (≤6 hours per night) and long (≥8 hours per night) sleepers showing 35% to 36% increase in risk.[68] However, other studies of both older men and women with actigraphy measures of sleep demonstrated no association of sleep duration and risk of cognitive decline.[69,70] In contrast, these studies showed that objective measures of sleep fragmentation (eg, sleep efficiency) consistently predicted both cross-sectional cognitive function, as well as prospective decline in cognition. Further studies are needed to better define the characteristics of healthy sleep that may prevent cognitive decline in older women, and to determine if treatment of sleep problems may slow the decline in cognition and development of dementia.

Snoring and Sleep-Disordered Breathing

SDB results in nocturnal hypoxemia and more fragmented sleep, both of which may have effects on cognitive function. Yaffe and colleagues[71] studied the association of SDB and nocturnal hypoxemia (assessed using overnight in-home PSG) with subsequent 5-year risk of developing MCI and dementia among 298 older women (mean age 82.3 years). In this study, older women with SDB (apnea-hypopnea index ≥15) had nearly a 2-fold increase in the risk of developing MCI or over 5 years of follow-up, whereas nocturnal hypoxemia was associated with a 1.71-fold increase in risk of developing MCI or dementia.[71] In another study, Chang and colleagues[72] used data from a large health insurance database in Taiwan to compare 5-year risk of dementia among adults aged 40 year and older with and without sleep apnea diagnosis at baseline. Among the 1414 subjects studied, presence of sleep apnea was associated with a significant 1.7-fold increase in risk of developing dementia. In this same study, sleep apnea diagnosis was associated with a 3.2-fold increase in risk of incident dementia in women aged 70 years and older.[72]

There is insufficient evidence for an association between snoring and risk of cognitive decline or onset of dementia.

Weakened Rest–Activity Rhythms

Tranah and colleagues[73] examined whether circadian activity rhythms (based on actigraphy) were associated with incident MCI and dementia over 5 years in 1282 older women. An approximately 50% adjusted higher odds of developing dementia or MCI versus those without any dementia or MCI was observed for those in the lowest quartile of amplitude and rhythm robustness when compared with those in the highest quartile. Timing of activity rhythms also predicted incident MCI or dementia. In particular, older women with delayed acrophase (>1.5 standard deviations of the population mean) had a significant increase in odds of developing dementia or MCI (OR 1.83, 95% CI, 1.29–2.61) when compared with the mean peak range (mean ± 1.5 standard deviations).

SLEEP AND OTHER AGE-RELATED OUTCOMES AND CONDITIONS

Disturbed sleep in older women, and hypnotics used to treat sleep problems, are independently associated with risk of incident falls.[74–76] Falls are common in older adults, and frequently lead to injury and increased disability[77] and mortality.[78] Further evidence suggests that poor sleep may contribute to decline in physical functioning among older women, independent of falls.[79] Sleep disturbance is also common in older women with chronic pain, and more recent evidence suggests that this association is bidirectional and that sleep problems may increase the risk of developing chronic pain.[80] Treatment of insomnia symptoms using cognitive behavioral therapy in older adults with osteoarthritis showed that short-term (2 months) improvements in sleep predicted longer-term improvement in chronic pain outcomes over 9 to 18 months.

IMPLICATIONS FOR CLINICAL PRACTICE

Given the high prevalence of sleep problems in older women, and the debilitating impact on quality of life and physical and mental health, it is imperative for health care professionals to identify, monitor, and treat sleep problems in this vulnerable population. Unfortunately, evidence suggests that, compared with other lifestyle behaviors, sleep problems have not been screened as frequently in family medicine clinics.[81] Special needs of older women should be considered in determining the best treatment options. In older women with sleep apnea, behavior modification, such as avoiding alcohol and certain medications, may be particularly important because these patients may be more sensitive to their effects on upper airway function during sleep.[82] Hypnotic medications are effective and commonly prescribed by physicians for treatment of insomnia but have been linked to adverse events in the elderly, including falls and fractures, adverse cognitive and psychomotor events, and daytime fatigue.[83] Therefore, the American Geriatric Society has recommended avoiding hypnotic prescriptions for insomnia in older adults.[84] Randomized controlled trails have shown that behavioral interventions, including cognitive behavioral therapy for insomnia, are effective in older adults[85] and should be considered as the first-line approach. Moreover, several studies also showed that exercise,[86,87] social activities,[88] and cognitive training[89] may also be beneficial for older adults with insomnia.

REFERENCES

1. Watson NF, Badr MS, Belenky G, et al. Recommended amount of sleep for a healthy adult: a joint consensus statement of the American Academy of Sleep Medicine and Sleep Research Society. Sleep 2015;38(6):843–4.
2. Roth T. Insomnia: definition, prevalence, etiology, and consequences. J Clin Sleep Med 2007;3(5 Suppl):S7–10.
3. Boehlecke BA. Epidemiology and pathogenesis of sleep-disordered breathing. Curr Opin Pulm Med 2000;6(6):471–8.
4. Carrier J, Semba K, Deurveilher S, et al. Sex differences in age-related changes in the sleep-wake cycle. Front Neuroendocrinol 2017;47:66–85.
5. Reyner LA, Horne JA, Reyner A. Gender- and age-related differences in sleep determined by home-recorded sleep logs and actimetry from 400 adults. Sleep 1995;18(2):127–34.
6. Ohayon MM, Carskadon MA, Guilleminault C, et al. Meta-analysis of quantitative sleep parameters from childhood to old age in healthy individuals: developing normative sleep values across the human lifespan. Sleep 2004;27(7):1255–73.
7. Foley DJ, Monjan AA, Brown SL, et al. Sleep complaints among elderly persons: an epidemiologic study of three communities. Sleep 1995;18(6):425–32.
8. Unruh ML, Redline S, An MW, et al. Subjective and objective sleep quality and aging in the sleep heart health study. J Am Geriatr Soc 2008;56(7):1218–27.
9. Mehra R, Stone KL, Blackwell T, et al. Prevalence and correlates of sleep-disordered breathing in older men: osteoporotic fractures in men sleep study. J Am Geriatr Soc 2007;55(9):1356–64.
10. Ancoli-Israel S, Kripke DF. Prevalent sleep problems in the aged. Biofeedback Self Regul 1991;16(4): 349–59.
11. Ancoli-Israel S, Kripke DF, Klauber MR, et al. Sleep-disordered breathing in community-dwelling elderly. Sleep 1991;14(6):486–95.
12. Ancoli-Israel S, Kripke DF, Klauber MR, et al. Natural history of sleep disordered breathing in community dwelling elderly. Sleep 1993;16(8 Suppl):S25–9.
13. Ancoli-Israel S, Martin J, Jones DW, et al. Sleep-disordered breathing and periodic limb movements in sleep in older patients with schizophrenia. Biol Psychiatry 1999;45(11):1426–32.
14. Kripke DF, Youngstedt SD, Elliott JA, et al. Circadian phase in adults of contrasting ages. Chronobiol Int 2005;22(4):695–709.
15. Buysse DJ, Monk TH, Carrier J, et al. Circadian patterns of sleep, sleepiness, and performance in older and younger adults. Sleep 2005;28(11): 1365–76.
16. Czeisler CA, Dumont M, Duffy JF, et al. Association of sleep-wake habits in older people with changes in output of circadian pacemaker. Lancet 1992; 340(8825):933–6.
17. van den Berg JF, Miedema HM, Tulen JH, et al. Sex differences in subjective and actigraphic sleep measures: a population-based study of elderly persons. Sleep 2009;32(10):1367–75.
18. Zhang B, Wing YK. Sex differences in insomnia: a meta-analysis. Sleep 2006;29(1):85–93.
19. Patel SR, Hu FB. Short sleep duration and weight gain: a systematic review. Obesity (Silver Spring) 2008;16(3):643–53.
20. Nielsen LS, Danielsen KV, Sorensen TI. Short sleep duration as a possible cause of obesity: critical analysis of the epidemiological evidence. Obes Rev 2011;12(2):78–92.
21. Magee L, Hale L. Longitudinal associations between sleep duration and subsequent weight gain: a systematic review. Sleep Med Rev 2012;16(3):231–41.
22. Xiao Q, Arem H, Moore SC, et al. A large prospective investigation of sleep duration, weight change, and obesity in the NIH-AARP Diet and Health Study cohort. Am J Epidemiol 2013;178(11):1600–10.
23. Lyytikainen P, Rahkonen O, Lahelma E, et al. Association of sleep duration with weight and weight gain: a prospective follow-up study. J Sleep Res 2011; 20(2):298–302.
24. Lopez-Garcia E, Faubel R, Leon-Munoz L, et al. Sleep duration, general and abdominal obesity,

and weight change among the older adult population of Spain. Am J Clin Nutr 2008;87(2):310–6.

25. Guo X, Zheng L, Wang J, et al. Epidemiological evidence for the link between sleep duration and high blood pressure: a systematic review and meta-analysis. Sleep Med 2013;14(4):324–32.

26. Cappuccio FP, Cooper D, D'Elia L, et al. Sleep duration predicts cardiovascular outcomes: a systematic review and meta-analysis of prospective studies. Eur Heart J 2011;32(12):1484–92.

27. Shan Z, Ma H, Xie M, et al. Sleep duration and risk of type 2 diabetes: a meta-analysis of prospective studies. Diabetes Care 2015;38(3):529–37.

28. Tan X, Chapman CD, Cedernaes J, et al. Association between long sleep duration and increased risk of obesity and type 2 diabetes: a review of possible mechanisms. Sleep Med Rev 2017. https://doi.org/10.1016/j.smrv.2017.11.001.

29. Stone KL, Ewing SK, Ancoli-Israel S, et al. Self-reported sleep and nap habits and risk of mortality in a large cohort of older women. J Am Geriatr Soc 2009;57(4):604–11.

30. Patel SR, Malhotra A, Gottlieb DJ, et al. Correlates of long sleep duration. Sleep 2006;29(7):881–9.

31. Krueger PM, Friedman EM. Sleep duration in the United States: a cross-sectional population-based study. Am J Epidemiol 2009;169(9):1052–63.

32. Grandner MA, Drummond SP. Who are the long sleepers? Towards an understanding of the mortality relationship. Sleep Med Rev 2007;11(5):341–60.

33. Ogilvie RP, Redline S, Bertoni AG, et al. Actigraphy Measured Sleep Indices and Adiposity: The Multiethnic Study of Atherosclerosis (MESA). Sleep 2016;39(9):1701–8.

34. Patel SR, Blackwell T, Redline S, et al. The association between sleep duration and obesity in older adults. Int J Obes 2008;32(12):1825–34.

35. Lauderdale DS, Knutson KL, Rathouz PJ, et al. Cross-sectional and longitudinal associations between objectively measured sleep duration and body mass index: the CARDIA Sleep Study. Am J Epidemiol 2009;170(7):805–13.

36. Appelhans BM, Janssen I, Cursio JF, et al. Sleep duration and weight change in midlife women: the SWAN sleep study. Obesity (Silver Spring) 2013;21(1):77–84.

37. Jennings JR, Muldoon MF, Hall M, et al. Self-reported sleep quality is associated with the metabolic syndrome. Sleep 2007;30(2):219–23.

38. Lyytikainen P, Lallukka T, Lahelma E, et al. Sleep problems and major weight gain: a follow-up study. Int J Obes 2011;35(1):109–14.

39. van den Berg JF, Knvistingh Neven A, Tulen JH, et al. Actigraphic sleep duration and fragmentation are related to obesity in the elderly: the Rotterdam Study. Int J Obes 2008;32(7):1083–90.

40. Xiao Q, Gu F, Caporaso N, et al. Relationship between sleep characteristics and measures of body size and composition in a nationally-representative sample. BMC Obes 2016;3:48.

41. Aziz M, Ali SS, Das S, et al. Association of subjective and objective sleep duration as well as sleep quality with non-invasive markers of sub-clinical cardiovascular disease (CVD): a systematic review. J Atheroscler Thromb 2017;24(3):208–26.

42. Lee SWH, Ng KY, Chin WK. The impact of sleep amount and sleep quality on glycemic control in type 2 diabetes: a systematic review and meta-analysis. Sleep Med Rev 2017;31:91–101.

43. Phillips B, Buzkova P, Enright P, Cardiovascular Health Study Research Group. Insomnia did not predict incident hypertension in older adults in the cardiovascular health study. Sleep 2009;32(1):65–72.

44. Bertisch SM, Pollock BD, Mittleman MA, et al. Insomnia with Objective Short Sleep Duration and Risk of Incident Cardiovascular Disease and All-Cause Mortality: Sleep Heart Health Study. Sleep 2018. https://doi.org/10.1093/sleep/zsy047.

45. Ioachimescu OC, Collop NA. Sleep-disordered breathing. Neurol Clin 2012;30(4):1095–136.

46. Al-Delaimy WK, Manson JE, Willett WC, et al. Snoring as a risk factor for type II diabetes mellitus: a prospective study. Am J Epidemiol 2002;155(5):387–93.

47. Shin MH, Kweon SS, Choi BY, et al. Self-reported snoring and metabolic syndrome: the Korean Multi-Rural Communities Cohort Study. Sleep Breath 2014;18(2):423–30.

48. Gottlieb DJ, Yenokyan G, Newman AB, et al. Prospective study of obstructive sleep apnea and incident coronary heart disease and heart failure: the sleep heart health study. Circulation 2010;122(4):352–60.

49. Shahar E, Whitney CW, Redline S, et al. Sleep-disordered breathing and cardiovascular disease: cross-sectional results of the Sleep Heart Health Study. Am J Respir Crit Care Med 2001;163(1):19–25.

50. Stone KL, Blackwell TL, Ancoli-Israel S, et al. Sleep disordered breathing and risk of stroke in older community-dwelling men. Sleep 2016;39(3):531–40.

51. Querejeta Roca G, Redline S, Punjabi N, et al. Sleep apnea is associated with subclinical myocardial injury in the community. The ARIC-SHHS study. Am J Respir Crit Care Med 2013;188(12):1460–5.

52. van Hilten JJ, Middelkoop HA, Braat EA, et al. Nocturnal activity and immobility across aging (50-98 years) in healthy persons. J Am Geriatr Soc 1993;41(8):837–41.

53. Tranah GJ, Blackwell T, Ancoli-Israel S, et al. Circadian activity rhythms and mortality: the study of osteoporotic fractures. J Am Geriatr Soc 2010;58(2):282–91.

54. Zuurbier LA, Luik AI, Hofman A, et al. Fragmentation and stability of circadian activity rhythms predict mortality: the Rotterdam study. Am J Epidemiol 2015;181(1):54–63.

55. Barry LC, Allore HG, Guo Z, et al. Higher burden of depression among older women: the effect of onset, persistence, and mortality over time. Arch Gen Psychiatry 2008;65(2):172–8.

56. Prather AA, Vogelzangs N, Penninx BW. Sleep duration, insomnia, and markers of systemic inflammation: results from The Netherlands Study of Depression and Anxiety (NESDA). J Psychiatr Res 2015;60:95–102.

57. Brostrom A, Wahlin A, Alehagen U, et al. Sex-specific associations between self-reported sleep duration, depression, anxiety, fatigue and daytime sleepiness in an older community-dwelling population. Scand J Caring Sci 2018; 32(1):290–8.

58. Patel SR, Sotres-Alvarez D, Castaneda SF, et al. Social and Health Correlates of Sleep Duration in a US Hispanic Population: Results from the Hispanic Community Health Study/Study of Latinos. Sleep 2015;38(10):1515–22.

59. Kalmbach DA, Arnedt JT, Song PX, et al. Sleep disturbance and short sleep as risk factors for depression and perceived medical errors in first-year residents. Sleep 2017;40(3). https://doi.org/10.1093/sleep/zsw073.

60. Roberts RE, Duong HT. The prospective association between sleep deprivation and depression among adolescents. Sleep 2014;37(2):239–44.

61. Fernandez-Mendoza J, Shea S, Vgontzas AN, et al. Insomnia and incident depression: role of objective sleep duration and natural history. J Sleep Res 2015;24(4):390–8.

62. Maglione JE, Ancoli-Israel S, Peters KW, et al. Subjective and objective sleep disturbance and longitudinal risk of depression in a cohort of older women. Sleep 2014;37(7):1179–87.

63. Furihata R, Hall MH, Stone KL, et al. An aggregate measure of sleep health is associated with prevalent and incident clinically significant depression symptoms among community-dwelling older women. Sleep 2017;40(3). https://doi.org/10.1093/sleep/zsw075.

64. Maglione JE, Ancoli-Israel S, Peters KW, et al. Depressive symptoms and circadian activity rhythm disturbances in community-dwelling older women. Am J Geriatr Psychiatry 2014;22(4):349–61.

65. Smagula SF, Ancoli-Israel S, Blackwell T, et al. Circadian rest-activity rhythms predict future increases in depressive symptoms among community-dwelling older men. Am J Geriatr Psychiatry 2015;23(5): 495–505.

66. Ancoli-Israel S, Vitiello MV. Sleep in dementia. Am J Geriatr Psychiatry 2006;14(2):91–4.

67. Shokri-Kojori E, Wang GJ, Wiers CE, et al. Beta-amyloid accumulation in the human brain after one night of sleep deprivation. Proc Natl Acad Sci U S A 2018. https://doi.org/10.1073/pnas.1721694115.

68. Chen JC, Espeland MA, Brunner RL, et al. Sleep duration, cognitive decline, and dementia risk in older women. Alzheimers Dement 2016;12(1):21–33.

69. Blackwell T, Yaffe K, Laffan A, et al. Associations of objectively and subjectively measured sleep quality with subsequent cognitive decline in older community-dwelling men: the MrOS sleep study. Sleep 2014;37(4):655–63.

70. Blackwell T, Yaffe K, Ancoli-Israel S, et al. Poor sleep is associated with impaired cognitive function in older women: the study of osteoporotic fractures. J Gerontol A Biol Sci Med Sci 2006;61(4):405–10.

71. Yaffe K, Laffan AM, Harrison SL, et al. Sleep-disordered breathing, hypoxia, and risk of mild cognitive impairment and dementia in older women. JAMA 2011;306(6):613–9.

72. Chang WP, Liu ME, Chang WC, et al. Sleep apnea and the risk of dementia: a population-based 5-year follow-up study in Taiwan. PloS One 2013; 8(10):e78655.

73. Tranah GJ, Blackwell T, Stone KL, et al. Circadian activity rhythms and risk of incident dementia and mild cognitive impairment in older women. Ann Neurol 2011;70(5):722–32.

74. Stone KL, Ancoli-Israel S, Blackwell T, et al. Actigraphy-measured sleep characteristics and risk of falls in older women. Arch Intern Med 2008;168(16): 1768–75.

75. Stone KL, Ensrud KE, Ancoli-Israel S. Sleep, insomnia and falls in elderly patients. Sleep Med 2008;9(Suppl 1):S18–22.

76. Stone KL, Ewing SK, Lui LY, et al. Self-reported sleep and nap habits and risk of falls and fractures in older women: the study of osteoporotic fractures. J Am Geriatr Soc 2006;54(8):1177–83.

77. Gill TM, Murphy TE, Gahbauer EA, et al. Association of injurious falls with disability outcomes and nursing home admissions in community-living older persons. Am J Epidemiol 2013;178(3):418–25.

78. Ensrud KE, Ewing SK, Taylor BC, et al. Frailty and risk of falls, fracture, and mortality in older women: the study of osteoporotic fractures. J Gerontol A Biol Sci Med Sci 2007;62(7):744–51.

79. Goldman SE, Stone KL, Ancoli-Israel S, et al. Poor sleep is associated with poorer physical performance and greater functional limitations in older women. Sleep 2007;30(10):1317–24.

80. Finan PH, Goodin BR, Smith MT. The association of sleep and pain: an update and a path forward. J Pain 2013;14(12):1539–52.

81. Sorscher AJ. How is your sleep: a neglected topic for health care screening. J Am Board Fam Med 2008;21(2):141–8.

82. Feinsilver SH, Hernandez AB. Sleep in the elderly: unanswered questions. Clin Geriatr Med 2017; 33(4):579–96.

83. Glass J, Lanctot KL, Herrmann N, et al. Sedative hypnotics in older people with insomnia: meta-analysis of risks and benefits. BMJ 2005;331(7526):1169.

84. By the American Geriatrics Society Beers Criteria Update Expert Panel. American Geriatrics Society 2015 Updated Beers Criteria for Potentially Inappropriate Medication Use in Older Adults. J Am Geriatr Soc 2015;63(11):2227–46.

85. Irwin MR, Cole JC, Nicassio PM. Comparative meta-analysis of behavioral interventions for insomnia and their efficacy in middle-aged adults and in older adults 55+ years of age. Health Psychol 2006; 25(1):3–14.

86. Benloucif S, Orbeta L, Ortiz R, et al. Morning or evening activity improves neuropsychological performance and subjective sleep quality in older adults. Sleep 2004;27(8):1542–51.

87. King AC, Oman RF, Brassington GS, et al. Moderate-intensity exercise and self-rated quality of sleep in older adults. A randomized controlled trial. JAMA 1997;277(1):32–7.

88. Naylor E, Penev PD, Orbeta L, et al. Daily social and physical activity increases slow-wave sleep and daytime neuropsychological performance in the elderly. Sleep 2000;23(1):87–95.

89. Haimov I, Shatil E. Cognitive training improves sleep quality and cognitive function among older adults with insomnia. PLoS One 2013;8(4): e61390.

Printed and bound by CPI Group (UK) Ltd, Croydon, CR0 4YY

03/10/2024

01040304-0020